When
Illness
Strikes

When Illness Strikes

Let Edgar Cayce Help You Manifest Your Healing Response

ELAINE HRUSKA

A.R.E. Press • Virginia Beach • Virginia

Copyright © 2004
by Elaine Hruska

1st Printing, June 2004

Printed in the U.S.A.

A.R.E. Press
215 67th Street
Virginia Beach, VA 23451-2061

Library of Congress Cataloguing-in-Publication Data
Hruska, Elaine
    When illness strikes : let Edgar Cayce help you manifest your healing response / Elaine Hruska.
        p.   cm.
    ISBN 0-87604-491-7 (trade pbk.)
    1. Holistic medicine. 2. Cayce, Edgar, 1877-1945. 3. Healing. I. Title.
R733.H76 2004
615.5—dc22

                                        2004013244

Edgar Cayce Readings © 1971, 1993, 1994, 1995, 1996
by the Edgar Cayce Foundation.
All rights reserved.

Cover design by Richard Boyle

Contents

Introduction

WHAT DO WE do when we become ill or, worse yet, are given the disheartening news of a life-threatening illness? Do we go numb with shock, continue our daily activities, ignore the sickness, and move into denial? Or do we surrender to the moment, allow emotions to arise and flow, seek guidance and comfort through prayer, and begin to make lifestyle changes? Are we even aware that how we respond to this interruption in our routine, whether slight or serious, may possibly determine its successful outcome?

Much as we might long for a convenient "how-to" explanation on ways to deal with our discomfort, such a handy tool is not easy to come by and probably doesn't even exist. Why? One reason is that we are unique individuals *who have* a specific disease or illness; hence, patterns and protocols will vary to fit our individualized needs, personalities, and growth experiences. Our uniqueness does not allow for a one-size-fits-all mentality. We are infinitely variable beings springing from an Infinite, Loving Creator. Secondly, the disease process itself is seldom understood, even by specialists and experts in their fields. The course of any illness can take surprising twists and turns during its manifestation, and the degree of severity can fluctuate from person to person. On the other hand, I recall a remark that Dr. C. Norman Shealy, a neurosurgeon and founder of a pain management clinic, made during a lecture at A.R.E. headquarters: "Doctors and scientists are always studying diseases, so we really know very little about health!"

What makes a person healthy? Not necessarily the absence of a disease process, for our bodies are in continual warfare with both inner and outer environmental bacteria plus other assaults to our physical system. So how do we really maintain our health or revert to it when sickness strikes us? How can we travel the road back to health after an illness has manifested or taken root?

There are no simple and easy answers. Yet we have a body of information contained in the Edgar Cayce readings, over 9,000 of which discuss health issues, to assist us in our search for clues. No doubt, the psychic nature of this information adds an unusual dimension to this source; nevertheless, its helpfulness and veracity continue to demonstrate positive effects. We also have the lived experiences of numerous people who have journeyed this path and have shared their insights with us—through books, tapes, interviews, or Internet access. Their pioneering struggles and efforts inspire all those who may follow in their footsteps. Thirdly, we have the breakthroughs in research studies that point toward a fuller understanding of the body/mind connection. The efforts of these scientists have done much to contribute to a more holistic image of ourselves.

Indeed, the wealth of information is tremendous—and plentiful. But is there a thread running through this knowledge and experience that can assist us in healing when the crisis of an illness occurs? With the insights and advice given to individuals in their Cayce readings, the experiences of recipients and practitioners of healing, and some examples from contemporary scientific research, we can discover a more holistic, healthful way of facing any lack of adequate energy, a momentary illness, or the onslaught of a debilitating disease. These avenues provide us with the tools to use to face the challenges that a sickness may present.

Note to the Reader: The accounts of healing presented throughout this book in some cases have been altered slightly to protect the individual's identity, but the basic story line is true. The names, however, were changed throughout, even though some individuals gave me permission to use their stories.

The Edgar Cayce readings are catalogued numerically. Each recipient of a reading was assigned a number to provide anonymity. The first set of numbers refers to the individual or group who received the reading;

the second set represents its place in a sequence. For example, in reading 294-3, "294" stands for the person's name, while "-3" means this was the third reading given for that individual.

When the readings were computerized, the body of the reading was referred to as the "text." Any notes, letters, background information, related articles, etc., were also placed with the text of the reading. Stylewise, "R" means reports and "B" means background. To locate this information easier these letters were used. For example, "202-1, R-5" means that in reading 202-1 under reports (R), item number 5, can be found that particular quote.

The language of the readings can be quite challenging. Rather than try to paraphrase, I felt it was better to quote the text verbatim. Oftentimes reading the quote several times may be required to grasp its meaning.

The readings were given for individuals, yet they carry a universality of content. With the physical readings, however, it is important that the information not be used for self-diagnosis or self-treatment. Any medical problems need the supervision and advice of a health care professional.

Preparing the Soil: Understanding the Basics

. . . into the soil of human experience go the activities of every individual in its dealings, its associations and its reactions to the mental, the material and the spiritual aspect of every soul's experience. 1391-1

All that is for the sustenance of life is produced from the soil . . . Every man must be in that position that he at least creates, by his activities, that which will sustain the body—from the soil; or where he is supplying same to those activities that bring such experiences into the lives of all. 3976-19

Upon what character of soil seek ye to prepare, even in thine own life and heart and body? 3660-1

Our Body's Destiny

OUR PHYSICAL BODIES are wonderful, intriguing instruments. They are capable of handling a wide variety of stresses and strains, enduring a great amount of pressures and tensions, and transporting our souls throughout the spiritual journey we call life. Generally our bodies operate so well that we often take them for granted until a crisis hits and they become too overwhelmed with a stressed load. How we think

about our bodies and how we respond when they are no longer operating optimally may determine the outcome of the ensuing crisis.

According to the Edgar Cayce readings, our physical body has a destiny, which lies with us in the choices that we make. Our body is the
temple of the living God, having the potential of being glorified and
spiritualized according to how we use our free will. "It is with right
thinking and right acting that we keep the holy temple pure." (*ASFG*,
Book II, p. 196)* So it becomes necessary for us to care for our temple,
eating and thinking properly, "so that nothing can enter that will in any
way defile or defame the abiding place of the Most High." (*ASFG*, Book
II, p. 196) Then purified and glorified, "it may be of priceless value when
returned to its Maker." (*ASFG*, Book II, p. 197) We remain responsible
agents throughout our earthly sojourn for the care and nurturance of
our bodies, keeping them fit and sound channels through which our
souls may manifest.

Definition of Terms

Before we explore further the holistic dimensions of the human body
and its relationship to healing, let us first clarify the use of some words
that we will be using. Probably the driest, most uninteresting section of
any book is the definition and explanation of terms. Tedious as this
effort may be, it is nevertheless fundamental to a fuller understanding
of the concepts presented and events related in the text. In the area of
healing, with the dangers of misinformation and confusion, it is even
more important that one understand the meaning behind the terms
used.

The verb "to heal" originates from the Old English word *healan* (akin
to the German *heilen*) meaning "to make whole." Another derivation is
the word *hal*, which means "sound, healthy," and is our English word
hale; that is, "sound in body; vigorous and healthy." Notice that in addition to the usual connotation of *heal*—"to restore to health; free from
ailment . . . to effect a cure; mend"—is the concept of holism: to make

---

*Quotations from *A Search for God*, Books I and II, are taken from the 50th Anniversary
Edition (A.R.E. Press: Virginia Beach, Va.), 1992.

whole or sound. This concept also reflects the healing philosophy of the Edgar Cayce readings: that the balance among our physical, mental, and spiritual aspects creates the wholeness, unity, and oneness we desire for optimum health. These ideas will be discussed more fully in chapter 2.

Healing vs. Cure

A rather important distinction, usually overlooked, is the difference in the meaning of the terms *healing* and *cure*. They are not the same. So often when we discuss the healing aspect of any disease process, we are inclined to think of it as a reversal of the illness, a restoration to our previous level of health, a return to our "normal" state. Of course, elimination or cessation of illness is the desired and even expected outcome, and may in effect be part of the healing process. But the description of this process is really covered by the term *cure*, which means that the physical progression of a disease has been successfully controlled or abated. Even when physical symptoms may be "cured," however, the underlying emotional and psychological effects might remain, making it probable that an illness will recur. The Cayce readings also echo this sentiment: " . . . healing of the physical without the change in the mental and spiritual aspects brings little real help to the individuals in the end." (4016–1)

A holistic philosophy of healing could entail even the death of the ill individual. For some this makes it appear as if the battle for health has been lost and the sickness has won. But a holistic philosophy sees death as a transformative event, with the real healing taking place at the person's demise, in the transitioning from one state of being to another. This particular meaning of healing reflects a broader, more expansive understanding of one's life purpose, so the death process is considered part of the healing event.

Throughout this book, though, the term *healing* as used by many individuals may refer specifically to the end of an illness and a restoration to health. When people say, "I'm healed!" what they usually mean is that the sickness, discomfort, tumor, or sore has disappeared and is no longer present. Because this frequently is the intended meaning, the term will sometimes be used with that definition in mind. Yet the precise meaning intended is *cure*.

The broader use of the term *healing* will be explored in chapter 2.

From Dis-ease to Disease

The Cayce information presents an interesting contrast between the terms *disease* and *dis-ease*. Occasionally people requesting a physical reading were told that the disease process had not set in yet, that what they were experiencing was rather a "dis-ease." In a number of readings Cayce explained the difference.

> When a physical body is at dis-ease, the pain or dis-ease is as a warning that some portion is in distress; and the body sends out the warriors within itself automatically to ward off. If there is lacking that which will supply the proper defense, or proper ammunition for the warding off of disorders, then conditions array themselves—as it were—against the better physical functioning of the body. Then organic disorders arise.   639-2

> . . . disease and dis-ease are different temperaments, or are the result of varied effects in the body. Disease is the effect of the correlation of disturbances such as to prevent recuperative forces being the more active. Dis-ease is rather a tendency or an inclination, because of excesses of this or that, or the lack of some activity in the body-forces.
>
> 2838-1

The process from the dis-eased state to one of disease is illustrated in several readings. A forty-year-old man complained of dizziness, frequent headaches, pains in the muscles around his shoulders, and a slight pain on the left side of his body. In a letter to Cayce he spoke of a "dull feeling, a feeling that there is something wrong somewhere." (531–2, B–1) Cayce explained:

> When these ["conditions that enable the organ to reproduce itself"] suffer from mental or physical disorders that make for repressions in any portion of the system, then first

> dis-ease and distress arise. If heed is not taken as to the warnings sent forth along the nervous systems of the body indicating that certain organs or portions of the system are in distress, or the S.O.S. call that goes out is not heeded, then *disease* sets in.   531-2

A different approach is expressed in the following:

> The body physically is made up of many atomic units, yet when one is not in accord with another trouble ensues, and when murmurings or dissensions arise from within, dis-ease—and finally *disease*—sets in.   996-11

> . . . there arises often . . . where the elements in system become unbalanced . . . giving improper incentives. Then the resultant force must be improper reaction which begins to take place, until the disturbances are created as to cause distress. First coming as dis-ease to a portion of a functioning system, then assuming the greater distresses as diseased portions through that of the gradual building up of conditions as are created by misdirected energies in system.
>   202-1

In the latter reading given on March 3, 1929, for a forty–four–year–old male who once had tuberculosis but recovered in three months, it would appear that some form of distress may be admissible, even normal, in any functioning body. However, as is evident from the excerpts just quoted, lack of attention to alleviating the distress or a buildup of toxic conditions misdirects energies in the system and leads to the setting in of a disease process. This person was later admitted to the Cayce Hospital "to be treated for nerve depression (hypochondria)." (202–1, R–5)

For one individual the reading seemed to indicate the possibility of different outcomes in the dis–ease process. This sixty–three–year–old male, who obtained the reading on October 23, 1929, had low vitality, poor eliminations that were causing toxic conditions, and cancer and anemia tendencies. The reading stated:

> **While these conditions at present do not cause disturbance
> sufficient to distress the body, other than for the body to be
> at dis-ease at times, allowed to run on may bring most *any*
> character of disturbance, dependent upon what cycle of
> functioning the poisons or the distresses, or the congestion,
> would attack.** 166-1

Overall, what these reading excerpts indicate is the importance of
paying attention to small aches, pains, discomforts, sneezing fits, sores,
or blemishes when they occur. While they may oftentimes be minor
annoyances, they nevertheless may be trying to draw our awareness to
an area that needs attention and care. How often have we heard the
comment that a stiff neck, sore lower back, cold or flu, or heart attack
came suddenly and without warning. It just appeared out of nowhere.
Perhaps, though, after some reflection, we might recognize the warning
signs that we were given: the dull headaches, the slight ache in our
back, the fatigue and sluggishness, or the heaviness in our chest. These
were the signals of "dis–ease" that our body was sending us, but we
took no real notice of them or dismissed them. Sometimes, of course,
these minor irritations go away on their own; our body takes care of the
discomfort through its own self–regulating mechanisms and self–healing ability. We are not meant to become hypochondriacs, worried about
every minor ailment, but need to maintain a balanced view of our
body's stresses and strains.

Some years ago I occasionally felt a slight pain (like a little pinch) in
the right side of my abdomen just below the rib. It would last about
two or three seconds, then go away—just long enough to get my attention. This happened only once or twice daily. When I mentioned it to
my chiropractor, he remarked that the pain was in the gall bladder area
and that if I would have tests run on that organ, they would probably
be inconclusive due to the lack of severity. "It's just too new," he said.
His suggestion to me was to drink American saffron tea several times a
day. (This tea was recommended a number of times in the Cayce readings for its beneficial effects on digestion; also for those with stomach
ulcers, psoriasis, and toxemia. It supposedly coats the stomach, thus
aiding digestion.) This I did for about four or five days. The pain disappeared and never returned. Because no tests were taken, I cannot state

with certainty that the gall bladder was the culprit that was later re-stored to its normal functioning. The incident is purely anecdotal, but the pain did leave and hasn't returned since.

Healing Crisis

Sometimes when people embark on a healing journey through try-ing a variety of remedies, they may have adverse reactions and begin to feel worse off than they felt previously. This has occasionally been re-ported at the A.R.E. Health and Rejuvenation Center, whether the mo-dality they had received is a steam bath, Epsom salts bath, massage, acupressure, colonic, or manual lymph drainage. Individuals may re-port flu-like symptoms, outbreak of skin blemishes, headaches, a slight increase in discomfort or pain, excessive fatigue, or nausea following the appointment. The effects often appear more pronounced the fol-lowing day, reverting later to a better feeling of health and well-being. Such a period has been described as a "healing crisis" and is often diffi-cult to predict. Clients frequently ask, sometimes a bit anxiously, "How will I feel after this treatment?"—especially if they have never experi-enced or received the modality before. One teacher told her massage class to answer the client, "You will feel a change," leaving open the nature of the possibility. In addition, the area affected by the reaction may also offer clues as to where the body needs the healing. (More about this process later.)

In the A.R.E. Library I overheard a conversation of a woman who had received an acupressure treatment at the A.R.E. Health and Rejuvena-tion Center. "The next day I felt as if a Mack truck had run over me," she said. "But the day after that I felt like a million dollars. I had a new body!"

Disconcerting as it may be to experience such a shift, it is not un-common or even critical. Yet if we don't recognize this possibility, we might give up just before the benefits begin to appear. The readings often warned people about such situations, but also encouraged them to continue with their treatments. Here are several examples:

> . . . if this is done as we have given here relief will be brought to the body, and the body will get better, at present

you see the body is getting worse.   304-1

... as we find, while conditions are serious, they need not necessarily be uncontrollable. While conditions must in some respects be worse before they are better, there has been the correct interpretation of the disturbances and there needs to be only those precautions, as following through with the suggested applications.   5327-1

(Q) Any suggestion to help combat frequent insomnia?
(A) You won't have any trouble sleeping after the third period of series of these treatments! Before that it may be a little bit worse, but after that it will be better.   3442-1

Sometimes the reading explained what was happening physiologically to create the disturbance.

... the condition has been such, as the adage might be put, the body at times feels worse to feel better; for as changes take place in the correction of functioning of organs, and where the physical forces have been [forced] by natural conditions to function under stress and strain, and these conditions are being broken up, there is naturally then the warring of the conditions as to *which* portion is to function during the change. This produces often restlessness, the inability to sleep, and the weakness and shortness of breath. These are *results*, then, of changes taking place.   5514-2

(Q) Why do all my symptoms seem worse instead of better ... ?
(A) As indicated, the body is really better; though there is the need for creating some inflammation that there may be better assimilated from the active forces within the body those elements which will aid in strengthening the nerve plasms of the body.   2094-3

In another reading Cayce said that the process could go either way:

much better or much worse "depending upon how the administration of the conditions for correction are kept up." (5514-2) He advised the person not to overtax the system by improper diet or activities since "either can bring *detrimental* effects to the system." It may be that when a body is reestablishing its attunement, it tends to be more sensitive. Hence, if we misunderstand this heightened sensitivity, we might not see the good that is slowly being effected.

Some of the treatments undertaken for maintaining or restoring health may increase one's toxic level; however, if you are already near toxic overload, you may feel worse. At the A.R.E. Health and Rejuvenation Center we often encourage clients to drink more water following their appointment, as this will help flush the buildup of toxins from the system. In general the readings recommended six to eight glasses of water daily for good health and maintenance, whether or not you are experiencing a healing crisis.

Conclusion

"Our bodies are only channels through which our souls may manifest the attributes of the spirit of truth in a physical plane." (*ASFG*, Book II, p. 199) To enable and assist our bodies to carry out their divine purpose in the earth, we shall consider in more detail in chapter 2 the philosophy of healing from the Cayce perspective. The groundwork of preparing the soil—clarifying terminology—will now give way to sowing the seeds: viewing the holistic dimensions of the human body and its relationship to healing.

Sowing the Seeds:
Holistic Concepts from the Cayce
Readings

Know this first and foremost: All healing of any nature must be of God; for God . . . alone is life, is health, is good . . .
1427-1

In giving those things, conditions or elements that may be of assistance or aid to this body, it would be well that the body mentally know and realize—in its mental consciousness—that all healing of every nature must arise from one source, the Giver of life, the Sustainer of all.
464-13

For, as ye understand and know, health is the gift of the Creator . . . in Him is health.
2574-1

Applying the Concepts from the Readings

TWO-THIRDS OF the over 14,000 psychic readings from Edgar Cayce are designated "physical readings" as they deal with the health concerns of those requesting information. A consistent holistic philosophy permeates this material, making application a rather simple and straightforward process, in the sense that, though given for specific individuals with their own unique health problems, the readings nevertheless contain a universality of meaning and purpose, an underlying principle to be worked with and followed as a regimen for treatment.

When you find yourself facing a health concern and would like to follow a Cayce treatment, there are several possibilities open to you. One, of course, is to study the readings themselves that cover your particular ailment. A listing of diseases and health concerns is contained in the Circulating File Index, medical section; each File, which can be purchased or ordered on loan, compiles in booklet form most of the readings on a certain illness or disease. Then determine from the various suggestions given which ones you yourself might follow.

Another more limited resource is the Research Bulletin, each of which documents a disease along with a commentary, representative readings, and a statistical abstract classifying causes and treatments of the disease. This is helpful if you would like to note the most often recommended remedies for that particular ailment and be guided to your decision about the course to follow.

The A.R.E. also offers for purchase individual research protocols—binders of standardized health packages on nearly fifty specific illnesses, which explain the process of following the recommendations suggested in the readings plus how you can participate in research on remedies for that disease.

Another helpful suggestion was one given often by Gladys Davis Turner, Cayce's longtime secretary. She recommended that the sick person study the series of readings of those individuals with the same or similar ailment. While poring over each one, notice which reading reflects your own particular symptoms, its closeness to your age, the same sex, etc. Which reading seems to mirror as near as possible your own body? Then follow the suggestions Cayce gave for that person; if necessary, omitting any remedy whose use truly does not fit in with your symptoms or which you feel intuitively is unnecessary to include. This process would help you wade through a perhaps excessive amount of information and narrow your search to a more manageable level. Then follow the recommendations consistently and persistently.

Before getting into more specific regimens for working with a health condition, let us look at certain principles and ideas which will serve as a basis in handling an illness or a disease process.

Source of Healing

On this particular point—the source of healing—Cayce was very consistent. Over and over again the readings insisted that healing comes from the God–force within. This includes healing of any nature— whether physical, mental, or spiritual. Here are some examples of those statements:

> For, as has so oft been given, *all* healing forces and influences are constructive and are thus of the Divine influence.
>   1363-2

> . . . let the body *know* this:
>   Not palliatives, but healing that is sincere—of whatever nature, whether spiritual, magnetic, mechanical, even drugs, electrical, heat, or whatever application—to be of real aid for the body—must bear the imprint or stamp of the universal or divine. No matter in what sphere or plane a soul may find itself, this law is ever the same!
>   Construction and constructive influences can only emanate from *good*. *Good* can only emanate from God.   366-1

> All healing of every nature comes from the *divine* within that body, or the body applied to such methods or manners of healing.   1861-4

To emphasize again this important concept, Cayce, after advising Mr. [1844] to cultivate such attitudes as hopefulness and thankfulness, stated that "all healing of *any* nature—*all* healing—must come from the divine; else there is no healing." (1844-3)

What does it mean that "All healing comes from the divine within . . . " (3312-1)? What is the nature of this healing source? How does it operate? What part, if any, do specific applications play in alleviating the symptoms of a disease? The following excerpt, which serves as a representative sample of a number of similar readings, may provide a clue:

> Know that all strength, all healing of every nature is the changing of the vibrations from within—the attuning of the

> **divine within the living tissue of a body to Creative Energies. This alone is healing. Whether it is accomplished by the use of drugs, the knife or what not, it is the attuning of the atomic structure of the living cellular force to its spiritual heritage.**   **1967-1**

This oft-quoted excerpt condenses a lot of information into just three sentences. It mentions vibrations and attunement, body tissues and atomic structures. It also seems to downplay the applied treatments—drugs, surgery, etc.—seeing them as mere aides to the healing process.

The reading defines healing as "the changing of the vibrations from within." This includes "all healing of every nature"—without exception. Any type, form, or occurrence of healing, what passes for healing, is a change in vibrations from within the person.

What is vibration? According to *Webster's New World Dictionary*, it is a "rapid rhythmic movement back and forth; quiver." In its plural form vibrations are "emotional qualities or supernatural emanations that are sensed or felt by another person or thing." Many of us have probably used at one time or another this latter form when describing someone we've just met as one having "good vibes" or a place we've recently visited as having "bad vibes." Vibrations underlie almost every aspect of nature: heat, sound, and light are created by the vibrations of atoms. In our bodies each electron, atom, molecule, cell, tissue, or organ vibrates in a unique pattern, forming a dynamic network that extends not only throughout the body but even beyond the body as well. However, in the healing process the Cayce readings are speaking about *inner* vibrations: "Know that all healing forces must be within, *not* without!" (1196–7) These inner vibrations may represent a variety of forms: those created by and emanating from the body's physical structure, or they could even include a range of attitudes, emotions, feelings, and sensations. So there exists quite a lot of activity going on inside us, and all this energy is vibrating and oscillating at different rates or different frequencies. Our physical body—at the atomic level, at least—is composed, then, of different kinds of vibrating energy, making each of us a unique energy system.

These energy patterns can be measured and are used today as diagnostic tools. For example, the electrocardiogram (EKG), routinely used by doctors on yearly exams of their patients, measures the electrical energy coming from the heart. By interpreting the patterns of this energy, physicians can determine the health of the heart. So this vibrational approach to medicine is not new; what *is* new is viewing the body not as a sophisticated machine—as Newtonian physics does (based on the work of Sir Isaac Newton)—but as a complex energetic system. As such, like other living organisms, our bodies are dynamic, open, self-organizing, and able to maintain form and function through self-renewal. (This concept of the body is part of a new scientific worldview that is gradually gaining acceptance by modern medicine.)

In reading 1967-1, quoted above, the changing of the vibratory patterns is done "from within"; in other words, it involves "the attuning of the divine within the living tissue of a body to Creative Energies." What is meant by "attuning"? The dictionary defines it as "bringing into harmony or agreement." The word is commonly used in the readings to explain the process of meditation and is an adequate descriptive word for that process. When we meditate, we are attempting to align ourselves with our divine source, to listen to God, to still and quiet our minds so that we can be open to our higher self.

One example of how this focused consciousness can influence, even restructure, physical reality is the "Maharishi effect" documented by transcendental meditation researchers. In certain cities where advanced TM teachers were conducting large meditation sessions the crime rate dropped to very low levels while the sessions were in progress. Studies had shown that the crime rates were high before and after the sessions, but very low during the sessions. This drop demonstrated a statistically significant effect during group meditation, even though the meditators were simply trying to create a harmonious consciousness within themselves and were not intending to reduce crime. The experiment indicates the powerful effect we can produce in bringing about a positive change. If making this attunement can lower crime rates, can it not also affect "the living tissue" in our physical bodies?

Attunement also involves awareness of the natural processes going on within our bodies and allowing ourselves to become fully conscious of what's happening and how our bodies are responding. It has been noted that many of the books about curing a disease are written by lay people who due to their experiences became quite knowledgeable about their sickness and the effects of specific treatments. Frequently they knew more than the physicians treating them, becoming practically experts on their disease. Cayce might refer to this as an increased awareness of creative or God forces, "the divine within," which produces the healing. In the following reading he indicated how the attunement could be achieved; in this case the attunement would be used in service to others:

> There is within each individual entity the soul, the mind, the body. By those rituals within self, and magnetic power, there may be produced that which may have an influence upon others. For, as the Master gave, "He that receiveth a prophet in the name of a prophet receives a prophet's reward."
>
> That does not indicate as to whether such is done to the glory of self, to the honor of the individual, or to the glory and honor of God. For, it is the ability of each soul, by faith, to receive that as may be a pronouncement from another soul. This is part of the universal law.
>
> Yet the promise has been, "I go to the Father—and greater things ye shall do in my name. For I will bear witness of you—that love me and keep my commandments."
>
> This is the sure way, the pure way—this is the way individuals may so attune their bodies, their minds, their souls, to be healers, to be interpreters, to be ministers, to be the various channels of blessings to others.   3019-1

Attunement requires not only a belief pattern based on faith—that we can do "greater things" and receive the "prophet's reward"—but also a compassionate, loving quality and an adherence to the "commandments." The readings emphasized the importance of keeping and obeying universal laws, of working within their framework, and applying them in one's daily life. Herbert Puryear, longtime A.R.E. speaker who was quite original in his interpretation of the Cayce philosophy, stated in a lecture that he had suggested that his minister preach on the topic of obedience. He had never before heard this topic expounded upon from the pulpit. Years later, he was still waiting to hear it!

If obedience is a difficult route to follow, having a greater conscious-ness or awareness of ourselves, our thought processes, what makes us tick, may be even more arduous. But there is a sense of hope given in the following reading:

> **Let the mental forces be applied in that direction in first understanding self and self's relation to every individual, knowing that the compliance to natural physical laws, and the laws of the Creator, gives that incentive for the very best development in the physical life, knowing there is an advocate with the Father, and same as made manifest through self and self's application to His divine commands.**
>
> **4771-1**

As was mentioned in chapter 1, we have the capacity to make choices about our lives and how we wish to live, and whether or not to comply with physical and divine laws. Making the commitment to follow and obey these laws means that we on some level recognize the presence of the divinity within us—even in our very cells, with their atomic and subatomic particles. In fact it is "the arousing of the divine within each cell of the body" (2964-1) that creates the healing. Understanding and believing that we have a divine presence, a higher force, residing within us helps us build in our consciousness the climate of a healing pattern, as Mrs. [2574] was advised to do in others:

> **(Q) How may I best develop my gift of healing, and use it more effectively for mankind?**
> **(A) By more and more arousing the awareness in the mind of others of His presence with them.**   **2574-1**

Coincidentally, Mrs. [2574], whose occupation was listed as Christian Service volunteer, was told in this past-life reading that at the time of Jesus she was the mother of Lucius (one of Edgar Cayce's incarnations) and the sister of St. Luke. A note from Gladys Davis Turner, dated March 27, 1963, stated that "she has been active in service as the reading indi-cated, not being bound by orthodoxy, cult or denomination, but rather a walking advertisement of God and Christ." (2574-1, R-2)

Role of Treatment Applications

We have at our disposal today an extensive variety of modalities for treatment—both traditional and complementary. Such methods include spinal manipulation, homeopathic and naturopathic medicine, hydrotherapy, massages, drugs, surgery, energy work, electrotherapy, herbs, traditional Chinese medicine, vitamins, and so on. Many of these are mentioned in Cayce's physical readings as recommendations for treatment. Often the modalities were to be used in a series and/or combined with other suggestions. So their use at certain stages in one's illness presupposes an understanding of one's body, a concept mentioned earlier, as well as knowledge of the particular outcomes to be expected by taking or using the remedy. A reminder: Because the readings' recommendations were for specific individuals, *do not use any treatment modality or attempt to change your prescribed medication until you have enlisted the advice of your health care professional.*

The representative reading, 1967-1, quoted earlier, states that the attunement which creates the healing occurs "Whether it is accomplished by the use of drugs, the knife or what not . . . " While each modality has a specific purpose to effect a particular outcome, its use entails certain qualifications which are linked to the body's overall healing process. One reading states:

> For after all, all *healing* is from the divine within, and not from medications. Medications only *attune* or accord a body for the proper reactions from the elemental forces of divinity within each corpuscle, each cell, each muscle, each activity of every atom of the body itself.   1173-6

A well-known axiom from the readings is that our cells have consciousness; they are aware and are influenced by our thought patterns, as expressed in "Mind is the builder." (This idea will be presented briefly in the next section of this chapter and more fully in chapter 4.) One reading states that "each cell is as a representative of a universe in itself" and that the "applications are merely to stimulate the atoms of the body."

(4021-1) Each of us, having the three-dimensional consciousness of body, mind, and spirit, participates in the creative process that is healing. Another reading expressed it this way:

> **For who healeth all thy diseases? Only when any portion of the anatomical structure of a human being is put in accord with the divine influences, which is a portion of the consciousness of an individual entity, may real healing come. Without it, it is nil and becomes more destructive than constructive.**   **5083-2**

The recipient of this reading was a forty-four-year-old physician and surgeon who obtained the reading on May 24, 1944. He later became a cooperating doctor with A.R.E. and stated that he derived great benefit and insights from the information contained in Cayce's readings.

On the A.R.E. premises, whose headquarters building is actually the former Cayce Hospital—now housing the Health and Rejuvenation Center and the Cayce/Reilly School of Massotherapy, plus other offices—one can hear lots of discussion on health issues: what remedy would be best for what ailment, what protocol should someone follow with a certain disease, and how does one apply and use a particular remedy. There appears to be an almost overwhelming amount of health advice—solicited or unsolicited. One Search for God Study Group participant, who also was a member of the A.R.E. staff, laughingly remarked how one could not sneeze or cough without getting from co-workers three or four different suggestions on how to waylay the oncoming cold or flu or allergic reaction. Helpful advice is readily available—and plentiful—with probably castor oil (applied externally) being the most often recommended remedy. In fact, the joke at A.R.E. is: When in doubt, use castor oil. Have an unusual sore, blemish, pain, or ache? Put castor oil on it. Called the *Palma Christi* (the palm of Christ) in medieval times, it has been shown time and again to be highly effective in relieving and alleviating a number of discomforts and dis-eases.

Each remedy—whether a castor oil pack, a spinal adjustment, a particular herbal tonic, one of the Cayce-recommended appliances, or a massage with peanut oil—does have a specific use and purpose. Sometimes this was stated in the person's reading, sometimes not. One individual was told that application of the suggested remedies would "only assist in alleviating the distressed areas and in adding to the system the influences that may—through constructive forces—materialize in active forces throughout the body." (1363-2) Cayce added that Mr. [1363] should remain as cheerful and optimistic as possible under the circumstances.

This reading, 1363-2, the second for a forty-four-year-old male, was given on July 29, 1937. Referred to as a "check reading" (that is, a follow-up to the previous one), this second reading added to his regimen a series of osteopathic manipulations as well as colonics, if needed. He had been ill since 1924, with a diagnosis of sciatic rheumatism, which worsened until he was completely paralyzed from the waist down. Later the diagnosis was changed to transverse myelitis. Several months later he regained the use of his legs, but had never fully recovered. In 1931 he was bothered by numbness in his right arm and side of face, had a sinus operation, was admitted to the Veterans Hospital, and received another diagnosis of moderate hysteria. As his right arm was useless, he had to give up his job as a telegraph operator but accepted the position of depot agent and learned to use his left hand. In 1936 he was readmitted to the hospital and told that his condition was worse, there was nothing to be done, and a wheelchair would be needed soon, as the motor nerves were practically destroyed. "Isn't it possible that they are all mistaken and each on the wrong track?" he asked in a letter. (1363-1, B-1)

His first reading, given on May 4, 1937, over two-and-a-half months before his check reading, said that his condition was not transverse myelitis, "but rather an infectious force," and that the complex condition could be overcome with consistent and persistent application. The suggested treatments were intended "to get rid of the excess poisons that are existent in the system and still not so deplete the body as to cause inability of activity . . . " (1363-1) His regimen was quite extensive: castor oil packs for three evenings; next day a series of Zilatone tablets; next morning, an enema; rest the following day; castor oil packs again for three days followed by Eno Salts for a week; wait three or four days, then packs again. Continue whole routine for thirty days. Then Wet-Cell Appliance with gold every day for thirty minutes for thirty days;

after the series of Zilatone and Eno Salts are finished, take Ventriculin with Iron every afternoon; massages with pure olive oil on the rest days between packs. Also given were dietary recommendations and an affirmation for meditation while on the appliance. After sixty to ninety days of these treatments he was to ask for a check reading.

On May 28, over three weeks after the reading, he had a rather severe heart attack. On June 19 Cayce wrote to [1363]'s wife encouraging her to continue the regimen, especially the packs, massages, and Wet–Cell Appliance. Shortly before the second reading was given, [1363]'s wife wrote to Cayce:

> I believe [1363] has been showing some improvement, although it is hardly noticeable to one who is with him all the time. He has not had a heart spell for the past three weeks. The day he received his first reading he was suffering from a severe sore throat followed in a few days with almost complete loss of feeling in the left side of the head and face and extending down to his left hand. That was the first time he had had a sore throat for several years. This has since almost disappeared. His bowel condition has improved, although it is not normal yet, but nearer so than for years. He doesn't seem so nervous and sleeps and eats well. What seems to bother him more than anything at present is worry over the fact that he is unable to work since the severe heart attack he suffered on May 28. He is still extremely weak in his lower limbs and weather changes always affect him.
>
> 1363-1, R-3

She submitted some questions for the check reading.

The second reading was guardedly hopeful: " . . . there are decided changes for the better . . . There is still much to be desired . . . " (1363–2) The uneasiness felt from the heart attack would be relieved by a series of gentle osteopathic treatments, and the colonics would help to purify the system because of the excess toxins being eliminated. To combat the tendency to hysteria, the reading suggested exercises outdoors as much as possible. "Not by overtaxing, but have these purposes for the activity; and these will not only make for the changing of the attitude but aid in

the physical activities." (1363-2) The recommended exercise was walking; as the reading stated, it would help him not only physically but
would also improve his attitude. The reading ended on a positive note:

> **Know that while this condition of the body is long stand-
> ing, and it has affected the body in the deeper senses, there
> is not the necessity nor the need for the body *remaining* in
> an inactive condition.   1363-2**

No more follow-up information was available for this case study, so
we do not know the ultimate outcome. We have only a comment from
his wife's letter (June 15, 1937) that "[We] Have been following instructions for his treatment closely . . . " (1363-1, R-1)

The reason for presenting this much detail at this time is to acquaint
the reader with an idea of how much could potentially be involved in
pursuing and following the suggested regimen of treatments in a given
Cayce reading as well as the orderly sequence in which they were to be
done. Some regimens were not this involved; others more so. Many of
the readings' supplements contain little or no follow-up information or
responses to subsequent questionnaires, so it is frustratingly difficult to
learn of the outcome. However, the book *Edgar Cayce on Healing* by Mary
Ellen Carter and William A. McGarey, M.D., published in 1972, relates
the stories of twelve people, many of whom were patients in the Cayce
Hospital, who received physical readings. A number of these people
plus family members were also available for personal interviews for
this book. Each regained his/her health as well as a different perspective on life by following the suggestions outlined in the reading.

In concluding this section on the role of treatment modalities, we
can state that while each particular application has its special meaning,
use, purpose, function, or vibration, each is actually assisting the body
to make its attunement to the divinity within. Another way of stating
this is that any healing remedy or method is attempting to create an
experience of oneness, with the hope of stimulating a similar response
in the body. Whenever you gather together the materials for a potato
poultice for your eyes, plug in the heating pad to warm up your castor
oil pack, or set aside organic apples for your three-day apple diet, you

are participating in a positive, active way in your own cure. You may even feel a shift of attitude as you perform these tasks, which demand more time and personal involvement than simply popping a pill. It is this self-care and nurturance which will facilitate the proper attunement, balance, and vibratory changes that are necessary for healing to occur.

The Triune Approach to Healing

Before we consider in more detail the readings' view of healing, it would help to first understand their approach to the nature of reality and the nature of humanity. What we believe about our reality and about how we function as human beings—from both consciously and unconsciously held beliefs—influences our actions and attitudes and permeates our words, thoughts, and emotions. It enhances what we bring to each moment, to each experience, in our daily lives.

According to the readings, the first principle is oneness—oneness of all force, oneness of all things. This principle reminds us that we are all connected to each other; there is a force which binds us together and keeps us in communication with one another. We become aware of the operation of this principle when we receive a phone call from a friend or meet someone shortly after we thought about that person. Or we need an article of clothing or an ingredient in a recipe or a part for our malfunctioning automobile and someone shows up unexpectedly with the needed object. Though these incidents may seem rare or unusual to us, they may indeed be the fabric of our ordinary lives lived "in the flow"—not really so extraordinary after all, but part of our common, everyday experience.

When the One Force manifests, though, it manifests in three dimensions. According to the readings, we humans are spiritual beings moving in a three-dimensional awareness. "Thus it is helpful for us in understanding oneness if we are willing to work with triune concepts—whether of the dimensions of time, space, and patience; or of the Father, Son, and Spirit; or of ourselves as physical, mental, and spiritual beings." (*Covenant*, Vol. 2, No. 12, p. 1) One reading states it simply:

> ... there is the physical body, the mental body, and the soul or spiritual body. They each have their environs. They each have their attributes. But they are *one*.   2812-1

The reading continues to explain that these three aspects impinge upon the part of the body which is out of attunement:

> Each influence, then, has to bear upon that particular phase of the consciousness not wholly in accord. Thus, though there may be mechanical or medicinal applications for the welfare of the physical body, these are to attune the body to that consciousness which makes or brings it aware of its relationship to the spiritual or God-force.   2812-1

Cayce, frequently drawing upon his knowledge of and expertise in the Bible, next mentions the encounter of Jesus with the man born blind. (See John 9.) Jesus had mixed His own spittle with dirt, making a type of mud or clay mask, and placed it upon the man's eyes. This had the effect, according to the reading, of bringing "the awareness of the presence of the Creative Force or God to those granulated lids, in the experience of that individual." In another encounter (Luke 17:14-19) Jesus instructed the ten lepers to present themselves to the priest. This action "brought the awareness, the attunement of body, mind and soul to the oneness of purpose." (2812-1) In other words, in these instances it took both an external influence, applied with purposeful intent and prayer, plus action upon the recipient's part (to visit a spiritual leader) that brought the attunement necessary for the healing.

How these three aspects—the physical, mental, and spiritual—work together and influence one another is key to understanding our work and our health in the material world. One formula found extensively throughout the readings by which a great deal can be conceptualized or explained is: "The Spirit is the life, mind is the builder, and the physical is the result." The first part of this formula speaks of the One Force; this is the Spirit, the life force, sustaining us and maintaining our total existence. The next part—mind is the builder—reminds us of mental patterns created by our thoughts, leading to those attitudes and emotions that can best foster healing. And the physical is the result of what we have built at the mental level that has been energized by spirit. A number of readings describe the relationship among these three aspects. Two examples follow:

> **In considering the physical, mental and spiritual relationships—it would be necessary that the premises be declared from which any reasoning or application of measures would be taken, that the body may gain the better concept of the relationships that the mental and the physical bear with the spiritual forces, in relationship to healing of any nature.**
>
> **The body finds itself in a material world of three-dimensional proportions. That which manifests in the mental is from or of a spiritual nature, but the results in the material or physical manifestation depend upon the spirit with which the activity is prompted.**
>
> **This is the law, that was begun when it was first indicated, "God said, Let there be light, and there was light." This was not as an activity from the sun, or light as shed from any radial influence, but it was the ability of consciousness coming into growth from the First Cause.   2528-2**

> **. . . only the higher vibrations set up by material conditions for the body [may] bring about better coordination between the physical, the spiritual, the mental body; for the triune remains—the physical, the mental, the spiritual—and to make one whole, each must function in *its* portion of the whole. Not to the detriment one of another, but that each be coordinating one with the other.   4735-1**

This concept of a triune pattern is repeated extensively throughout this material, not just in the physical readings. Balancing and coordinating each aspect is necessary for health maintenance. Understanding the relationship among all three and how they influence one another can promote true, life-giving healing, since they all are necessary components for a healthful life.

When we experience a so-called physical illness—a flu or cold, an upset stomach, constipation, diarrhea, a headache—or mental illness, such as depression or anxiety, we may not necessarily consider its spiritual component or even that there exists a relationship among all three aspects. We become preoccupied—perhaps rightly so—with taking care of the physical disturbance: gargling with Glyco-Thymoline for our sore throat, drinking peppermint tea for our upset stomach, applying a castor oil pack for intestinal problems, doing head and neck exercises to alleviate our headache. We may attempt visualization or meditation or focusing on constructive, positive thoughts to calm our anxieties or relieve our depression. We seem to know instinctively that we are working with meeting certain conditions in our bodies and they need to be addressed in a particular order. This dilemma was similar to what Mrs. [4308] experienced.

> **(Q) Should the body take care of the physical first and then the spiritual?**
> **(A) As given, meet the needs of the physical conditions of the body through the physical at present. Meet the needs of the spiritual, the mental, through the spiritual and the mental. Apply then those physical needs for the body at present, applying *through* the spiritual those of the mental and spiritual nature for the physical and mental as given, each through its own sphere, and each are as *one* in application to the body.**   **4308-1**

Not mixing physical with spiritual applications is reiterated in the following reading, along with the underlying principle of oneness and the sense of relationship that each part of the body has to the whole:

> **There is a vast difference . . . between applying physical laws to spiritual conditions and spiritual laws to physical conditions. While all is one in a life, yet each in its own sphere; for well has it been given that the foot does not find fault with the body that it is not the eye, nor the eye that it is not the hand; yet each in its own sphere necessary for the full accomplishing of that which may be attained by the whole.**
>   **1982-2**

One final reading to conclude this section offers practical advice on choosing the means toward achieving healing, again using Jesus as the model.

(Q) Please advise how I can realize my desire for healing to come without physical remedies. Is it possible for me to demonstrate this?

(A) Anyone may demonstrate that which is really desired, if the entity is willing to pay the price of same!

As we have indicated so oft, when there are disturbances in the physical that are of a physical nature, these need to be tended to or treated, or application made, through physical means. There is as much of God in the physical as there is in the spiritual or mental, for it should be one! But it was as necessary, when the Master demonstrated, to use that needed in the bodies of individuals as curative forces as it was in the mental. To some He gave, "Thy sins be forgiven thee." To others He applied clay. To others they were dipped in water. To others, they must show themselves to the priest, offering that as had been the mental and the material law.

These are one. Understand them as one, yet do not attempt, at all times, to heal with word when mechanical or [other] means are necessary to attune some disturbed portion with the mental and the spiritual forces of the body.

Remember, the spirit is ever willing; the flesh is weak.   69-5

One example of applying the right remedy for the illness or injury was given in a health lecture by a naturopathic physician. She stated that if you suddenly fractured a bone in your arm or leg, it is not the time to take herbs or homeopathic medicine. Go to a hospital emergency room to have it set and a cast put on. The natural remedies can be applied later to aid in the healing, but conventional treatment is excellent in many respects, such as in setting broken or fractured bones.

Becoming aware of our threefold nature and working with these aspects is both complex and simple. It becomes a challenge to maintain the balance within ourselves at all three levels: in the physical body, the mental body, and the spiritual body. The word *body*, we come to realize, refers not just to the material aspect: There is more to us than meets the eye. Taking these concepts into consideration we will arrive, as one reading states, at "understanding why life manifestations in the flesh are necessary, and what an experience at any period is for, or what it is all about." (864-1)

Conclusion

"Spirit is the life, mind is the builder, and the physical is the result." This formula can be our byword as we attempt to meet our needs for healing at each level and as we apply remedial procedures to attune our body to its spiritual source. Having sown the seeds by presenting some basic principles from the Cayce readings, we can delve in a more detailed way into how to nurture ourselves through a practical application of these concepts.

3
Nurturing the Soul Body: Spirit Is the Life

The manifestation of spirit in materiality is to use what it has and to do the best it can with same!　　　　　　　*1527-3*

For the whole of the experience of an individual entity in a material plane is the coordinating and cooperation of Creative Forces from without to the divine within, as to keeping an activity that may bring into manifestations health and happiness.　　　　　　　*1158-8*

The spiritual is that portion of same, or that body, that is everlasting; that is a portion of all it has applied in its mental experiences through the sojourns in the environs of which the entity or soul or spirit body is a part.　　　　*826-11*

Creating an Inner Balance

EDGAR CAYCE, WHO died in 1945, has been called the father of the modern–day holistic health movement. Holism implies an inter–connectedness among body, mind, and spirit. These three aspects are so intertwined that an imbalance or dis–ease in any one will also affect the other two. Keeping this in mind, we realize that overcoming illness and achieving good health require an overall program that may include a healthful diet, physical therapies, spiritual ideals, positive attitudes, and proper medical care. It also involves self–responsibility, taking charge of our healing process by helping our body to mend. This need for self–responsibility can take several forms, from becoming an active participant in our own healing to analyzing the causes of our imbalance and working to set them aright. How did we get out of balance? What created our lack of attunement? These sorts of questions can only be answered by ourselves. Often, when looking closely at our lives, we may see what is causing our distress and what we need to do to put ourselves back into balance.

About one year after I had moved to Virginia Beach and started employment at the A.R.E., I returned to my apartment after work feeling the effects of an oncoming cold: scratchy throat, feverish, slight headache, tired—generally, miserable. I lay down in bed and began to ponder why this was happening. After all, my diet had been pretty good—lots of fruits and vegetables (alkaline–reacting foods); not too much meat (acid–reacting). I was familiar with the readings' statement that a cold cannot exist in an alkaline environment; hence, the improvement in my diet. So I could pat myself on the back, knowing that I was doing OK in the food department. But what else? I recalled a comment made by Elsie Sechrist, who knew Cayce personally and had had readings from him. During our Search for God Study Group meeting one evening Elsie had described how sometimes colds manifest as a result of withheld emotions or responses; for example, not speaking up when it was appropriate or necessary, perhaps because you were afraid of what other people might think. For some reason you chose to keep your response inside, creating what she described as a toxic condition. The increase in toxins, then, creates in your body the cold symptoms. I reflected on this for a while, then gradually began to review my day. Eventually I remembered a conversation in which that very thing occurred! Someone obviously did not have all the facts and viewed a situation incorrectly. I knew a piece of information the person did not, but chose to keep it to myself. Either I did not want to be bothered by revealing the detail or was timid or fearful about releasing it. So I kept quiet.

Wow! This caused my cold. How remarkable! This was indeed where the cold started! But wait a minute. It was really such a minor incident, no big deal. How could such a small thing as this cause me to feel so ill? Gee, I told myself, you must be *really* sensitive if such a tiny incident as this makes you sick. I equated sensitivity with caring and loving—something really positive. But for me it was a negative, creating my miserable, ill feelings. I continued to berate myself for my oversensitivity. Then it hit me. If my sensitivity was so powerful that it produced the sickness, couldn't I also use it to reverse the process and create healing? Why not? I stopped my self-condemnation and began to look at my sensitivity as a potential force for good. Yes, it is powerful and I can use it to make myself well.

While this was taking place, I also revisited in my mind the incident that had occurred earlier in the day. Patterns began to emerge. Yes, I am at times too withdrawn. It's true I don't speak out when I really need to, when it's really appropriate. After acknowledging this failure, I began to forgive myself, resolving to try to do better in the future. There was no self-condemnation this time, just simply an acceptance of my fault and a promise to try to improve. I fell asleep, halfway expecting to call in sick in the morning. But I awoke completely symptom free. No trace of the cold at all. It had totally reversed itself. What a lesson in one's innate power to heal oneself!

No doubt many of us have had similar experiences. We may have consciously or unconsciously created for ourselves the road back to health.

David (not his real name) was busy setting up programs on psychic development in his town when he came down with a severe case of conjunctivitis or pinkeye. Being a college student with little income, he went to the public health clinic for help. After waiting around all day, a young intern finally examined him and stated, "You have conjunctivitis." "That's what I told you six hours ago when I arrived," David answered. Not being able to do anything for the eye, the intern sent David home. David's study group was to meet that evening, so he quickly called around for someone else to head the meeting and asked for prayers for his condition. Later that evening about the time the group would be starting the meditation, David lay down to get into a receptive mood. He fell sound asleep. Hours later he awoke. The conjunctivitis was completely gone.

We can speculate on what occurred to produce this healing effect. On some level an attunement was made that brought the body into better balance. One reading states:

> For the bodily functionings of an animating body . . . with the powers, the abilities of discernment into the activities of spiritual influences within the body, should and may create within the system all influences necessary for the keeping of an equal balance. True, when conditions have reached such proportions at times . . . it becomes necessary to use outside influences. But *know*, as has been given, *all healing* must be and *is* of a deeper source than just the administration of a drug, of the knife, manipulative forces or vibrations that may be created! For all such measures merely create that environment through which the active forces and principles of an active body may gather their forces and influences for the destruction of that which should be eliminated—the elimination of that which has been used or destroyed within the body.
>
> Thus, as has ever been, all power, all force that is of a constructive nature, emanates from the spiritual influences.
>
> Hence the attitudes of the body, in its mental and in its spiritual way and manner, come to be a portion of the Whole.   1158-3

Again we are reminded of the interconnectedness among our bodily systems and that all healing comes from the inner divine source. External applications assist in the attunement; in this case, they help to eliminate "that which has been used or destroyed within the body"—in other words, toxins or poisonous substances produced within our bodies that can be the cause of disease. These obviously need to be gotten rid of in order to maintain a better healthy condition.

Making the Attunement

In chapter 2 we discussed briefly the concept of attunement. Defined as "bringing into harmony or agreement," it is mentioned numerous times in the readings, sometimes along with the verbs *adjust* or *correlate*, to help explain and clarify its meaning. Turning the dial on a radio to reach exactly the precise position where the signal can be picked up and the broadcast clearly heard is one illustration of attunement. Adjusting the pegs on a violin or guitar to match the pitch of a musical scale is another. Evidently there is a tuning or a shift which necessarily occurs that helps to bring "the activities of the bodily functions to nature and natural sources! All healing . . . is the adjusting of the forces that are manifested in the individual body." (2153–6) But how do we make the attunement in order to achieve the desired healing?

Many religious traditions encourage a regular practice of prayer and/or meditation. It is this daily discipline, according to the readings and other spiritual sources, that provides the basis for understanding our relationship to our Creator and fosters an environment that is conducive to healing. Because of the readings' repeated emphasis on the importance of meditation for soul development, the A.R.E. has committed itself to educating and encouraging seekers to learn and practice it. Books, courses, tapes, and conferences on this subject have been offered throughout the years. A half–hour meditation period beginning at noon is part of the work day for staff, volunteers, and visitors, making A.R.E. one of the few companies that *pays* its employees to meditate! Added to the twenty–four lessons that comprise *A Search for God* (Books I and II) is a "twenty–fifth" lesson on meditation, as requested by the readings themselves. "We must learn to meditate just as we learn to walk or talk or to develop any physical attribute." (*ASFG*, Book I, p. 11) While approaches to and forms of meditation will vary with individuals—and it is not within the scope of this book to offer these—to seek a higher state of spiritual consciousness is the aim and purpose of meditation. It is also the surest and safest way to self–understanding.

Cultivating a regular practice of prayer and meditation helps us to understand what in life is truly worthwhile and valuable. Prayer has been defined as talking to God, while meditation is listening to God. "In prayer we speak to God, in meditation God speaks to us." (*ASFG*, Book I, p. 2) One complements the other. Prayer is considered the basis for meditation in that we demonstrate a willingness for guidance and help, then maintain "an attitude of waiting, of silence, of listening, to be able to hear the still, small voice whisper within, and to know that all is well." (*ASFG*, Book I, p. 3) Through both we develop a fuller expression of consciousness and come to an awareness of what in our lives separates us from this more complete union of body, mind, and soul. Another way of describing these effects is through the raising of vibrations. Because illness causes various discordant vibrations in our bodies, with prayer and meditation we can fine-tune our bodies, raise the rate of vibration to a higher level, and become more sensitive to these positive influences that bring us the healing we seek.

In the Prayer Group series of readings, the following question was asked: "Is it possible to give any advice as to how an individual may raise his own vibrations, or whatever may be necessary, to effect a self-cure?" A portion of the lengthy reply follows:

> **By raising that attunement of self to the spirit within, that is of the soul body . . .**
>
> **Oft in those conditions where necessary ye have seen produced within a body unusual or abnormal strength, either for physical or mental activity. From whence arose such? *Who* hath given thee power? Within what live ye? *What* is Life? It is the *attuning* of self, then, to same. *How?***
>
> **As the body-physical is purified, as the mental body is made wholly at-one with purification or purity, with the life and light within itself, healing comes, strength comes, power comes.**
>
> **So may an individual effect a healing, through meditation, through attuning not just a side of the mind nor a portion of the body but the whole, to that at-oneness with the spiritual forces within, the gift of the life-force within each body.**   **281-24**

Making the effort, then, to live a prayerful, meditative life is well worth it, bringing us joy, peace, and true happiness and healing that cannot be found elsewhere. Herbert Puryear, who developed and taught courses on meditation, often encouraged audiences to learn to meditate. Then when a crisis hits, one has a resource, a spiritual tool, at hand upon which to draw. It's too difficult to learn to meditate, he stated, *after* the disease, the divorce, or the death of a loved one occurs. It's harder to pray and meditate in the midst of turmoil. But if one has already developed a familiar routine, a habit, of regular, daily prayer/meditation, it is easier to rely and call upon this inner source of strength when one most needs it.

Additional Benefits of Meditation

Dr. Mehmet Oz, a cardiovascular surgeon who is director of Columbia Presbyterian Heart Institute, offers an optional program of massage, yoga, and meditation to every patient who comes to Columbia Presbyterian Medical Center in New York for heart surgery. In addition to using the most sophisticated tools that modern medicine can provide to replace his patients' diseased hearts with healthy ones, Dr. Oz also relies heavily on what he refers to as "an ancient Eastern technique—meditation." (*Time*, January 20, 2003, p. 71) The reason he does that is, he says, because it works. Though some patients may be a bit self-conscious and unwilling, often the prospect of surgery motivates them to attempt something new and different. The patients buy a specially prepared ninety-minute cassette tape that contains gentle New Age music along with a calming voice directing them to remember a place where they felt comfortable and happy. A significant percentage of his patients choose to participate. The results? Better pain management and reduction of anxiety. Even in randomized trials in which some patients got tapes with sham mantras (meaningless scripts of random phrases) and some received the legitimate voice/music tapes, the results were the same. "What we've discovered is that the words don't matter. The patients who do the best . . . are the ones who use the tapes, real or sham."

What is going on physiologically? When we are under stress—whether facing surgery or taking an exam—our fight–or–flight response is activated, flooding the body with cortisol, a stress hormone produced in the adrenal cortex, and resulting in the shutting down of the parasympathetic nervous system. The parasympathetic system works in opposition to the sympathetic system, which is concerned with the body's response to alarm: increased heart rate, rise in blood pressure, pupils of the eyes dilated. The parasympathetic system's function includes slowing the heart beat, constricting the pupils of the eyes, and stimulating certain digestive glands; in other words, returning the body to an orderly state after the alarm has passed. Studies demonstrate that meditation, at a hormonal level, can counteract the fight–or–flight response of the body's sympathetic nervous system.

At a molecular level, meditation has been shown to slow metabolism in red blood cells. Hence, patients undergoing surgery experience less operative bleeding than those in a control group who were given placebos and who did not meditate. It has also been demonstrated that meditation suppresses the production of cytokines. These are proteins whose presence is usually associated with any kind of increased immune response when people are stressed–out; for example, students who are taking exams.

Yogis and monks, while meditating, are able to manipulate their bodies' metabolism and redirect their bodies' energies. Dr. Elmer Green, known as the father of clinical biofeedback, is a scientist with a life–long interest in healing and spirituality. He worked at the Menninger Foundation as a teacher of biofeedback and, always curious about the cosmos, investigated the yogis of India, observing and testing them during their meditative states. He discovered that they had the ability to control their heart rate, slowing it down or speeding it up—even choosing to make their heart skip a beat. In other experiments scientists witnessed Buddhist monks, sitting in the high Himalayas and melting the snow around them with the heat thrown off their bodies during meditation. In addition the cold towels draped over their backs and shoulders were warmed, evidently because the monks could direct the heat from the core of their bodies to the external surface to warm the towels and melt the ice. According to Dr. Oz, this drop in the internal metabolic rate during meditation is well documented.

In his book *Why God Won't Go Away* Dr. Andy Newberg of the University of Pennsylvania described brain–imaging techniques he used to document changes in blood flow in particular regions of the brain while subjects were engaged in prayer and meditation. "This could be the link between religion and health benefits such as lower blood pressure, slower heart rates, decreased anxiety, and an enhanced sense of well-being," he stated. (*Parade*, March 23, 2003, p. 5)

Other studies have indicated that meditation can reduce arteriosclerosis (hardening of the arteries), especially in African Americans with high blood pressure. Those who suffer from various anxiety disorders can get relief from meditation through lowered stress levels, reduced blood pressure, and slowed heart rate. Also, there is growing evidence that a meditation program can have a positive, sustained effect on chronic pain and such moods as depression and anxiety. Lastly, in a rather dramatic example from initial research, meditation combined with changes in diet may slow the progression of tumors in prostate-cancer patients.

No doubt, experiments will continue in this field and new ground will be broken, with further discoveries for treatment and prevention being made. The beneficiaries of this research will be the patients themselves, who will explore the power of this inner resource and find in it a most effective solution. If meditating for fifteen minutes twice a day can reduce your visits to the doctor over a six-month period, saving the health-care system $200 a patient, as found in one study, then it is well worth the time and the effort to pursue it.

Power of Prayer

Prayer is one of the most ancient expressions of religion. As a human act of communication with the holy or sacred—whether with God or gods and goddesses—it is cherished in all cultures throughout recorded time. Theologians have divided prayer into five categories: adoration, confession, petition, praise, and thanksgiving. Hand gestures, body postures, even dance steps of all kinds may often accompany the religious expression of prayer. It has been defined as conversations with God (Neale Donald Walsch), the raising of the mind and heart to God (*Baltimore Catechism*), religion's primary mode of expression (William James), or an "intimate friendship, a frequent conversation held alone with the Beloved" (St. Teresa of Avila). It can take as many forms as there are personality types, so it remains highly individual in its expression.

One example of the powerful effect of prayer is the case of Tina, who had been diagnosed with a cyst on her ovary. Because the cyst was close to rupturing and thus life-threatening, her surgeon wanted to remove it as quickly as possible. But Tina, who was living in an ashram at the time, resisted, did not want the surgery, so kept putting it off. A woman at the bank whom Tina spoke with was a believer in the evangelist Oral Roberts and gave Tina his card with the telephone number for prayer requests. Tina was not a follower of Oral Roberts, but called the number anyway. The woman who answered took Tina's name and address, prayed a short while with her, then hung up. As Tina walked away from the phone, something told her to lie down. So she entered her bedroom and lay down. Suddenly she realized she could not feel her arms or her legs; they seemed to have become numb. But in the rest of her body—her torso, neck, and head—she felt waves of heat flowing up and down. This sensation lasted for about twenty minutes before subsiding. She got up and felt that she was healed. She had also lost her appetite and wound up going on a three-day fast. Four days after the incident she returned to the surgeon for a checkup and he confirmed that the cyst was no longer present. It had disappeared.

How does prayer work? Today science can tell us *that* prayer works, but cannot really tell us *how*, according to Larry Dossey, M.D. His books, *Healing Words* and *Prayer Is Good Medicine*, describe scientists' attempts to measure and evaluate prayer in the healing process. One study that caught Dossey's attention was conducted by cardiologist Randolph C. Byrd in the 1980s at San Francisco General Hospital. Byrd, a practicing Christian, after much prayer designed his ten-month experiment as a scientific evaluation of the role of God in healing. It involved 393 patients who were admitted to the coronary care unit and were randomly assigned by computer who would be prayed for: 192 would receive prayer from home prayer groups, 201 would not. It was a double-blind study, meaning that the nurses, interns, physicians, and family members did not know which patients were receiving prayer. Various religious groups were used. They were given the patients' first names only and a brief description of their diagnosis and condition. They were to pray each day for the patient, but not instructed on how to pray. Each patient, then, had five to seven people praying daily for him or her.

The results were published as "Positive Therapeutic Effects of Intercessory Prayer in a Coronary Care Unit Program" in *Southern Medical Journal* (July 1988, pp. 826–829). They showed that the prayed-for patients were (1) five times less likely to require antibiotics and (2) three times less likely to develop pulmonary edema; (3) none required endotracheal intubation (an artificial airway inserted into the throat and attached to a mechanical ventilator), and (4) fewer patients died. In the first three results the statistics were not overwhelming, and in the last the number of deaths was not statistically significant. The published results, however, created a sensation; the study was sharply criticized and needed improvement in many ways. Key variables, such as physician and nursing skills, are difficult to eliminate. Prayer is easier and more feasible to study when the subjects are nonhuman living systems, such as plants. However, though inconclusive and inherently ambiguous, the study does strongly suggest a therapeutic effect of distant, intercessory prayer. Dossey comments: "If the technique being studied had been a new drug or a surgical procedure instead of prayer, it would almost certainly have been heralded as some sort of 'breakthrough.'" (*Healing Words*, Harper Collins, San Francisco, Calif., 1993, p. 180)

Author of *The Faith Factor*, Dr. Dale Matthews of Georgetown University would concur. "If prayer were available in pill form, no pharmacy could stock enough of it." (*Parade*, March 23, 2003, p. 4) According to his estimate, 75 percent of the studies in spirituality have confirmed health benefits.

Probably hundreds of scientific investigations into faith and healing are being conducted, representing a new frontier for medical research. Professor Diane Becker of Johns Hopkins, who has received two National Institutes of Health grants to conduct research on prayer, stated: "We are not out to prove that a deity exists. We are trying to see whether prayer has meaning to people that translates into biology and affects a disease process." (*Parade*, March 23, 2003, p. 4) Not long ago this premise would have been looked upon with a great deal of skepticism. No research foundation was willing to fund or review a protocol with "prayer" in the title, but now acceptance from the medical community has slowly grown along with some solid scientific data on the impact of prayer. Research studies done at a number of medical centers, for example, have shown that prayer and faith speed recovery from depression, alcoholism, hip surgery, drug addiction, stroke, rheumatoid arthritis, heart attacks, and bypass surgery.

Because of the scientific culture that we live in today, it is necessary to prove the effectiveness of what many people have instinctively known all along; such as, the success and power of prayer. Some scientists speculate, however, that it is the peaceful, calm state that prayer fosters that may lead to beneficial changes in our cardiovascular and immune systems, making prayer a potent healing force. "It boosts morale; lowers agitation, loneliness, and life dissatisfaction; and enhances the ability to cope in men, women, the elderly, the young, the healthy, and the sick," adds Dr. Harold Koenig, director of Duke University's Center for the Study of Religion/Spirituality and Health. (*Parade*, March 23, 2003, p. 4) So prayer—whether for oneself or others—affects the quality, if not the quantity, of life, he surmises.

Throughout the centuries prayer has been used in a wide variety of ways by a wide diversity of people. Singer/songwriter/author Judy Collins, who has been in the recording business for over forty years, credits folk music to leading her to a deeper prayer life.

> I think prayer is the strongest antidote there is for negativity and fear. In my own work, I rarely start to write a song without first going to the prayer place within. It is essential for my own stability and emotional health to do that . . .
>
> [After mentioning surviving the tragedy of her son's suicide, she states:] We all have challenges, and we just need to know there are tools that help us overcome them. Prayer is a powerful tool by which we can maintain a strong connection with that greater force than ourselves . . .
>
> . . . our own inner guide knows what is going on and what is ours to do. It's an inside job and takes a lot of prayer, a lot of work, and a lot of trust, but that is when the real healing comes through.
>
> (*Daily Word,* January 2003, pp. 10-11)

The Cayce readings would concur. Not only is an attitude of trust and hope needed, but also a sense of purposefulness (a redemptive aspect) to the difficulties we are experiencing. The following excerpt is indicative of a number of similar readings that express these same sentiments:

> Let the body . . . be in that attitude of putting self—in a
> meditative, prayerful mind—into the hands, into the arms,
> into the care of the Savior. Not merely as trusting, not as
> merely hoping, but as relying upon the promises; and make
> them cooperative, co-active. Be used for something; not only
> good but good *for* something; that ye may bring into the
> experience of others—even by thine own ability to suffer—
> the glorious knowledge of the working of the Christ Con-
> sciousness within the individual mind.   528-8

Doreen, who was raised Catholic, always enjoyed the Monday
evening novenas to the Blessed Virgin Mary in her parish church. Now
married, she'd already lost two children during pregnancy and was in
danger of losing another. Her doctor ordered her to bed where she
prayed several times a day the novena prayers she'd learned as a child.
The baby, a girl, was delivered safely and considered a "miracle baby"
by the doctor who knew how close Doreen was to losing her. The daughter is now married and recently celebrated her fortieth birthday. Doreen
has great faith in those novena prayers though she no longer attends
church. In any emergency or extreme difficulty she always resorts to
those prayers and invariably a successful outcome is attained. She has
no doubt in their efficacy to achieve results.

For a thirty–eight–year–old car salesman who was struggling with
alcoholism, a second reading was obtained on December 21, 1937. Those
concerned about him asked what they could do to prevent him "from
indulging in stimulants" and received this startling answer:

> They can pray like the devil!
> And this is not a blasphemous statement, as it may ap-
> pear—to some. For if there is any busier body, with those
> influences that have to do with the spirit of indulgence of
> any nature, than that ye call satan or the devil, who is it?
> Then it behooves those who have the interest of such a
> body at heart to not only pray for him but *with* him; and in
> just as earnest, just as sincere, just as continuous a manner
> as the spirit of *any* indulgence works upon those who have
> become subject to such influences either through physical,
> mental or material conditions!

> For the *power* of prayer is *not* met even by satan or the devil himself.
>
> Hence with that attitude of being as persistent as the desire for indulgence, or as persistent as the devil, ye will find ye will bring a strength. But if ye do so doubting, ye are already half lost.
>
> For the *desires* of the body are to do *right!* Then aid those desires in the right direction; for the power of right *exceeds*—ever and always.
>
> Do that, then.
>
> Like the devil himself—*pray!*   1439-2

The readings assure us that with the proper attitudes of sincerity, earnestness, and persistency the strength to overcome any obstacle will be provided. In the case of Mr. [1439] the degree of persistency should equal "the desire for indulgence," the craving for a drink that he was struggling with in this lifetime. According to the follow-up notes provided by Gladys Davis Turner, it was not known if he actually conquered his addiction, though this second reading seemed to indicate that he certainly had the desire to do right.

From the perspective of the Cayce readings, it is prayer that helps us prepare for meditation, as mentioned earlier; in prayer we begin the process that leads us into the stillness where we meet the Divine. It is "the concerted effort of our physical consciousnesses to become attuned to the Consciousness of the Creator . . . the attunement of our conscious minds to the spiritual forces that manifest in a material world." (*ASFG*, Book I, p. 2) Prayer and meditation, then, can be considered focal points for nurturing our spiritual body. They help to ground us and make us more aware of our abilities "to overcome [those] conditions that disturb the body . . . " (543-19) The readings counseled people not to neglect their spiritual side and even to pray for a cure if one is ill or for any human need. Daily prayer and meditation periods were encouraged as part of the healing process, but the results were to be left to God.

Reading the Scriptures

Scripture reading was also heartily endorsed; often it was mentioned

as a regular therapy added to the ill person's regimen. Frequently recommended selections include Exodus 20, Deuteronomy 30, the Psalms,
John 14–17, and the Book of Revelation. Sometimes a simple admonition was given:

> . . . search ye the scriptures daily. For in them ye have prom-
> ises that are *thine!* In them ye have hope, in them ye have
> the promise of life, of eternal life, of the water of life, of the
> bread of life, that makes man free; free here and now—of
> disease, of disturbance in the various centers . . .
> [Use] that thou hast daily in hand, and the next step may
> be given thee.   2994-1

The Scriptures were to be read and prayed over, with the intention of
making them applicable and personal today. They can thus become
part of one's regular prayer/meditation period, to be reflected and acted
upon consciously in one's daily life. This is not, then, a passive approach to life's problems and challenges, but a participatory movement
toward application of what one knows. A well-known Cayce phrase is:
"In the application comes the awareness." The Cayce readings are, therefore, a strong proponent of individuals being active participants and of
putting into practice what they know to be true. Insights come as a
result—insights perhaps into how the disease process got started, what
caused it, and how to reverse it.

It is well known that Edgar Cayce himself loved to read the Bible. In
fact, he reportedly read it clear through, from cover to cover, each year
of his life. How many ministers and clergy can claim that achievement?!
In addition, during most of his adult life, Cayce was a popular Sunday
school teacher, whose students often mentioned that he made the stories from the Bible come alive for them. Because of his thorough
grounding in the Bible, it is no wonder—as many students of the readings observe—that biblical quotations and allusions are scattered like
seeds throughout the readings, as well as his advice and encouragement to many to read "the Good Book." One person even asked about
which version of the Bible was the most accurate in meaning. The question and answer follow:

(Q) What present printed version of the Bible gives the nearest to the true meaning of both the new and old Testaments?
(A) The nearest true version for the entity is that ye apply of
whatever version ye read, in your life. It isn't that ye learn
from anyone. Ye only may have the direction. The learning,
the teaching is within self. For where hath He promised to
meet thee? Within the temple! Where is that temple? Within!
Where is heaven or earth? Within! Meet thy Savior there.
For He hath promised, "I stand at the door—open. If ye
open, I will enter and sup with thee." Again, "If ye will
open I will come in—and I and the Father will abide with
thee."   2072-14

Again application is advised, with the learning coming then from
within the individual, in the inner temple where the Savior has promised to meet us.

Church Affiliation

While the readings neither give authority to nor endorse any particular church organization or ecclesiastical structure, they did counsel
some individuals to affiliate with a church. Edgar Cayce himself grew
up in the Disciples of Christ (Christian) Church, but joined the First
Presbyterian Church when in the 1920s the family moved to Virginia
Beach, as there was no Disciples of Christ congregation established in
the Beach at that time.

One woman who asked, "Should I affiliate with any particular church
organization?" was advised: "A particular church organization is well.
For it centers the mind." (3350-1) Another woman asked: "Is there any
indication of what church I should join and associate with?" The reading answered:

Remember, rather, the church is within self. As to the organization, choose that—not as a convenience for thee but
where ye may serve the better, whatever its name—let it be
thy life proclaiming Jesus, the Christ.   3342-1

A man who asked how he should "meet the opposition in my church activities" was advised not to condemn himself or others, that those in service to the church "are seeking, as well as thou." He was also told:

> **Render unto the church that which is the church, whether in creed or in organization, but render unto God, unto Christ, the *service* that is His in whatever field of activity thou goest. In meeting it in this manner will ye unseat those that would ride over thee in *any* opposition.**   **556-1**

The ideal of service was also mentioned in another reading for an osteopath who asked if it would help his professional practice if he attended a church and, if so, which one. He was told:

> **This is rather irreverent, my son. For, to be sure, to do good that good may come from same is well. But to question self—if there is the answering from within, that due reverence to the spiritual forces would arise from thine service and thine activity with an organized service, then through such and from such must come, of course, the greater *ability*, opportunity, to be of service to thy fellow man. Would be *well*, if the promptings come from within. If the promptings come that such may be used as a steppingstone for thine own self alone, not so well; for thine heart and soul cannot be in same if it be for material gain alone!**
>   **657-3**

Cayce's own example and several readings' excerpts would indicate the advisability—even wisdom—of church affiliation and participation. Not only would it be well for spiritual support, but also give one the opportunity for experiences needed to be met. This concept is reflected in an excerpt from the Work Readings (254 series) when the question was proposed as to the proper way to handle those "interested in cults, isms, etc."

> **As He has given, it will ever be found that Truth—whether in this or that schism or ism or cult—is of the One source.**

> Are there not trees of oak, of ash, of pine? There are the needs of these for meeting this or that experience. Hast thou chosen any one of these to be the *all* in thine usages in thine own life?
>
> Then, all will fill their place. Find not fault with *any*, but rather show forth as to just how good a pine, or ash, or oak, or *vine*, thou art! 254-87

This sense of inclusiveness is prevalent as a theme throughout the body of the Cayce readings. By choice individuals face certain experiences necessary for personal growth. Recognizing and understanding this decision-making aspect of the soul and this freedom of choice we have as a birthright help us to refrain from fault-finding or criticism of others. An individual's spiritual development—whatever path he or she chooses to follow—is top priority and becomes the Truth for that person. And Truth is where heaven is, according to one reading given to the original members of the Search for God Study Group. The reading itself had asked where heaven is and this answer was provided:

> Within the hearts, the minds; the place where Truth is made manifest! Wherever Truth is made manifest it gives place to that which is heaven *for those that seek* and love truth! but a mighty hell for those that seek gratification of their own selves! And these are those things which become stumbling-blocks to many an individual that becomes more and more material-minded. 262-87

Earlier in the same section of this reading Cayce defined "the Holy Church" as "That which makes for the awareness in the heart of the individual." The excerpt continued:

> The Church is never a body, never an assembly. An *individual* soul becomes aware that it has taken that Head, that Son, that Man even, to be the intermediator. *That* is the Church; that is what is spoken of as the Holy Church.
> 262-87

The Church, then, is not equated with any institution or organization, but consists of those in relationship with "that Head, that Son, that Man [as] the intermediator." Regardless of our disagreements or discouragements with human–made institutions, the true church within us is the place where we may find answers "to many of those questions sought concerning the Spirit, the Church, the Holy Force that manifests by the attuning of the individual; though it may be for a moment." (262-87) This reading went on to explain what Jesus Himself stated, that Peter's answer to His question, "Whom say men that I am?" was revealed to him not through flesh and blood (ordinary human means), but that God the Father inspired Peter to answer, "Thou art the Christ, the son of the living God!" Insights and revelations flow from an awareness that is in touch with, in tune with, one's inner spirit. Answers to some of life's perplexing questions—what is the role of suffering; why are we ill—can be discovered in this same fashion, through contact with this "kingdom within."

Not surprisingly, according to dozens of research studies, regular church attendance can even be beneficial to one's health. People who pray frequently and participate in religious services stay healthier and live longer than those who rarely or never do. This was found to be true even when other factors, such as age, health, habits, or demographics, were considered. One six–year study at Duke University, consisting of 4,000 men and women of various faiths and all older than sixty–four years, found that the relative risk of dying was 46 percent lower for those who attended religious services frequently. Likewise, from a University of Miami study of AIDS patients, those who became long–term survivors were more likely to be involved in religious practices or engaged in volunteer work—again the service aspect that the readings so highly recommend.

One final note is this comforting reminder:

> **Know, as has been given, God looks on the heart, not on the outward appearance. A rose by any other name may be just as sweet. So may an individual by any name. What is the purpose? The church, the God-force, is within self; not in the name that may be added by man. That oft becomes the**

> stumbling stone to man. For to such there is limitation, and
> who can limit God? Who would limit the Master? Who
> would limit self, in God's direction?   3350-1

When the Divine Spirit introduces us to limitlessness, opening us to
a more heart-centered spirituality, we become further aligned to our
purpose, to carrying out our destiny, through the strength and insights
derived from this wellspring of spiritual energy.

Conclusion

Attunement creates for us the balance and harmony we need for a
more fulfilled, purposeful life. A commitment to frequent prayer, meditation, and Scripture reading along with an active church life helps us
to make that attunement and thus to nurture our spiritual body. Nevertheless, though spiritual beings, we live and work in a material world.
Chapter 4 will address one aspect of that world: our mind and its role in
nurturing our mental body.

Nurturing the Mental Body:
Mind Is the Builder

. . . if one would correct physical or mental disturbances, it is necessary to change the attitude and to let the life forces become constructive and not destructive. 3312-1

It is true then that the mind may heal entirely by the spoken word, by the laying on of hands, dependent upon the consciousness of the motivative forces in the individual body. 262-83

Then, Mind being the Builder . . . is the contact for the life forces in materiality or physical body. 1436-1

Mind as Healer

NOWADAYS MORE HEALTH care professionals as well as patients are recognizing that mental states and physical well–being are intimately connected, that the mind and body are not separate at all, but are part of a single system. An unbalanced, unhealthy body can lead to an unbalanced, unhealthy mind and vice versa: illnesses of the mind or long-term negative, nonconstructive thought patterns can trigger or worsen diseases in the body. This awareness is also reflected in the Cayce material. From Book II of *A Search for God* we read: "What we think, what we put our mind to work upon, to live upon, to feed upon, to live with, to abide with, that our soul body becomes. That is the law . . . " (p. 187)

In November 2002 in Washington, D.C., at a two-day national conference sponsored by the nonprofit Depression and Bipolar Support Alliance, audiences listened to the evidence linking depression with one illness after another. However, we know from everyday experiences that brain chemistry governs more than just the emotions. When your mind feels terror, for example, the resulting surge of adrenaline makes your stomach churn. Effects may be even more direct with the powerful chemicals in the brain (such as serotonin). These circulate not just in the brain, but all through the body. Because of this, effects are created and felt throughout the physical system. Since the research is preliminary, it is not well understood just how these brain chemicals known as neurotransmitters affect the course of an illness or disease. When serotonin is circulating in the bloodstream, for example, it appears that platelets are then less sticky, thus less likely to clump together creating blood clots that block arteries. So, to keep serotonin in circulation, doctors regularly advised patients who had suffered heart attacks to take a daily dose of children's aspirin in order to prevent blood clots.

Stress, both acute and chronic, can also be harmful to the physical body. The brain first detects a threat, then signals the body in the form of hormones and nerve impulses to go on alert and prepare for fight or flight. Muscles tense, the heart beats faster, arteries widen, the stomach stops digesting, the lungs ventilate faster, and the adrenals release stress hormones. Thus the body is prepared for action. When the threat has ended, the stress hormone levels drop. Ideally, when the danger has passed, the response turns off. But many people today are suffering from chronic stress in just trying to deal with the ordinary pressures of modern life. This constant emotional pressure continues the fight-or-flight response and weakens the immune system, making the body less able to deal with and overcome illnesses or making infectious diseases worse. Though useful in the short term, this flood of hormones can be subtly toxic in the long run. So any attempt we make in trying to reduce the level of stress—whether through meditation and prayer, as discussed in chapter 3, or by adopting a more positive attitude—could add up to many years of a significantly healthier life. These disciplines engage the mind, helping it to focus on the spiritual dimension of our lives, and at the same time creating a healing activity in the physical body. One reading described the work of the "mental body" as enabling an individual "to centralize or to agree within itself as to its hopes, its desires, and how it would use its abilities and its efforts." The reading cautioned against using the mind's abilities for selfish purposes, as then "there will be little use of any corrective measures" (3254-1); in other words, unless there was the proper, unselfish attitude, remedial treatments would be useless and the healing would not occur.

The Role of Attitudes in Healing

Tonya had been suffering from blackouts ever since she was ten years old. Now in her mid-thirties she was hoping to reduce or eliminate completely the amount of medication she was on to control them, as the side effects were bothersome and uncomfortable. So on her own she researched the Cayce readings and with her physician–husband mapped out a wellness plan that included dietary changes, a series of Epsom salts baths, some massages, tonics, and castor oil packs. She had recently quit her job so had more time now to devote to her health regimen. After pursuing her plan for nearly a year, she seemed to be making progress despite setbacks now and then. Surprisingly with the gradual reduction in her medication her blackouts were occurring less frequently—something really unheard of by her skeptical doctor. Learning more about her peculiar illness and searching the readings for other remedies to add to her wellness plan, she came across an article in an old A.R.E. publication on attitudes. Despite the progress she was making, she realized after reading the article how entrenched she was in her illness: her family and friends revolved their lives around it, making it almost a part of her personality. So it was difficult for her to imagine herself without this illness, so much a part of her it had become. Shortly thereafter she had a serious fall and injured herself. She then discontinued her plan and resumed her regular doses of medication, realizing that despite all the physical efforts she had made, she honestly was unwilling to change her attitude, and this reluctance was holding her back from progressing further.

Perhaps many of us can identify with this situation. We may choose

to carry out a certain number of treatments—a series of colonics, osteopathic adjustments, steam baths, a better diet—and feel we are on the path
to restoring our health. These physical applications may be necessary
and helpful for recovery to take place, yet if we intend to work with the
triune concept of the body, all aspects must be taken into consideration.
One Cayce reading reminded a sixty-three-year-old woman to:

> . . . **care for the physical, that the spiritual and mental may
> better apply those truths, lessons, as are being attained by
> the body through the application of spiritual truth to the
> nerve and blood supply of body . . . The physical and the
> mental and the spiritual are *one*, yet each must be dealt with
> in and through its own sphere . . .** 4308-1

In continuing, the reading again used Jesus as the model. At the end
of His forty days of fasting in the desert prior to His public ministry
(Matthew 4:1–11), Jesus was tempted by the devil to turn stones into
bread so that He could alleviate His hunger. Though Jesus answered,
"Man shall not live by bread *alone* but by every word that proceeds out
of the mouth of the Lord," yet He "[supplied] the physical needs to the
thousands to meet the physical conditions of the body and [supplied]
the needs of the spiritual to the individual man." Mrs. [4308] was advised then to "Apply those truths, those lessons as attained—in and
through those of the Master—in the life in the physical, in the spiritual, in
the mental." (4308-1) In a follow-up question, she asked about the order
to follow in making the applications. The question and answer, which
were given in chapter 2 but repeated here, follow:

> **(Q) Should the body take care of the physical first and then
> the spiritual?**
> **(A) As given, meet the needs of the physical conditions of
> the body through the physical at present. Meet the needs of
> the spiritual, the mental, through the spiritual and the men-
> tal. Apply then those physical needs for the body at present,
> applying *through* the spiritual those of the mental and spiri-
> tual nature for the physical and mental as given, each
> through its own sphere, and each are as *one* in application to
> the body.** 4308-1

Even though you may be following a particular health regimen that includes a number of applications, such as a dietary plan, medicine, exercise, manipulations, packs, etc., the mind and spirit can also be engaged: the mind providing the proper attitude and intention and the spirit adding a prayerful, meditative focus to the physical remedies. Chapter 3 already covered the topics of prayer and meditation, so here will be presented the mental aspects of attitude and intention.

Attitude: If we were to examine what it is that makes us really enjoy the company of another person, we might come up with the word *attitude*; or rather, the *quality* of the person's attitude. According to the dictionary, attitude is "a manner of acting, feeling, or thinking that shows one's disposition, opinion, etc.; one's mental set." Most of us like to be around cheerful, optimistic, joyful personalities. Their upbeat characteristics are almost contagious, lifting up those of us who come in contact with them. Their lightheartedness practically lingers in the atmosphere after they've left, and we may sometimes feel good about ourselves after being with them. Conversely, we find those with negative, pessimistic characteristics difficult to be around, their heaviness weighing us down; they seem to create a density even in the atmosphere about them. We are relieved—perhaps exhausted—when they leave our presence.

Some of the positive qualities of what we'd consider a "good attitude" was mentioned in a reading for a thirty–three–year–old woman who received her thirteenth reading from Cayce on December 7, 1940. At the end of her reading she asked for "further suggestions for the physical and spiritual improvement of this body." The answer came:

> **Keep the attitude that as the physical body is the manifestation of spiritual life and influence, it is to be used in a constructive manner as to bring hope and cheer into the lives of others. This is a reasonable service, as an appreciation, as a duty, as an opportunity for expressing the divine in self.**
>
> **Be expectant in the opportunities. These *will* present themselves in many ways.**   **808-13**

In a follow-up letter to Cayce on December 11, 1940, she commented: "I was certainly impressed with the answer to the last question. Wasn't it good?"

To a woman who, according to her reading, had "pathological conditions" as well as "psychic or psychological conditions that must be corrected," Cayce advised:

> . . . all animosity, all hate, all jealousy, must be eliminated from the mental self, and the hopes and the desires to be able to contribute to the welfare of those less fortunate than self. For, remember, unless we may learn to love that something in even those who have been and are our enemies, we have not begun to think straight. For the law of the Lord is perfect and it converteth the soul. And it is the soul that one would save.
>
> With that as the correct attitude—consider:
>
> Who healeth thine afflictions? who giveth life to those that would seek His face?
>
> That should be done first. 3254-1

Many years before contemporary medicine accepted the concept of psychosomatic illness Cayce was already referring to the mind's influence upon body and soul, and the effect of emotions and attitudes upon the physical body. Physical and mental imbalances could be corrected, he stated, by changing one's attitude. This would create a way or channel, then, for constructive—not destructive—life energies or forces to flow through the body, bringing balance and healing. When our bodies, as temples of the living God—as mentioned in the Bible—are kept in a proper state of health and attunement, then the mind can function better as well. That these systems interact is expressed in one excerpt from a reading for a young boy that was given on February 4, 1934, at the recommendation of Mrs. [255]. The child, suffering from tonsillitis and sinusitis, among other illnesses, was apparently also stubborn, so a question was asked about how to deal with this trait. The reading gave this explanation:

The stubbornness is not so much in self as it is caused by

the feelings in the body as resentments to the general conditions. A more healthy body will make a more healthy outlook. And do not say *don't!* Give the body things to do,
instead of saying Don't—do!   508-1

Over a month later in a letter dated March 16, 1934, Mrs. [255] told
Cayce: "[508] got over his trouble wonderfully, without having an ad-
enoid operation and is fine now." The connection was evidently made
between a healthy attitude and a healthy body.

Quite a large percentage of the physical readings offered some advice to the recipient regarding maintaining the proper attitude. In addition to cheerfulness and hope, an attitude of expectancy was also
important. Considering the number of exclamation points used in the
text of these readings, it seems that the sleeping Cayce was quite em-
phatic about the individual acquiring this particular mental set. Expectancy implies that a person has a considerable degree of confidence that
a certain event or outcome will happen, that something will probably
occur. Because of outward appearances—the physical manifestation of a
disease process—this expectation may be quite difficult to achieve; nevertheless, the readings continue to encourage seekers to *expect* a complete recovery, as demonstrated in the following for a twelve-year-old
girl who was suffering the effects of poliomyelitis. Her mother requested
this check reading and was present for it. Her daughter had made some
improvement through following the recommendations in the first reading, but the mother had further questions regarding "hastening her recovery." (2604-1, R-3) Among several questions she asked: "Will there be
a toe drag in the left foot?" Cayce's answer was:

If that's what is desired, if that's what is being sought,
there will be! If there is being sought, if there is being
expected a *complete recovery*, it will come—if there will be
done that as indicated!   2604-2

When the mother later asked for "any spiritual advice," this information was given: "Keep that same constructive attitude; not only being
good but good *for* something." (2604-2) Being good for a purpose was
stressed many times in the readings, and it no doubt helped to contrib-

ute to a more healthy physical body.

Another reading stated: " . . . do all with that *expectancy* of that which is desired to be accomplished in this body—and it will come to pass." (456–1) This attitude of a hopeful outcome, a frequent refrain in a number of physical readings, seems to point out the importance of focusing on the desired outcome, the end result, in order to create the conditions for it to occur.

After cautioning a forty–one–year–old man not to pity himself, Cayce told him: "Expect good health! Don't expect to remain ill! and you'll be better off." (5609–5) In a follow–up reading the same man asked, "How soon may I expect a complete cure?" Cayce answered:

> **Set the time for self, then do the things necessary to bring them about! and then expect to be well! How soon will he do these? and then we may find how soon he may expect to be well!** 5609-6

In a letter on August 24, 1932, Cayce himself (not in his trancelike state!) commented on [5609]'s question about how soon he should "expect a complete cure":

> **If the doctor applies the treatments properly, it has already been outlined as to how long it should take to make the correction. If you set the time, and the doctor sets the time, and there is builded in your whole system and mind that it should be corrected, you will no doubt see the results in that time.**
>
> **[Then came a note of warning and frustration.] Sometimes . . . even among the best physicians, according to the readings and according to the conditions that arise with individuals, they get overanxious or are desirous of keeping the patient as long as possible—and know more about it than the readings do themselves; consequently, they bring about harmful conditions rather than helpful.** 5609-6, R-2

Negative emotions and feelings—especially if indulged in over a long time period—can also bring about harmful conditions, as mentioned in a number of readings. Resentments, unjustified anger, hatred, worry, jealousy are all disruptive and toxic to the physical body, creating discordant vibrations that can harm, damage, or prevent the body's normal functioning. That attitudes do influence one's physical condition is stated repeatedly in the readings.

Some comments on anger are indicative of this influence. "For anger can destroy the brain as well as any disease. For it is itself a disease of the mind." (3510-1) There was some concern for this person, [3510], who seemed to be experiencing "a gradual deterioration of mental faculties" and was "fighting against the administrations being made." In another reading Cayce gave advice that he said was good for most people: " . . . don't get mad and don't cuss a body out mentally or in voice. This brings more poisons than may be created by even taking foods that aren't good." (470-37) Here a negative attitude seems to take precedence over or have more power than a poor diet. Note also that mental expressions of anger are just as harmful as verbal expressions!

One person wanted to know if his body was ridding itself, in a timely manner, of poisons that had been discharged into the bloodstream. The reading responded:

> **. . . it is getting rid of some, but when there is the ruffling of your disposition when there is any anger, it prepares the system so that it blocks the flow of the circulation to the eliminating channels. Thus you can take a bad cold from getting mad. You can get a bad cold from blessing [cursing] out someone else, even if it is your wife.   849-75**

Other physical conditions that can be brought about by negative attitudes are mentioned in this frequently quoted excerpt: "No one can hate his neighbor and not have stomach or liver trouble. No one can be jealous and allow the anger of same and not have upset digestion or heart disorder." (4021-1) However, we cannot deduce that because these physical disorders exist in someone that the person must be jealous, hateful, or angry. There could very well be other factors creating the imbalances; it is not our place to judge another or feel guilty because we may have that ailment. These reactions—judgment and guilt—can be self-defeating and purposeless, negating the good we are attempting to achieve.

Other attitudes that were to be eliminated were doubt and worry. Cayce told one woman: "He who doubts that the best will come to him with doing of that which is correct is already defeated. Don't blame others for what has happened or may happen. Do right yourself, physically, mentally and spiritually, and the best will come to you." (5203-1) One husband who asked: "How can I keep from worrying so much about my wife's health?" was told: "Why worry, when ye may pray? Know that the power of thyself is very limited. The power of Creative Force is unlimited." (2981-1) Again prayer and the cultivation of a positive way of responding will bring more helpful and healing results to the body. But how do we go about creating these positive effects?

Changing one's attitude is not a simple, easy task. Much like changing a habit, it requires persistence, consistency, and patience, attributes that are mentioned frequently in the readings. As one chiropractor noted, "It took us a long time to become ill, so getting well again won't happen overnight." It also takes effort and willpower to replace a negative attitude with a positive one. Some of these characteristics were noted in one reading given at the request of a nineteen–year–old woman who, at seven years of age, had been diagnosed with infantile paralysis. Both she and her mother questioned the diagnosis. She had tried chiropractic and Christian Science, but got no relief. The daughter wrote to Cayce, wondering about the curvature in her spine, her useless leg, and abnormal left thumb which prevented her from playing the piano. "I have an absolute faith in you and will follow your directions implicitly. I don't question my faith in you any more than I question the faith I have had in reincarnation since I was a child." (2968-1, B-1) Her mother, writing ten days later, mentioned the specialness she felt about her child: "I have never felt that her coming to this world was just a usual event. I wanted that child more than anything in life and my one and only prayer was that he or she would be a blessing in this world." (2968-1, B-2) The reading, given on April 21, 1943, stated in part:

> . . . these, as we find, may be materially aided. It will re-
> quire time, patience, persistence, expectancy on the part of

the body, and prayerful application of those things suggested that may create in the body-forces that necessary for
creating a greater number of energies or elements in the
energies of the body that are attuned to the divine conscience.

First, know this—in thy inner self:

Ye can be a channel of blessings to others, whatever may
be thy physical state—provided there is the application of
that which is known within self of the divine manifesting
through a material chamber.

Thy body is indeed the temple of the living God. Hold to
that. By might and main of the mind, attempt to make the
best, the most beautiful, the most acceptable temple according to thy concept of a living Christ Consciousness. Hold to
that. Let no one, in any manner, take that from you.

Then apply, in an expectant manner, those measures
which will aid the body-forces to create within self those
influences necessary for this building of the body to a beautiful temple to thy God.   2968-1

This very positive, uplifting message evidently was taken to heart.
On May 5, 1943, [2968]'s mother wrote to Cayce: " . . . we immediately
took steps to carry out your instructions . . . [The reading] bore out the
belief I have had since she took sick and we certainly are going to
cooperate and follow your suggestions regardless of the doctors." (2968–
1, R–2)

Follow–up letters indicated that the treatment recommendations were
carried out with successful results. The daughter wrote to Cayce after
her second reading: "I've been following your instructions faithfully . . .
My condition is really much improved. My leg used to be discolored all
the time, and for weeks now it has not been . . . I have implicit faith in
your instructions. Neither Mother nor I have any doubt or shadow of
doubt that you will help me. We are expectant and hopeful, if that
helps. Thank you again for all you have done for me and others." (2968–
2, R–1)

Comments such as these serve as a reminder of how often ill people
sought out Cayce as a last resort. They had either been given up on by
doctors—who might have been baffled or stumped by their patients'

conditions—or were simply not receiving relief from following their physicians' advice and treatments. These types of stories and letters throughout the background and research reports of many of the physical readings bear this out. However, the Cayce readings also referred seekers to physicians and therapists for help with their treatments. Harold J. Reilly, one of the first doctors of physiotherapy in the U.S., at one time estimated that Cayce had sent him approximately 1,000 patients—more than any other health practitioner. Reilly, who died in 1987 at the age of ninety-two, is still remembered for his contributions to the field of holistic health. In the 1960s he helped the A.R.E. set up its Therapy Department (now called the Health and Rejuvenation Center), donating equipment such as massage tables, a whirlpool tub, sitz baths, and a steam cabinet, heading the department, and personally training all the massage therapists who worked there. Shortly before his death, the Cayce/Reilly School of Massotherapy opened its doors, and today the A.R.E. continues to carry on Reilly's work by teaching his method of massage and healing. His book, *The Edgar Cayce Handbook for Health Through Drugless Therapy*, is based on his forty-five years of experience with the Cayce work and is used as a textbook in the school curriculum.

Another physician who treated individuals sent to her from the readings was Mrs. [1125], an osteopath. On June 23, 1937, she reported on the results, stating:

> It has been a pleasure to take these cases from Mr. Cayce. I wish that we might have both the physical and life readings in all these disorders as back of most of the physical is the mental and environmental influence.
>
> With sincere appreciation of Mr. Cayce's wonderful gift I wish to state that as far as my work has been with his readings the results have been 100%.
>
> It has been a privilege to have had the experience.
>
> 1125-2, R-1

In her second reading, given on February 2, 1937, she received not only advice for her sinus and weight problems, but much information on the relationship of attitudes to illness. Early on in the reading, she was told:

> True, we find there are pathological conditions that may be corrected for a better reaction. But without the causes or the attitudes of the body mentally, and without a better co-ordination of the ideals of the body in its relationships to material, to mental, as arise from its spiritual concept, made to be in better coordination, there can not be any real help; it will only produce or cause greater confusions later on.
>
>   1125-2

To begin her healing process through following the suggested treatments, she was advised to first work with her attitudes and then apply the "mechanical adjustments" (treatments with the Radio–Active Appliance) that were recommended. Some of the attitudes seemed to be "thrust upon" her, creating "resentments, animosities . . . hate—as well as anxieties. And hate to a body in a reaction is poison . . . " (1125–2)

> Then, to correct such an attitude—the entity should coordinate those ideals that have been and are a portion of the entity; not in what but in *Whom* the entity may believe, for its relationships to Creative Forces as are manifested in a material world.
>
> Then when this is done, we will find that in the place of resentment, animosity, hate or disagreements or confusion, we will replace with patience, long-suffering; enduring *all* things, not merely as passive but as an active way and manner!
>
> For as the body experiences, to give or to bring help physically, hope mentally to others, brings into the experience of the mental body the greatest boon for purposeful life as is experienced by the very *choice* of the entity as to a profession!   1125-2

She was encouraged to take this more positive attitude into all the relationships in her experience.

The reading continued to describe the effects of her attitudes on her physical body: "pathological and psychological conditions" that created an excess of lymph in the soft tissues of her face, resulting in poor circulation.

Thus we have then a deflection in the segments or ganglia along the upper dorsal [thoracic] and cervical that—by the very activity of emotions, the very activity of pressure itself—prevents the normal circulatory forces.

Hence we have those tendencies for cold, those tendencies for the sniffles at times, those tendencies for the desire to clear the throat, the filling up of the sinus, of the soft tissue; those inclinations for such reactions in the body.

Now to remove the pressures alone and not to change the attitudes—have we helped to the fullest extent?   1125-2

After a regimen of treatment was outlined, with reminders throughout that attitudes can create poisons or toxins in the system, she was given this advice:

Do these, consistently, persistently, keeping the mental attitudes *proper*—and we will bring normal forces; and a life of activity and service that makes the experience of the entity *so much more* worth while!   1125-2

Realizing that she is being helpful and of service to others, bringing them health, hope, and strength when they "have lost their hold upon the better things in a material experience," will help her to overcome her own physical difficulties, the reading promised.

In surveying just a handful of the physical readings, it may be surprising, considering how ill some of the recipients were, to detect a tone of optimism and hope in the text of the readings themselves. Often, too, in the follow-up letters sent by Cayce (not in his sleeplike state, but awake) or by Gladys Davis Turner, his secretary, to answer or clarify some questions or statements in the readings, the tone was again one of deep concern and care for the seeking individual with a sincere desire to serve him or her. Typical of these sorts of letters is one that Cayce wrote on July 22, 1943, in answer to [2968]'s letter, whose reading excerpts were quoted earlier:

I think I would keep up the treatments until about between the first and middle of September before I would have a check-up again. Of course, we are glad to make this at any time you wish it, for our whole purpose is to try to help and, of course, in being on the ground we sometimes may be prone to put it off when we should be a little quicker about it. I am glad to know that you are feeling better. I feel that you will really improve. You are going to have periods, of course, when apparently there isn't any change, then you will have times when you will feel a little better, but you just keep to it and I feel sure you will really get results. Let us hear from you at any time that you feel like writing and know that we are very glad to have your feelings in the matter. Of course, we are busy, but never too busy to try and be of help.   2968-2, R-2

One final note about attitudes involves the readings' stress upon their overall importance in achieving health. A number of times it was suggested, as alluded to in several earlier quoted excerpts, that the mental attitude be dealt with first before even attempting a physical treatment; otherwise, very little would be accomplished or changed for the individual. One typical reading stated:

. . . if anything is to be done in the way of correcting or eliminating the causes of the disturbances, much in the mental and spiritual must be considered by the body first. For, there will be little to be gained by making physical applications without there being a change in the mental attitude and spiritual purport of many of those conditions about the body.   3194-1

In this same reading some specific attitudes were mentioned that needed correction.

First, as we find: Change the attitude of the body, spiritually and mentally. Do not be so pessimistic about self, conditions, or others. Do not give expression to nor hold to, nor entertain malice, injustice, self-righteousness, or those things that cause such great amounts of anxieties through the body.   3194-1

To another individual other attitudes were pointed out:

> **When the body becomes so self-satisfied, so self-centered as
> to renounce, refuse, or does not change its attitude, so long
> as there is hate, malice, injustice, those things that produce
> hate, those that produce jealousy, those that produce that
> which is at variance to patience, long-suffering, brotherly
> love, kindness, gentleness, there cannot be healing to that
> condition of this body.** 3124-2

Sometimes poor health, general malaise, or simply a painful condition accompanies a negative attitude. A thirty-five-year-old tavern
owner had a number of complaints: a rapid pulse, stomach and intestinal problems, a general sickening feeling, pains in his back and under
his heart, and an abdomen that was sore to the touch; X-rays taken
revealed nothing. He asked what would give him a new interest in life
and was told:

> **Change the attitude towards life. Be interested more in cre-
> ative influences and in spirituality, and there will be a better
> interest in life.**
>   **Of course, the change of the general conditions physi-
> cally will have much to do with the attitude. For with a
> constant pain, or cramping pains and disturbance through
> alimentary canal, the general interest in life becomes such
> that the body appears rather peeved with most everything.**
>   **Do as indicated and we will make better conditions for
> the body.** 4064-1

Another woman was told in her reading not to feel sorry for herself
because she was having difficulty walking without some assistance:
" . . . think how much better this is than no limbs at all, or those that are
constantly in pain! And the body will find that it has much to be thankful for." (3642-1) To a sixty-seven-year-old man Cayce recommended an
optimistic attitude and suggested wherein the fault lay if results were
not achieved.

(Q) How long will it take to cure the condition?
(A) Remember, the condition is both pathological and psychological. To take the properties as outlined and not
change the attitude towards the surroundings and the conditions will be *little* worth while. Become more *optimistic* in
the outlook upon conditions surrounding the body; knowing that, if self is spended in doing the best service for that
the body worships (whether of the spiritual or mental nature), the results if not in keeping with that desired is self's
own fault! If the ideal is set in the spiritual things, and the
results are not in keeping with that meted out, the fault is
then in the manner in which the ideal is kept.   592-1

The setting of ideals has been mentioned already in several readings
and will be discussed in the next section of this chapter, as it is a mental
exercise and is related to the healing process.

Intention: When we are determined to do a specific thing or act in
some specified manner, we are using intention. We may even have a
plan or design in mind and aim to carry it out, with the use of intention.
"Purposeful behavior" is another description of intention. Surprising
and sometimes powerful results can occur when we hold a particular
plan or design in mind, then proceed to fulfill it. A number of contemporary healers refer to their use of intention prior to conducting healing sessions. (More about this later in chapter 7.)

In place of *intention*, the readings often use the word *intent*, a rather
formal term which connotes more deliberation; or the word *purpose*,
which again implies a greater resolution or determination to carry out a
set plan. In a dream interpretation reading a fuller definition was presented for these terms: "Something desired to be done, something desired to be accomplished, something to be desired to give the correct
impression to individuals." (487–6)

What qualities or characteristics make up a proper intent and purpose? From the Work Readings series we find: "The intent, the purpose,
is to serve, rather than to gratify [one's] own personal intent or gain . . . "
(254–34) Other short excerpts give additional information:

... ye are judged according to thy *spiritual* intent and purpose. And as these become a part of the activity through the directing in that way and manner, the ways will open . . .
622-4

So long as the intent and purposes, the real desires of the heart are prompted by the spiritual truths latent and manifested within, ye may carry on and grow in grace, in knowledge, in understanding.
2090-1

The stress should be upon the spiritual purposes, the spiritual intent. For, remember, only good, only the spiritual lives on. Temporal things perish with the body.
2612-1

The ideas and ideals, then, and the application of self in the material relationships, should be in keeping with that which is ever constructive in the experience, and never of the material or the mercenary nature as the first cause; for, as the intent is manifested, each soul, each entity lives and moves and has its being in the Creative Forces.
2058-1

Purpose and intent, then, are intimately connected to the spiritual realm; they represent a striving toward a fulfillment in what is considered the higher range of existence where truth and goodness lie. Purpose and intent also relate to how the treatments or physical remedies are to be applied. While this notion will be explored in chapters 5 and 7, here are a few examples from the readings that exemplify this use:

In the applications, do not apply just to be gotten through with—but with the purpose, with the intent, with the desire, with the application to *accomplish definite* conditions for the body! and these will be accomplished in this way and manner!
389-2

(Q) How long before satisfactory eye condition will be achieved, and how much time should be given daily to its aid?
(A) Fifteen to twenty minutes about twice a day should be

the time given to same, unless there is the ability for the body to lay aside other impending or pending conditions.

You see, in making such applications it is the concentration that aids the whole consciousness and thus aids the body. If it is done merely as rote, little may be accomplished. If it is done with a purpose, and with the intent that goes with same, then much more should and will be accomplished. In six weeks there should be all the change as would be desired.   1158-22

(Q) Will the treatments as outlined relieve the insomnia?
(A) That's the intent and purpose!   1343-2

So, if I am using an abdominal castor oil pack because I want to prepare myself to receive a colonic in a few days, my motive for doing the series of packs would be not only to have a better colonic, but also to help relieve the stress in my colon caused by constipation. Because I know and understand that the Cayce readings recommend castor oil packs for a variety of physical discomforts, my overall purpose in using the packs might be to help alleviate the congested condition in my colon, to assist the liver in its detoxifying function, to soften the muscles in my abdomen and relax them, or to increase lymph flow in the area. I might even try to *see* all these occurring while under the pack. These conditions will also help to prepare my body for the impending colonic irrigation, creating more beneficial results from that treatment.

The power of intent is also reflected in what is known as "the placebo effect." A placebo is some type of harmless, nonmedicated pill, tonic, or some other substance given as a legitimate "medication" or "medicine" to placate the patient or humor him or her so that the one taking it thinks it will have beneficial and salutary effects; hence, the translation from the Latin: "I shall please." Experimental research studies utilize placebos as controls in order to test or determine the efficacy of a particular medicine or procedure. Certainly placebos demonstrate the power of purpose and intent, for how can an ill person take a pill or follow a procedure that has no real health–inducing value to it and receive the desired cure? It seems miraculous!

A former A.R.E. employee convinced her mother to try a castor oil pack. The packs can seem complicated and rather messy to apply. First, a piece of wool flannel, three to four thicknesses, is soaked with the castor oil (cold-pressed), then heated on a heating pad with a layer of plastic in between to protect the pad. When it is warm, the wool flannel is placed on the abdomen, usually on the right side where the liver and gall bladder are located. The plastic cover goes over it, then the heating pad, and finally a large bath towel encircling the body to stabilize the layers. The heat from the pad drives the oil in deeper. After an hour or so, it is removed and the abdomen rinsed off with a cloth soaked in warm water with a dash of baking soda added. The mother decided to try the pack and received such marvelous results she began raving about it to all her elderly friends, getting them to try it as well. One day the daughter overheard her mother's description of the procedure and was horrified to learn that she was wrapping the castor oil pack *entirely* in the plastic and putting the *plastic* against the skin—not the flannel cloth. How was any of that oil being absorbed? Was a little leaking through the plastic? Yet her mother was getting such good results!

A teacher of lymph drainage therapy told this story about one of his students. The student could only attend part of the class as she was scheduled to work in a hotel overseas in the Middle East. But she really wanted to absorb as much as she could before she left. After learning a simplified neck routine, she left for her month-long job, really excited about practicing on others. Hotel employees and visitors were willing recipients of her short, but effective procedure, and word quickly spread about her wonderful neck routine. People reported feeling so much better, illnesses were reversed, and she was achieving quite a notoriety. After her return home, she reported on her fantastic success to her instructor. Curious, he asked her to demonstrate on him exactly what she'd done. To his horror, all the moves were backwards, done in the *opposite* direction; in other words, instead of draining the lymph toward the neck nodes, she was reversing the flow, technically causing more congestion. Yet this didn't seem to be happening, considering clients' responses to it. How could this be? The procedure, though done incorrectly, was nevertheless achieving remarkable, beneficial results.

In these two instances, the enthusiasm and service-oriented attitudes of the providers carried great weight, no doubt covering up the "multi-

tude of errors" committed. In cases such as these it's difficult to under-
estimate the power of intent.

One final comment on intent includes its relationship to setting ideals:

> **(Q) Any further advice?**
> **(A) As we find, and as indicated—especially in the analysis**
> **of self as to the intent and purposes—there should oft be**
> **the analyzing of the purposes, hopes, fears, aspirations—in**
> **the light of what is thy ideal.**   **1947-5**

The Role of Ideals in Healing

The shortest chapter in the two-volume *A Search for God* books is Lesson III, "What Is My Ideal?" Despite its brevity, however, the setting of
an ideal is considered, according to the readings, highly important *for
everyone*, as exemplified in this frequently quoted excerpt: " . . . the most
important experience of this or any individual entity is to first know
what is the ideal—spiritually." (357-13) So what exactly is an ideal?

An ideal is "a mental concept or that conceived as a standard of
perfection . . . something beyond and above us toward which we build.
[Ideals] are either consciously or unconsciously the bases for the motivating forces in our lives." (*ASFG*, Book I, p. 37) We all have ideals in the
sense that there is something against which we measure ourselves, like
a yardstick placed alongside a wall and a pencil mark made to denote the
growing height of a child. Though we may be unconscious of exactly
what it is, it nevertheless becomes the spark that ignites us, motivating us in
our actions, thoughts, and speech, as well as in our dealings with others.

We can have a spiritual ideal, a mental ideal, or a physical ideal. A
spiritual ideal, mentioned in the reading excerpt, describes the spirit or
motive with which we do these things—again what lies behind our actions or the quality with which we carry on our activities. Phrases such
as school spirit, team spirit, the spirit of a company or an organization,
or free spirit give an indication of what is meant when the quality of
such a group or person is being described.

By consciously setting an ideal for ourselves—whether physical, mental, or spiritual—through using the imaginative forces of our mind, we

are helping to reawaken patterns of healing within our bodily system, setting in motion a more healthy pattern for the cells in our physical system to function; in other words, we are feeding our mind a better mental diet. This diet may serve to realign our desires to perhaps change those patterns that led to our illness, to replace destructive with more constructive attitudes, so that we can serve our God and others in a selfless, more productive and useful way. All these results have to do with setting the intent and following through on the application of that ideal. Two readings summarize this process:

> In these directions, then, we find that—with the setting of the ideal in the activities of self, with the mental trained and attuned in those conditions or thoughts that bring more activity in the direction of the ideal set—there would be the better balancing; for, as we have often given, those that make for the better coordination of a well-balanced mental, spiritual *and* physical may develop the more, accomplish the more, making greater success—either from the mental, the material or the spiritual angle of their experience.   2733-3

> Know, however, that it is what the will does about that which is set as its ideal in a mental, in a material or in the physical experiences as well as the spiritual—and then having the courage to carry out that ideal—makes the difference between the constructive and creative forces or relationships and those that make one become rather as a drifter or a ne'er-do-well, or one very unstable and unhappy.
> 1401-1

Besides being "a drifter or a ne'er-do-well . . . very unstable and unhappy," one who does not set or hold to an ideal or is without an ideal "never is at peace with self" (1538-1) and is a "wanderer." (323-1) Success in life, the readings maintained, is "a mental state of any individual, and depends upon the ideal that is set . . . " (1437-1) Once a choice has been made and a path chosen, "the way in which that sought must be accomplished, is *in* keeping with that *ideal* that is held, is set before self." (1089-3)

The readings encourage self-analysis, self-examination, and self-un-
derstanding in order that one become more attuned to one's inner life;
discover innate desires, abilities, and talents; and to gauge whether one
is making progress spiritually or regressing. In one of the Study Group
series of readings, obtained on October 2, 1932, an aspect of self-under-
standing with regard to ideals was offered:

> **When one has set the ideal, and knows what the ideal repre-
> sents, and then knows self measured by the ideal, one sees,
> is aware of that lacking or that overdone in self, and plucks
> it out, and beholds *not* the mote that is in his brother's eye
> but considers rather the beam that is in his own eye.**
>
> **262-29**

The choices that we make, what we do about those experiences or
influences that come to us, related to what we've set as our standard or
ideal, "becomes that which produces or brings the soul development."
(1207-1) Holding to that standard of measurement, that pattern—and
living it—is growth-producing, especially in the spiritual realm. We want
to create a life for ourselves that is not just materially based but one
that is "beyond the purely material things . . . For these that are of the
earth-earthy rust and corrupt. But those that are founded in the spirit
of life and truth take hold upon the very throne of mercy and peace
and harmony and justice and long-suffering and brotherly love; for
they are *of* God—and thus are everlasting!" (1125-1)

Being in the material world, however, we *are* prone to conflicts between our impulses and our desires, and these create what the readings
call "contending influences." But "if the ideal is set, if the ideal is held, if
the ideal is made the point of harmonizing or measuring or holding to
as the gauge, the guide, the rule, these will make for developments in
the proper way and manner." (443-6) This description is probably what
we think of as the real purpose of an ideal: the balance or anchor that
we need to bring some stability into our lives, especially if we're confronted with a severe or life-threatening illness. It's often amazing how,
in the midst of a health reading, Cayce would weave a comment about
setting ideals into the text, tying this practice along with the physical

recommendations. When one person asked near the end of his reading if there were any further physical conditions to correct, the reading stated that these conditions were very good, just some weakened condition referred to earlier was causing a "drain upon the system." Without missing a beat, the reading continued:

> Keep before the mental body that that will ever be *constructive* in its nature; for the mind *is* the builder, the spiritual or the ideal is the life. If the ideal is set in material things, these do rust, they do corrupt. If the ideal is set in heavenly things, in spiritual things, they grow brighter by use, they grow more harmonious by their age and attunement, and build in the material body, the material experience of the body, that which is *satisfying* in that it brings contentment.
>
> 912-1

To a forty-six-year-old woman who was having problems with poor eliminations, the reading mentioned even setting an ideal for this condition, but not getting overly stressed out about it. The question and answer follow:

> (Q) What can be done for elimination now and will condition be cured permanently?
> (A) These can be changed a great deal by the diets as indicated: Raw foods often, as the foods which tend towards better eliminations: figs; pie plant (this prepare in the different forms), senna leaves, senna pods, all of these may be parts of the diet at various periods. We will find as the ideals are set, what are thy ideal eliminations? Once a day, twice a day or the activities of the liver, activities of kidneys, the activities of digestion and assimilation and the drosses which should be eliminated. Do not lay such a great stress on these that you find mind applying self as, "I can't do this and I can't do that or I can't do the other," but being rational and normal in keeping with conditions which develop. 3051-6

Making the best of any situation and bringing to any relationship what one would consider as ideal represent the highest that one can accomplish, bringing into one's life contentment and happiness, as expressed in the readings.

Setting the Ideal: After being convinced of the importance of having ideals and working with them, we have several options as to how to go about choosing our personal ideals. Ever practical, the readings suggest this written exercise: Make three columns on a sheet of paper. At the head of each write *spiritual, mental, physical.* Then, using thought and prayer, "[begin] with the spiritual (for all that is in mind must first come from a spiritual concept) [and write down] what is thy spiritual concept of the ideal, whether it be Jesus, Buddha, mind, material, God or whatever is the word which indicates to self the ideals spiritual." (5091-3) Does the word or phrase you have chosen sum up to you what you wish to live by, to emulate, or to become? Other suggested words or phrases which could indicate the spirit by which you choose to live might include *peace, love, channel of blessings*, or *service.*

Under *mental*, write down "the ideal mental attitude, as may arise from concepts of the spiritual, in relationship to self, to home, to friends, to neighbors, to thy enemies, to things, to conditions." (5091-3) What is the ideal attitude you'd like to have toward each of these? For example, if my spiritual ideal is "love," then how I might demonstrate this ideal toward my friends or a certain acquaintance would be with an attitude of appreciation; in relation to myself, an attitude of patience; in relation to my job, an attitude of industriousness. These attitudes (under *mental* ideal) are expressions of how I might choose to manifest my chosen spiritual ideal "love."

Under *physical*, list specific activities or actions to take related to the above. For example, toward my friends or a particular person to show appreciation I might write them or him/her a thank-you letter or try to give frequent verbal compliments; to express patience with myself I might stop and take three deep breaths whenever I feel rushed or stressed; in my job I might work at meeting deadlines on time to demonstrate an attitude of industriousness.

Once written down, look at them and study them, suggest the readings. You may need to erase them from time to time and replace them with new ones as your own desires of what you'd wish to attain change.

In A.R.E. workshops on ideals, a slightly different format for listing ideals has been taught. Instead of three columns, there are three concentric circles. Visually this format may be slightly easier to work with, but the process is the same. In the center circle would be placed the word or phrase denoting one's spiritual ideal; in the next circle one would write in the ideal mental attitudes; the outer circle, which could be divided into sections, would list the areas or persons in one's life that one would focus on to apply the ideals: work, self, friend, home, spouse, church, job, and/or neighbor. It could be a few areas or as many as one wants to work with, but each would be an important area of special concern. In the divided sections one would also write in the actions to be performed in order to apply in a practical way the mental and spiritual attitudes.

This exercise is not necessarily easy, the readings admit. When one man asked what his ideal was, Cayce refused to give it, saying that the man "must answer for self," using his will, and that he alone knows what he should hold as the criterion. "Then, *whatever* is set in self the body should work toward . . . If the body's ideal is set in that which is *right* in the sight of its ideal, or by the measurement of that it holds as its criterion, as its ideal, *that* it will develop to. That must be set by self." (4866-2)

One advantage of this exercise is that we become conscious and more aware of what we are striving toward; we also have a concrete idea of how to put this into practice. In doing this we are operating on a higher level, using our will, our birthright, to choose, with thought and prayer, what we wish to hold as our standard of measurement or perfection. Also in doing the exercise we are not only attempting to merge our physical and mental ideals with our spiritual ideal—in the example given, the spirit of love permeates our attitudes and actions—but attempting to bring our lives into a better balance, bringing our daily acts, words, and thoughts more in alignment with a higher purpose. By creating this oneness in ourselves, we are helping to create better coordination in all aspects of our lives, making for a more harmonious physical body; for "As we seek, we find; as we knock, we are heard." (*ASFG*, Book I, p. 40)

A Word About Emotions

Although closely linked to attitudes, emotions as a topic were not specifically addressed in this chapter. Yet they are an important component in the healing process, particularly as we become more aware of them. These intense feelings—with both physical and mental manifestations—can help us tune in to our body's inner wisdom, giving us guidance as to our needs and stresses. They have been described as the driving energy of the body, seeming to arise occasionally out of nowhere, surprising us sometimes by their intensity and clarity. According to the Cayce information, emotions are rooted in our past lives in the earth plane, our sojourns from one incarnation to another—as stated in these representative excerpts from individuals' life readings:

> **In giving the biographical sketch, the interpretations of the record are with the intent to make more understandable and practical in application the urges and experiences that arise, which . . . find manifestation in the emotions of the body.**   **1468-4**

> **. . . the influences from the sojourns in a material or physical environment make for the emotions that arise. 1486-1**

> **As we find, such astrological influences or urges arise through the innate mental forces; while the emotions arise from the sojourns of the entity in the material plane.**
> **1620-2**

The readings sometimes use the descriptive terms "physical emotion," "mental emotion," or "spiritual emotion," indicating the area or playing field where the motion or vibration is carried out; also that "the emotions may affect the physical, the mental and the spiritual body, here and now." (2647-1)

Seekers who are serious about being on the spiritual path often have difficulty with emotions, labeling some "good" and others "bad." It's just not spiritual to express anger, they say. However, the readings do not concur. Here is one example:

> For, no emotion, no desire that may be a part of the entity's experience is in itself bad; but that use to which it may be put, that purpose for which it may be sought becomes the *thing* itself that brings the type of disappointment that may have been a part of the experience. 369-16

In the case of anger, the readings repeatedly stated, "Be angry, but sin not." So it's the *use* we put to the feeling, what we *do* with it, that makes for destructive behavior. The readings also cautioned against gratifying one's emotions in a selfish way, but the emotion itself is judged to be neutral.

Another unique way of understanding emotion is to notice the division of the word: "e" plus "motion"; that is, energy in motion. So it can be thought of as simply a movement of energy, being carried in our physical, mental, and spiritual bodies.

To a fifty-one-year-old woman who had had an unsettled childhood with lots of fear and now was suffering from periods of frustration and melancholia this physical description was given:

> Remember, all activity or emotion in the body is as a vibratory reaction from one portion of the body to another. It is as a system of sensitivenesses, that with any tautness as may come from an upset digestion, upset animation—as conditions that arise from dis-ease of any nature through the system—causes the nerve impulses from ganglia to be magnified. 3002-1

The interconnectedness of body and emotion was also expressed in this reading excerpt:

> The emotions of the body . . . are as electronic energies. This again is a name, until the individual entity experiences that there is the heart beat and pulsation, there *is* the respiratory activity of the lungs to purify the body-flow of life, blood, fluid, *with* a glow from the emotions controlled through the centers or lines of the nervous systems for both positive and negative natures. 263-13

Another reading advised a woman to engage in "physical bodily exercises [to] bring the full flow of blood force through all functioning
organs, and through the action of the physical portions of the body, [so]
that every muscular force, nerve force, nerve plexus, may find a mode
of manifesting its emotion." (4376-1)

Mental and spiritual emotions were described as deeper emotions
latent within the individual. They often arose from artistic endeavors in
one's past life—such as music, dancing, sculpting, painting, etc.—that
were showing up as inclinations in the present life. So these particular
types of emotion have a close connection with creativity and imagination.

As mentioned earlier, emotions have a part to play in the overall
healing process, especially as we become conscious of their presence.
They help us to center upon our innate divinity, which is where true
healing begins. Several readings referred to this characteristic:

> . . . the very fact of consciousness itself, the very fact of an
> awareness of self and self's emotions, is an expression of the
> awareness within of the divine and of His (God's) hope for
> thee. And if He be with thee, what matters what others
> think or say—in the material world?   2647-1

> That thou art in physical consciousness—with the aware-
> ness of emotion of love, of hate, of jealousy, of brotherly
> love, of kindness, of patience, should indicate to thee that
> thy heavenly Father is mindful of thee. Then know, nothing
> in heaven or hell may separate thee from the love of God
> save thine own self!   3063-1

Emotional outbursts can seem overwhelming, and their strength and
intensity too great at times to cope with, yet the readings express the
hope of engaging the will in helping us deal with this power. Several
excerpts describe this process:

> . . . know that no urge, no sign, no emotion—whether of a
> latent mental nature or of a material or emotional nature
> finding expression in the body—surpasses that birthright,

> *will*—the factor which makes the human soul, the human
> individual, *different* from all other creatures in the earth,
> from all manifestations of God's activity! 2172-1

> . . . there is no urge, no emotion, that may not be altered
> through the *will* of self, either for the good or for the woe;
> for the will is that gift of the Creator which makes the soul
> of man equal with the abilities of a creative force, and thus
> the son of God. 2301-1

One man, due to his experiences in a prior incarnation, had the desire this lifetime to help free souls from being bound by any sect built
on fear. Cayce referred to this urge "as a key to the whole of the entity's
experience" and commented on the workings between fear and will:

> . . . fear is—as it ever has been—that influence that opposes
> will, and yet fear is only of the moment while will is of eter-
> nity. Hence fear takes hold upon the emotions, while will is
> deeper-seated into the soul, into the warp and woof of the
> very being of an *entity* in its entirety; finding expression to
> be sure in the lowest of the emotions, yet is prompted by
> the creative force itself. 1210-1

A woman who served others by lifting their emotions in "creative
influences . . . whether in song, in dance, in art, or in music" was told
that these were "expressions of the emotions of body, the emotions of
the soul." However, there are two sides to this expression:

> When these are of the constructive nature, no greater chan-
> nel is open for the material manifestations of spiritual
> truths; yet no channel may be made lower in bringing self-
> indulgences than in the expressions of same. 871-1

Again, it's the use and purpose of the emotion that makes the difference between destructiveness and creativity.

One way of working with emotions is to acknowledge their impact
upon our physical bodies. Though the process is not fully understood,
emotions have a way of becoming encased or entrapped in our flesh—

something that has been recognized by bodyworkers through the application of touch, the results of which are often described as emotional releases.

As a child, I learned that whenever I noticed a bruise on my body and wondered where it came from, I could softly massage it just to the point of a slight pain and gradually I'd remember the scene that caused it. It could be that I rounded a corner in the hallway too quickly and bumped my shoulder against the wall or I whacked my leg with a baseball bat during a game. Years later I was living on the top floor of a three-story apartment. I kept my portable massage table on the landing outside my bedroom door and did one or two outcalls a week. One morning I awoke with a pain in my left deltoid muscle in my upper arm. Curious about it, I began to rub it, thinking about all sorts of possibilities. Had I strained it while exercising? Did I pull a muscle? No. Finally it came to me: I'd done an outcall the day before and had carried my massage table up the two flights of stairs. But I'd done this many times before without any resultant pain in my arms. What was different this time? Then I distinctly remembered how angry and frustrated I felt while carrying the table. Really annoyed at something that had happened, I struggled upstairs with the table, telling myself I was tired of doing this, it was too much of an effort, feeling unappreciated, etc., etc. I really carried on about this while at the same time lifting my table up to the landing. Those intense feelings had settled in my arm, causing what felt like an ordinary strained muscle, but the excess intensity of feelings exacerbated the weight on the muscles, creating the pain. I was astounded by that! Just to check it out, the next few times I carried that massage table, I tried to reflect on positive, uplifting thoughts. No pain at all; everything was just as usual as when I'd carried it before.

Just how much sickness and pain are really the result of simply an injury or an injury plus the intense feelings is difficult to differentiate; the two seem inseparable. But the circumstances indicate the positive use of emotions in bringing an increased awareness or sensitivity to ourselves: we become more conscious of our mental activities—our thought processes—as well as our physical activities. Much like, as described in chapter 1, the healing crisis in which the embedded emotions may draw our attention to an area of our body that needs the healing.

These processes will be elaborated upon in the next chapter where the origin of illness will be considered.

Conclusion

"Healing begins when our desires, choices, and subsequent applications move in the direction of being in harmony with the Whole." (*Covenant*, Vol. 2, No. 2, p. 1) Through the activity of the mind, since it is the builder, we can start this process by reinforcing constructive attitudes, seeing the physical applications that we are receiving as having their proper and desired effect, setting an ideal and working toward it, and allowing our emotions to bring us to an enhanced sensitivity toward our bodies. With these efforts as a solid foundation, we can begin to look at their results through the nurturing we give to our physical bodies.

5
Nurturing the Material Body: The Physical Is the Result

Thy body is indeed the temple of the living God. There He hath promised to meet thee . . . the physical body is a pattern of the universal consciousness.　　　　　　　　2787-1

. . . the physical body is the material representation of the soul or spiritual forces in this material world.　　　99-8

Keep the body not only in the way of being better physically but better physically for a better mental and spiritual purpose.　　　　　　　　1968-9

Origins of Disease

TO BE PRESENT here in this three-dimensional world we need our physical body. It is through our body that our nonphysical parts—mind and spirit, which give us our greatest pleasures and make us human beings—can function and operate. In order for these aspects to carry on their work optimally, they need a balanced, healthy channel. Unfortunately due to the stresses of modern living, we have inadvertently put our body out of balance. Without realizing it, we may have been driving ourselves too much, concentrating on creating this imbalance rather than focusing on balance. We might have worked hard, to the point of exhaustion, to get where we would like to be, to make the money to pay for the material goods we wish to possess, and to enjoy the pleasures that life has to offer. But if we don't feel well or are tired most of the time due to the toxic, unhealthy conditions we've created, pleasures of any sort would be difficult to enjoy, and our body eventually suffers the effects of our neglect and abuse. If we find ourselves faced with coping with a long-term illness, we may wonder just how did we get here. What brought all this about? Since, according to the Cayce readings, our physical bodies are the result of all that we have been, is it possible to trace our steps, our thought processes, back in time in order to discover a link to our present material state? Doing this exercise could be both beneficial and challenging!

Spirit vs. Flesh: In chapter 4 some reading excerpts were quoted which implied a connection between a particular negative attitude and a physical disorder. In other readings Cayce mentioned various origins of general disturbances or distresses that the physical body was experiencing. To one woman, after stating that "all forces, all power as manifested in materiality, whether as related to the physical body or to those things outside the body, have their inception in Good—or God," he went on to say that "what is disturbing in a physical body—mentally, physically, spiritually—arises from a misconstruction of good." (1309-1) Perhaps another way of expressing this same concept is found in the Study Group Readings series in answer to the question: "Would the conflict between spirit and flesh cause one to be affected physically, to become tired or even ill?" The answer began: *"Relatively* so." Then Cayce explained that dis-ease was the natural result of being "at-variance to the divine law! Hence it may truly be said that to be at-variance may bring sickness, dis-ease, disruption, distress in a physical body." (262-83) A further elaboration on this source of dis-ease is given in the following question and answer:

> **(Q) What is disease and the purpose of the germs produced . . . ?**
> **(A) Disease arises from, first, dis-ease—as a normalcy that *is* existent and yet becomes unbalanced. Disease is, or dis-ease is, a state at variance to the ideal or first cause or first principle. Then, in its final analysis, disease might be called sin. It is necessary to keep a balance.**　　　**2533-3**

This reply echoes a rather strong statement given in another reading: " . . . all illness comes from sin. This everyone must take whether they like it or not; it comes from sin whether it be of body, of mind, or of soul, and these manifest in the earth." (3174-1) Revising our definition of sin and its expression, seeing sin as a separation from God, an error, misjudgment, or "missing the mark"—rather than the breaking of a moral or behavior code—may make better sense. "There are laws, then, as govern the physical, the mental, the spiritual body . . . The abuse of a physical law brings dis-ease and then disturbance to the physical organism, through which mental and spiritual portions of the body operate," states reading 1947-3. Another reading affirms, "As has been given of old, when there are disturbing or harmful or detrimental influences, there is error at the base or the cause of same." (1527-1)

The word *sin* may not appeal to many types of people, but when viewing it from a broader definition it could simply mean, as expressed in one reading, knowing what to do, yet not doing it. This leads to "mental attitudes that will later produce for the body-physical, as well as the body-mental, an environment or surrounding that would become more and more aggravating." (257-199) So there is a process that is being enacted and lived out which over time can create disharmony and imbalance in us.

In another reading given for a forty-nine-year-old housewife, whose religious affiliation was listed as Christian, these aggravating conditions were described as "hurts to the self-consciousness; and these create what? Disturbing forces, and these bring about confusions and faults of every nature." Then the reading added: "For the only sin of man is *selfishness!*" (987-4) This statement came in part in answer to her question: "What is my worst fault?" and the reading responded: "What is ever the worst fault of each soul? *Self—self!*" (987-4) Undaunted, she followed up by asking how she could overcome this fault. Cayce's answer reiterates a number of positive attitudes and the living out of the "fruits of the Spirit":

> . . . **showing mercy, showing grace, showing peace, long-suffering, brotherly love, kindness—even under the most *trying* circumstances.**

> For what is the gain if ye love those *only* that love thee?
> But to bring hope, to bring cheer, to bring joy, yea to bring
> a smile again to those whose face and heart are bathed in
> tears and in woe, is but making that divine love *shine*—
> *shine*—in thy own soul!
> Then *smile*, be joyous, be glad! For the day of the Lord is
> at hand.
> Who is thy Lord? Who is thy God?
> Self? Or Him in Whom ye live and move and have thy being
> . . . ?   987-4

Anyone remotely familiar with the philosophy of the Cayce readings knows the importance of service to others that is repeatedly emphasized. From the information given to this woman, [987], on equating selfishness with sin, it appears that living a life that is self-centered or prompted mainly by self-interest, showing little or no concern for the welfare of others, is in direct contradiction to a life of service that demonstrates loving care of and helpful assistance to others. Of course, there needs to be a balance here, too. Living *totally* in service to others is not healthy either if one neglects care of one's self or one's family to whom one is also responsible. We need to include ourselves as recipients of that selfless service, taking care of ourselves so that we can be better channels of blessing for good. Dr. Harold J. Reilly was a good example of this: He exercised one hour a day so that he could devote eight hours to his patients. In a similar vein, a woman, who was one of the original members of the Search for God Study Group, was told:

> Make the body fit for the channel first! Then the spiritual
> may have the *opportunity* to manifest through; for . . . few
> people, few individuals, may be able to manifest with a liver
> in bad shape, or suppressions in any portion of the system
> . . . These make for conditions wherein the mental forces are
> *unable* to manifest properly. The *physical* must be fit, and
> the *spiritual* forces may manifest the better.   295-3

To another woman, a thirty-year-old singer who was struggling with seasonal hay fever and asthma, Cayce, after praising her for her beautiful voice and personality, "gifts to the body," gave this advice, harkening back to ancient biblical history:

> **Remember, then, in meeting the difficulties (that disturb the body), that His first injunction to man was to *subdue the earth*.**
>
> **This, then, interpreted in the practical experience of individuals in a material world—through neglect, indifference or non-care by many an individual entity or soul, those influences have been loosed that are to be subdued—yet—in man's experience.   2812-1**

In addition to "neglect, indifference, or non–care" as potential origins of disease, the reading mentioned that some experiences often "cause disturbing forces in the material or physical body." These were noted as "a race influence, heredity, environment." (2812–1) The reading did not elaborate on the meaning of these sources.

Eight days before she obtained this reading given on September 11, 1942, [2812] wrote to Edgar Cayce, describing her difficulties and how she had been working with them. Through changing her attitude she had already begun to make some improvement, as she approached her condition on the physical, then mental and spiritual levels.

> **For some years now I have been completely and wholly interested in the guidance and work of the spirit. I have studied the Bible and all the reputable literature that has been available to me on this subject and on many occasions have had demonstrations that were altogether wonderful. So it is with complete faith and openness to receive that I come to you at this time.**
>
> **First of all the problem of immediate importance is this condition that medicine calls hay fever and asthma that has appeared each and every August since I was around eight or nine years old. I have gone to other climates several years and at those times always the condition has been lighter. I have been given the scratch test to determine exactly what causes the trouble and have been given so much serum—**

seventy some shots in all—that now the doctor refuses to give me any more—the last shot almost having taken my life. I have tried just about everything possible—however, let me explain that these treatments were all given me several years ago. Since developing the mental and spiritual side of my life I have almost entirely done away with medicine . . . this year I made up my mind that this condition was no longer going to hold any power over me and so I started to work. I have studied, fasted, and made my Bible my constant companion. The time for my trouble to begin came and went and I was fine—then a few days ago it started much different than ever before, but enough to make it impossible for me to continue with my work as a singer . . . it is because of this physical difficulty that each fall of the year when everyone has been starting on their winter's work I have been sitting around waiting for my voice to clear. With God's help I know that this no longer has to be. So this is the first thing I want you to tell me about.

Then there are several other things I would like to have you assist me with. One being that I am five foot three-and-one-half inches tall—rather small boned and though I'm not considered a large woman at all I am much too large from my waist down. Especially for my work my hips and legs are too large. Everything I have ever done to lose weight has failed to have any effect on them, but has succeeded in making me look sick in the face and upset me otherwise. So, if you can advise me with this, it will be a tremendous help.

[She also asked for advice on a family tendency toward broken surface veins and what to do for graying hair, bloodshot eyes, moles on her body, and "any other condition that you find in going over me . . . "]   2812-1, B-1

Recommendations in her reading included a series of mechanical adjustments with specific vertebrae named to assist the osteopath with the treatments, an inhalant for throat and nasal passages, and massages. After six months of carrying out these treatments, she was to leave them off for two to three months. She was also given this prayer or affirmation to use in her meditations and while applying the remedies:

Father-God! In Thy promises to Thy servants Thou hast prom-
ised to hear, through Thy Son in the earth. I, Thy handmaid,
come seeking, that Thou would create in my body, in my mind,
in my hopes and purposes, that Thou wouldst have me be—in
body, in mind, in soul. Use me, Lord, wholly in Thy service.

2812-1

The affirmation expresses a firm faith in the Divine and a desire to be a willing channel of service. Unfortunately no follow-up information exists on her case. We have only the record of her own attempts and the changes already being made from those efforts. It would be a matter of curiosity as to what was occurring in her life around ages eight and nine that seemed to be the onset of her asthma and hay fever. This is something that could be explored by [2812] if she so desired.

Two other sources of disease remain to be discussed: conditions from the past (karmic) or strictly pathological (purely physical) reasons. The latter will be dealt with first.

Pathological Causes: There are instances in the Cayce readings in which for some people the disturbances they were experiencing were considered *purely physical*, even though reactions from them might create imbalances elsewhere in the physical body or even in the mental realm in the form of hypochondria or other psychological conditions. Here are some examples:

(Q) Is the extreme nervousness and sleeplessness a purely
physical thing that can be remedied with medicines?
(A) Purely physical. [Osteopathic adjustments to specific areas
were recommended to correct the imbalance.]   3261-1

(Q) Is there a spiritual cause or significance for his lip and
palate affliction, or is it purely physical?
(A) . . . this is more a purely physical condition or mishap—
and not a karmic condition or a working out of something
from the past.   2814-1

This question-and-answer exchange appeared in a life reading, given on September 15, 1942, for an eight-month-old boy. Probably the condition referred to was a cleft palate. Although the rest of the reading focuses on his past lives (he was the reincarnation of the French dramatist Molière [1622–1673]) and his latent talents and abilities, there was one brief reference to his physical condition. The reading stated that it had "little to do with what is termed karmic; but rather with that having to do with purely physical or accidental conditions in physical manifestations in its period of gestation." (2814-1) Usually with birth injuries or defects, prenatal conditions, inherited tendencies, or very early onset of a disease process, we tend to label them "karmic" because an infant's close proximity to his or her past life allows easy carryover into the present lifetime. But this was apparently not the case here. Something happened in the womb while the fetus was developing, a "purely physical or accidental condition," that resulted in "his lip and palate affliction."

To continue with other examples of a "purely physical" nature:

> **(Q)** What can I do about a disturbing noise that is in my ear (or is this purely physical, requiring physical treatment)?
> **(A)** Purely physical and not karmic. Remove the stress by head and neck exercise. Have . . . corrections osteopathically made in the 3rd cervical to the 1st cervical and 4th dorsal. 5346-1

> **(Q)** Is there any reason in my past for my weak back and lack of vitality?
> **(A)** None as indicated here. This is purely physical, but if there is used those properties to keep a better alkalinity in the system, we find that this would lend towards suppressing and removing the heaviness and tautness there, and will contribute to the better eliminations, thus bringing better strength and vitality to the body. Use on the back, then, the Glyco-Thymoline Packs; small crash towels [coarse cotton or linen cloths with a plain loose weave] or about three thicknesses of cotton cloth saturated in Glyco-Thymoline and applied for an hour at the time, once each day. 1533-2

(Q) What causes me to grit my teeth when sleeping?
(A) These activities are from purely physical causes, coming from the condition in the digestive system. Take occasionally those properties that will cause better assimilation, such as the combination of Willow Charcoal with Honey; and a few drops of Elixir of Lactated Pepsin after the heavier meal of the day—and this effect will disappear.   2746-2

(Q) What mental or spiritual condition brought [my gall bladder attacks] about?
(A) Neither a mental [nor] spiritual, but rather a purely physical reaction. And . . . keep away from meats!   3008-1

A thirty–three–year–old woman wrote to Cayce about a hereditary condition: hair loss. She had given up on receiving any help from physicians and, according to a series of letters she'd written, her condition was worsening. Several years previously she had taken electrical treatments to stimulate the scalp, but they didn't help. "Though I am pretty, this fact [of losing my hair] makes me very self–conscious and unhappy . . . Also my praying has not helped. I am perfectly healthy otherwise. I do so much hope you will help me in finding a cure for me." (4086-1, B-1) Several months later, as the condition was worsening, making her almost bald on the top of her head, she stated: "I am afraid to look ahead . . . What can I do to cure myself from my trouble?" (4086-1, B-3) Right away in the second paragraph of the reading Cayce addressed her concern:

As we find, general conditions in a manner are very good, yet there are disturbances that cause a great deal of anxiety to the body. These, however, are more in the purely physical, than that having to do with the body as an entity. For these are rather the activities in the reflexes in the sensory and sympathetic nervous system, and arise from the body attempting to improve in a selfish manner upon what nature had intended for the body to be.   4086-1

She was advised to take a series of Calcidin tablets (primarily a source of calcium and available iodine in tablet form), massage pure hog lard into her scalp, eat raw salads, fix soups made from the peelings of Irish potatoes, and take high enemas (colonics). When she asked if giving birth seven months ago had worsened her condition, Cayce said it only aggravated it. The real source of the problem was the "too much drying out of the scalp . . . to improve upon nature." Then he added: "Be natural. You'll be much more attractive." (4086-1) No follow-up information is available.

Nervousness, insomnia, cleft palate, ear noises, weak back, fatigue, gritting one's teeth, gall bladder attacks, and hair loss all had purely physical causes, according to these reading excerpts. We can only surmise that, despite a purely physical origin, these effects could have been the result of an imbalance somewhere in the body, an incoordination between or among the systems of the body—not aided or abetted by mental or emotional influences. Was the breaking of a law at the physical level, then, somehow responsible for these *purely physical* disturbances?

Karma: Another source of disease to be considered is described by the readings as physical karma. Nearly 300 cases were designated as such, manifesting in a wide variety of illnesses: from acne, anemia, cerebral palsy, epilepsy, and eye disorders to mental illness, MS, Parkinson's, paralysis, poliomyelitis, and TB. Reflecting mistakes of a past life that were to be met now, these conditions were called "karmic"; that is, a cause-and-effect reaction or reaping the effects of what one has sown. A karmic condition also implies a "working out of something from the past," as stated in a previously quoted excerpt (2814-1), though the "past" could conceivably refer to a past action in this present life.

In a lecture on hypnosis delivered at the A.R.E. the speaker related the story of a man who was allergic to freshly cut grass. Healthy otherwise, the man sought help from a hypnotist who regressed him to when the allergy first began. As an active three year old, he was cavorting around the backyard one day while his father was mowing the grass. The youngster got dangerously close to the mower and the father, alarmed, pushed the boy out of the way and spanked him. Though the child was not hurt by the lawn mower, the potential for injury so upset

the father that he spontaneously reacted in that way. So began the allergy. During the hypnosis session, however, when the man understood
his father's rather negative response and could see the purpose behind
it—ultimately meaning to protect rather than harm him—he no longer
was troubled by freshly cut grass.

Another example of how helpful, even healing, it can be to link one's
physical ailment with its initial stage of disease is the experience of
Margaret, a "senior citizen", who was troubled for over twenty years
with painful, crippling arthritis. At the urging of a friend, she finally
attended a two-week program at a stress management clinic where she
engaged in various exercises, including meditation and reveries. Near
the middle of the second week she announced to the attendant physician, "I no longer have arthritis." Startled, the physician asked her how
she knew this. She replied, "When you've had arthritis for as long as I
have, you *know* when you no longer have it!" Then she related her story.

As a result of the past week's reveries and reflections, insights into
certain patterns in her life emerged. About five years into her marriage,
she found out that her husband was having an affair. But the couple
had two small sons to raise, so she postponed confronting him and
seeking a divorce. I'll wait until they're older, she promised herself. They
became teenagers. I'll wait until they graduate. Sometime after graduation came the Vietnam War and both boys enlisted. I can't do it now
with all the uncertainty of war. War ended, and the boys returned home
safely. I'll wait until they're settled. And on and on, she continued to
find excuses to delay the divorce, despite her husband continuing his—
by now—series of affairs. Connecting this unfulfilled promise she'd made
early on with the onset of this eventually crippling arthritis, which held
her nearly physically immobile as well as emotionally restricted, she
made a decision to confront her husband and seek a divorce. The arthritis left her.

From the standpoint of reincarnation, however, the reason behind a
physical trouble may have developed in a prior lifetime, where an excess of some kind would implant a weakness in one's psychic pattern.
This weakness would then be reproduced in the body of the person,
perhaps even carried over several lifetimes, until the lesson was learned
and the weakness worked out.

We may have a tendency to assume that if no sure cause of a disease pattern can be determined in our present lives, then it must be related to something in our past incarnation or previous life on this earth plane. These possibilities have been demonstrated quite effectively for many people through past–life regression therapy. Since we no longer have a reputable psychic like Edgar Cayce to point out to us the influence of our previous existences, we may have to rely on this form of therapy or other avenues, such as dreams and reveries, to understand the origin of our health concern.

According to a case from the readings—one of nearly 300—a fourteen–year–old boy had had a past–life influence that was causing him physical problems in his present life. Over the course of fifteen years he received a total of nine readings. The first one, given on August 29, 1927, was a life reading in which Cayce made a reference to his health condition:

> . . . one strong of body—yet with those inclinations and tendencies toward those physical defects or physical disabilities that afflict the body as tending toward that of the digestion, or of the internal system. Hence the body should be warned against indulging in any of those conditions that might tend to bring about troubles that would be as afflictions in the physical, under that strain and stress of the digestive system.   **641-1**

A notation made by Gladys Davis Turner indicated that both his mother and sister "corroborated this digestive weakness, saying he had always had a weak stomach, couldn't eat as the other children did." (641–1 Reports) In a follow–up memo after his second reading she indicated that he had followed the recommended treatments and, as a consequence, "the night–sweats disappeared, also the headaches, tiredness, and disagreeable reactions, and his adolescent years were normal." (641–2, R–1) It wasn't until his sixth reading given on December 3, 1940, that the young man, now twenty–seven years old, inquired about the karmic implications of his digestive problem:

(Q) What circumstances of a past sojourn brought about

my present weakness of the digestive system, and why?
(A) The overindulgence through the French as well as the
Persian experience, with too much of the activity of the acid-
producing forces in the system.

Hence in the present, as indicated in the physical reactions from the mental and spiritual, there needs to be kept
that of *uniformity* as well as consistency, in thought, speech
and foods.   641-6

What was he doing in those incarnations? In France he was an escort
and protector of the monarch Louis XIII, engaging in many of the ex-
cesses—too much rich foods—of the court life at that time. He also chose
the wearing apparel for the king, setting the dress standard for that
period. (Interestingly in his present life [641] was a uniform salesman,
quite involved in his work and quite successful.) For his Persian incarnation not much detail is given. He was a court physician (the time
period was not certain; perhaps it was during the reign of Croesus in
the sixth century B.C.) and, according to the reading, he gained and lost.
He lost through the "misapplication of self to that that the entity stood
for." (641-1) Yet acidic conditions due to some overindulgence messed
up his digestive system, and this weakness was carried over into his
present lifetime.

According to his letters, he continued to have stomach problems and
had difficulty regulating his diet, despite attempts to follow the readings' recommendations. A follow-up notation made on November 1,
1974, revealed that he had had surgery to repair an inguinal hernia and
to help ease a spastic colon. He had also been treated for an intestinal
condition bordering on ulcers, though X-rays showed nothing. Along
with chronic constipation, he had much pain and discomfort from food
not agreeing with his system. The author of these notes speculated:
"Could all these remaining, recurring symptoms be the physical karma
of neglect during his business pressure years [as a uniform salesman],
based on the original karma (prenatal condition) mentioned in his life
reading . . . ?" (641-7, R-7) It may seem that given this long period of
time he should have been able with treatment to overcome this condition. But something that has been built up over several lifetimes cannot
be wiped out easily, especially if the weakness is strongly imprinted in

the individual's psychic pattern itself. In the February 1960 issue of *The Searchlight*, Dr. Harold Reilly comments:

> . . . if [one] continues to dissipate for an entire life, with-
> out taking corrective measures, you would not expect,
> would you, to see [that person] emerging in another life
> with a brand-new body, perfect in all parts and functioning
> as if it had never been misused? . . . if you believe in reincar-
> nation with its law of karma—an eye for an eye and a tooth
> for a tooth, as you sow so shall you reap—you must include
> the body in that plan. (p. 5)

In some instances the karmic pattern of an illness may have a double source, as shown in this question–and–answer exchange:

> **(Q)** Is the ill health I have been experiencing the past years
> the result of mistakes of a past life or is it due to something
> amiss in this present life?
> **(A)** Both. For there is the law of the material, there is the
> law of the mental, there is the law of the spiritual. That
> brought into materiality is first conceived in spirit. Hence
> as we have indicated, all illness is sin; not necessarily of the
> moment, as man counts time, but as a part of the whole
> experience. For God has not purposed or willed that any
> soul should perish, but purgeth everyone by illness, by pros-
> perity, by hardships, by those things needed, in order to
> meet self—but in Him, by faith and works, are ye made
> every whit whole.   3395-2

This question was asked in a life reading. The recipient of the reading was a sixty–three–year–old editor of religious publications who had suf-fered from facial paralysis, headaches, and arthritis, which confined her at times to a wheelchair. Even before she received this information she commented in a letter: "I am now quite convinced that no former life need necessarily have had anything to do with my illnesses of the past few years, for there have been enough of inhibitions, fears, and worries in this present life, which I carried with me such a long time, to account for the kind of body I have now. I think all these were quite unnecessary—but if I had to have the results in order to bring this awareness home to me—then I accept them with thankfulness." (3395–1, R-1)

Her positive attitude was also reflected in her first reading in which she asked for guidance for her physical condition. Near the beginning of the reading Cayce stated:

> **As we find, these are wonderful experiences for this body, even in the suffering and in the trouble—if the body will only accept it as such. Ye have taught, ye have preached it in thy literature and thy activities, as to how and as to what spirituality, practically applied in the life of the individual, should create for its environ, if the mental and body-mind is the builder of the body. Why not try practicing it in self?**
>
> **These are not harsh words, nor meant to be harsh, but the lack of proper eliminations is the source of infection that causes arthritic tendencies. In the natural consequence of the mind, in reason, this should indicate to such a wonderful, a beautiful mind as this entity, the lack of self-control, the holding back in self of those things that should be stressed in mind, in body. These are indications of the nature of disturbance in the mental self, if the soul-purpose is in the right direction. And who could question here the purpose of this entity?   3395-1**

Besides offering her encouragement, the reading stated the physical source of her illness: poor eliminations leading to an infection that created "arthritic tendencies." One can only wonder if this same condition could apply to all or maybe similar arthritic cases.

Her good spirits continued to sustain her, despite a three-week hospitalization due to a fall because of her stiff knees. "I've had a lot of help from the verse, 'He will give His angels charge over thee—lest thou dash thy foot against a stone'—and most of the time this works, but about once a year something seems to happen to block the effectiveness of this. Perhaps even so, some good comes from it—I'm given time to *think.*" (3395–1, R-1)

In confirming the appointment for her life reading she wrote on January 5, 1944, about the progress she was making in her spiritual life. For some years she considered herself a "nominal Christian," then was influenced in 1939 by Glenn Clark (founder of Camps Farthest Out, a college professor, and spiritual writer), "And my life has been very different since then. There isn't much excuse for the years I wasted for I was always surrounded with Christian influences . . . Of course, all along I thought I was being a Christian but I didn't have the enthusiasm nor inner life that I have now. If I had all along had this, I'm sure I would not have the wrecked body I have now. But we can only go on from the place where we are . . . " (3395–1, R–1) Both her father and husband had died, her son and daughter were now running the business, yet "I'm hoping to be restored to greater usefulness." (3395–1, R–1) She still retained an interest in her spiritual progress and desired to know what changes she needed to make in her "present habits of thinking and living." (3395–1, R–1) Her physical reading contained these comments:

> **Then, in bringing about proper attunement of soul-purpose, mind-activity, the body results should be creative and helpful, just as the attempt in the mind structure here to create that environ for others. Can one teach greater truths than one practices in one's own life? Yes, for out of the mouths of babes comes the wisdom of the ages. For the soul-purpose is set in the oneness of Creative Forces.**
>
> **Here we will find for this body that to attune body to mind, to purpose, would be the correct manner in which to attune all to a cooperative body-building influence.   3395-1**

In answering a questionnaire from Hugh Lynn Cayce (January 5, 1947), she mentioned that she'd lost the copy of her physical reading. "It may have been my own fault in not persisting long enough in carrying out the directions of the physical reading," she lamented. (3395–4, R–3) She felt that because her arthritis was of such long duration, her progress to heal it was slow, so she'd stopped trying. However, when she paced herself and rested from time to time, it didn't really bother her too much. She died about five years later.

Origin of Information

It is in making the attunement—whether through meditation, right thinking, or unselfish living—that insights come, revealing to us the origin of our distress and providing us with the clues and resources we can utilize to improve our condition. But how do we know that this is so? Cayce himself pondered the question in regard to his career as a "psychic diagnostician" (as he described his profession). Where and how was this information coming to him? His own reading provided some answers. In attempting to offer what would be beneficial "in correcting and in meeting the ills" of others, attention in the reading was first focused on the channel himself and his own preparation.

> Consider the fact that there was first the study, the meditation and prayer upon His Word, which brought that desire, that hope, that purpose to give self as a channel through which help might come to those who would in Him seek for the betterment of their physical forces and conditions.
>
> Then consider the vision, the spoken word: *"Ask! What seekest thou? What desirest thou to do?"* Then: *"Thy prayer has been heard."*
>
> The desire was that there might be the ability to help others who were ill—especially children . . .   294-202

These last two paragraphs refer to an event that has been recounted in the Cayce biographies. When Edgar was about twelve years old, he had an encounter with an angelic presence who asked him what he would like most of all. His reply was, "To be helpful to others, especially children when they are sick."

Once the channel was set and readied, those requesting the reading also had a role in their own preparation:

> First, there are those influences that arise in the minds of those who hear of such. Then there is set in motion *desire, purpose, aim.*
>
> Those that seek, then, attune themselves to that promise which was made to this entity, Edgar Cayce.   294-202

One of the Work Readings also described the seekers' part in the effort to obtain the information: "When an individual seeks for personal or bodily aid, it is part and parcel of that individual and is read by and through the real desire of the seeker." (254-95)

The intention and motivation of the one who requested the reading was therefore an important part of the process. Then when Cayce entered his trancelike state, laying aside his physical body as in sleep, his "*spirit-mind* [attuned] itself with the purpose of the seeker, [giving] that as may be helpful in the experience of any of those who seek to know better their relationships to their Maker." (294-202) In turn, the recipient or seeker attuned him/herself to the "promise which was made to this" channel, Edgar Cayce; that is, that Cayce's wish to help others was now being fulfilled.

After these comments a rather important statement follows: "Who knows better than the individuals themselves that which has hindered them from being physically, mentally, spiritually in accord with the divine that *is* life manifested in the body?" (294-202) Or, as stated in 254-95, quoted above, the information "is part and parcel of that individual" seeking. So we *do* know the source or origin of our illness, better even than any psychic. This information is stored within us, in our subconscious minds (according to a number of sources), where forgotten memories are kept hidden, suppressed thoughts and ideas are contained, knowledge not needed is held in abeyance, and maybe even details of former incarnations are shelved. This same concept is implied elsewhere in another reading, 3744-3, in which the question was asked: "From what source does this body EC derive its information?" The reply was:

The information as given or obtained from this body is gathered from the sources from which the suggestion may derive its information.

In this state the conscious mind becomes subjugated to the subconscious, superconscious or soul mind; and may and does communicate with like minds, and the subconscious or soul force becomes universal. From any subconscious mind information may be obtained, either from this plane or from the impressions as left by the individuals that have gone on

before, as we see a mirror reflecting direct that which is before it. It is not the object itself, but that reflected, as in this: The suggestion that reaches through to the subconscious or soul, in this state, gathers information from that as reflected from what has been or is called real or material, whether of the material body or of the physical forces, and just as the mirror may be waved or bended to reflect in an obtuse manner, so that suggestion to the soul forces may bend the reflection of that given; yet within, the image itself is what is reflected and not that of some other.

Through the forces of the soul, through the mind of others as presented, or that have gone on before; through the subjugation of the physical forces in this manner, the body [Edgar Cayce] obtains the information.   3744-3

Though this rather difficult–to–understand answer was recorded here in full to be studied and reread for better comprehension, survey lecturers at A.R.E. have given a more simple, straightforward explanation to their audience: When Edgar Cayce was giving a physical reading, his subconscious mind was *reading* the subconscious mind of the one for whom the information was being obtained. So all the information that was being revealed and taken down in shorthand by Cayce's secretary, all this was coming from within the individual. Cayce, as the channel, was simply responding to the suggestion. For a health reading the suggestion, usually read aloud by his wife, Gertrude, might be as follows:

"You have the body of [individual's name] before you, who is in [city and street address given]. You will go over this body carefully, examine it thoroughly, and tell me the conditions you find at the present time, giving the cause of the existing conditions, also the treatment for the cure and relief of this body. You will speak distinctly at a normal rate of speech, answering the questions as I ask them."

Cayce's usual response was, "Yes, we have the body here . . . " To Cayce the body appeared to be actually "here" even though he was in Virginia Beach and the seeker perhaps a thousand or more miles away.

His usual opening statement would cover the general physical condition of the body, such as:

> "Now, we find the body is very good in many respects. There are those conditions rather of which the body should be warned, and of some corrections that should be made, that there might be better functioning throughout the system, for the deficiency in the more normal functioning lies in the glands of the body. Now, these, then, are the conditions, physical, as we find in this body. First . . . "

Following this general introduction, Cayce would then proceed usually with a description of the blood supply, the nerve system, and the organs involved in the difficulty. Then he would offer detailed treatment methods for relief.

What is truly remarkable and needs to be kept in mind is that all this information was coming out of the subconscious mind of the one receiving the reading. It was not like a diagnosis that a contemporary physician would conduct on a patient: take a health history, make an examination, study the results of some tests, then conclude with a diagnosis. The sleeping Cayce didn't need these probes and tools; he went right to the source—the person him/herself—and from the person's mind came the stored information. What this implies, then, is that whenever we are ill, we not only know the cause, we also know the treatments for cure. All this needed information—the source of our illness and the procedures to follow for its cure—is within us, waiting to be tapped.

Some people may see this as a mixed blessing. Of course, we still reach out for assistance and advice from others, as Cayce complied by allowing himself to be a channel for this information. We may know of intuitive people to call upon for help in figuring out our health problem and what to do about it, yet the responsibility for implementing any of this advice still rests with ourselves. The thousands of people obtaining a reading from Cayce were not really any different from people today. They had hopes, dreams, heartaches, disappointments, frustrations, joys, sorrows. Some seemed really intent on following the suggestion from their reading as closely and as thoroughly as possible;

others gave up easily or made a partial try, then abandoned the effort. They seemed to lose the willpower and motivation necessary to follow through.

One story that I heard from Elsie Sechrist, as she and her husband, Bill, traveled around the world as A.R.E's international representatives, concerned a woman psychic living on an island in the South Pacific. This woman had developed into quite a reputable and accurate psychic, so much so that gradually a woman friend of hers grew more and more dependent on her for everyday advice. It was amazing how sound her suggestions were, so her friend came to rely on her and consulted her almost on a daily basis. Then the psychic died. The friend was devastated and completely lost; she had not learned how to develop her own inner psychic gifts or make decisions for herself based on her own thought processes. Her will, too, was weakened as a result of this dependency. Elsie's point was to make us aware of the importance of strengthening our own will to help motivate us not only to make plans for our self-development but to carry out and follow through with those plans. Then we would be in a better frame of mind to accept the information wherever it came from, since indeed it is the same information. The psychic was merely tapping in to what the other person already "knew" but perhaps was not consciously aware that she knew it.

Returning to Cayce's reading on himself regarding his source of information and its helpfulness to others, we find these concluding statements:

> As to why this or that information may be indicated oft to individuals through this channel . . . An individual who understands the pathology of a physical body is taken where he is, and is supplied that information which if applied in that condition existent will be helpful in his relationship to that he worships!
>
> God seeks all to be one with Him. And as all things were made by Him, that which is the creative influence in every herb, mineral, vegetable or individual activity *is* that same force ye call God—and *seeks* expression! . . .
>
> Hence those who seek in sincerity, in hope, in purpose, to *know*, receive; only to the measure that they manifest their

> **hope, their belief, their desire in a God-purpose through a promise made to a man [Edgar Cayce]!**   **294-202**

Recognizing ourselves as the main source of medical information whenever we are confronted with a health problem can be a truly empowering revelation. That we have this knowledge stored inside us and can access it may help us to strengthen our will to meet the challenge of doing whatever is necessary to achieve a cure. Also, the ability to cope with our illness, coming from our spiritual roots, will bring the openness we need to discover in a fuller sense the purpose of our discontent. These comforting thoughts were also included in Cayce's reading given on himself:

> **From whence comes that individual entity's ability to cope with the problems?**
>
> **Are ye not all children of God? Are ye not co-creators with Him? Have ye not been with Him from the beginning? Is there any knowledge, wisdom or understanding withheld if ye have attuned thyself to that Creative Force which made the worlds and all the forces manifested in same? Thinkest thou that the arm of God is ever short with thee because thou hast erred? "Though ye be afar, though ye be in the uttermost parts, if ye call I will *hear!* and answer speedily." Thinkest thou that speakest of another, or to thee?**
>
> **Open thy mind, thy heart, thy purpose to thy God and His purpose with thee.**   **294-202**

So struggling with this information is a twofold process, requiring our own analysis of the situation plus, because we are co-creators with God, accessing the Divine within ourselves. This powerhouse combination will assist us in effecting the results we desire.

The Role of Desire

In March 1944 Harmon Bro, Ph.D., who worked closely with Cayce for years and observed many readings being given, wrote an article for A.R.E. members entitled "Physical Readings: A Study of Their Source,

Contents, and Purposes as a Personal Preparation for Their Use." He, too, knew the powerfulness of these readings. Some people might ask, he speculated, that "if we can attune ourselves to God through such readings for information about our diseases, why not just get cured at the same time and be done with it?" (3901–1, R–7) After all, the purpose for obtaining the health reading was to get healed, wasn't it? That's why you were requesting the information? Bro provides this explanation for them:

> **The answer seems to be that we have to meet diseases for reasons, for our own growth. If the healing were done for us, if we had to exert no effort of understanding, achieve no realization of the source of our strength, what would be our soul's gain? We would have well bodies but keep our troubled souls.   3901-1, R-7**

The readings, he continued, "along with their marvelous accuracy and helpfulness, propound a hard teaching—'All sickness is sin.'" (3901–1, R–7) The definition of sin, as mentioned earlier, is broader than our usual perceptions of sin. Along with its many expressions recognized by the readings, sin is basically selfishness. Thus, as one reading states, it is necessary "to eliminate sin in the lives of individuals [requiring] oft the use of mechanical means of various forms . . . " (254–114) In addition to applying physical aides as treatments for healing, another necessary ingredient is that the recipient of the treatments *desires* to get well. We might conjecture that, of course, ill people wish to feel well again. So why is it when situations from healers were presented in the readings that this quality was recognized as important to the process?

One such example comes from the 281 series, referred to as the Prayer Group Readings because they were given for the Glad Helpers, a prayer/healing group that formed from the original Search for God Study Group members. Totaling sixty–five readings in all, given over a period of years from 1931 to 1944, they contain, according to Hugh Lynn Cayce, the oldest son of Edgar Cayce, "some of the finest and most provocative material that came through Edgar Cayce. Herein is to be found the heart of the philosophy of the readings combined with profound insights as to how it may be applied in everyday life." (*Meditation: Part I*, Vol. 2, Edgar Cayce Library Series, 1974, p. vii) As the Glad Helpers worked with these lessons, they began to raise questions about their own gifts of healing and the process itself. Working and praying as a group, they developed a prayer list, using affirmations and keeping special times during the day for healing prayer. Though the group members have changed over the years, they have met continuously as a group since 1931.

On December 3, 1931, a variety of questions was presented to "seek at this time a clearer understanding of the healing forces and their interaction through us as members of this group." One such question and answer, asked by member [2112], concerned a woman in Norfolk, Virginia:

> **(Q) [2112]: Could Carrie Everett, Colonial Ave., Norfolk, be healed through me? and in what way?**
> **(A) By gaining first that sincere desire on the part *of* Carrie Everett *to* be, *want* to *be* healed! . . . There must first be the *desire* on the part *of* Carrie Everett to be healed! *God* cannot save a man that would *not* be saved!** 281-3

In several readings this same idea is expressed. Used as a criterion and basis of any endeavor to help or aid others, this approach was recommended:

> **God may not aid him who does not desire or seek aid. He continues to put in the way of individuals, opportunities, and man may do only that. There can never be love, contentment, peace, happiness, forced upon any soul; for he that seeks, must believe that God *is*, and that He hears when being sought. So in the approach to individuals as one approaches same, this can only be as a soul is awakened to its own needs . . . Neither attempt to tell the divine how this or that is to be accomplished in human experience. Do that thou hast in hand; God gives the increase.** 5502-2

For an adult male another excerpt simply stated: "He must *desire* to be aided . . . " (1546-3)

Working along with desire is the will. Both are important in one's

connection with God. " . . . God Himself does not take away nor overcome desire. The *will* and desire are man's attribute, that make them
one with or separate them from His presence." (295-3)

One seven-year-old girl was suffering from a severe cold and cough.
In her reading, requested by her mother who was present, on February
19, 1943, this question was posed: "At my last illness, my mother and I
prayed together that I be healed, according to the promise of Jesus in
Matthew 18:19. [" . . . if two of you join your voices on earth to pray for
anything whatever, it shall be granted you by my Father in heaven."
(NAB)] Please advise if our attempt in this respect had any effect, as it
was several days before I got better. What should be the attitude when
the desire is for healing?" This answer, quoted in part, was given:

> There *is* the desire deep within every atom of the body. It is
> such that attunes the vibrations of body to the spiritual love,
> see? Not as the desire merely for affection, not as the desire
> merely for a demonstration, but that *self* be used by same.
> That should be the attitude . . . 2308-3

Embedded in our physical bodies—in every atom—is this yearning
for wholeness and oneness which fosters health and healing. For a fifty-
year-old woman, whose case was classified as multiple sclerosis, a distinction was pointed out between really wanting to be cured and merely
stating it.

> There will first have to be the arousing in the mental forces
> of the body, [2997], the *desire* to get better; the *wanting*—
> deep down in itself—to get better. Not merely the saying so,
> but the *wanting* to be better—and not be tormented by the
> conditions and the environs that have been a part of the
> experience of this tortured body! 2997-1

In a letter to Cayce on March 30, 1943, [2997]'s daughter wrote:

> While listening to the radio yesterday we heard a story of
> your wonderful power. As my mother has been an invalid
> for ten years, we were wondering if you could help us in any

way in her recovery. She first became stricken in her left arm
and leg, although she is not paralyzed. She is not able to do
much for herself and is only able to walk with someone
holding both her hands. She has such a drawing all through
her body and when sitting in her chair, her neck seems to
draw down so. Every little bit someone has to pull her arms
up over her head to relieve this drawing. There are six of us
children and we have had the faith that somewhere we
would find a cure for her. Perhaps you can help us.

                                                    2997-1, B-1

Her reading on May 10, 1943, recommended, among other treatments,
a series of Epsom salts baths, massages with peanut oil, and Atomidine
(a less toxic form of iodine to be taken orally). Vitamin B-1 or B-1 Complex was to be added later. Unfortunately there were no follow-up reports or check readings for this case.

Purpose: Desire is also related to purpose. The purpose for which one
desires to be healed is of paramount importance. A number of ill people
approached Cayce with the question of whether or not they would ever
be healed. In turn, Cayce would ask them why they wanted to be healed.
Was it to return to the same lifestyle or life patterns that led to the
illness? Many of us may wish to be healed for that very reason. We
want to return to a "normal" state, to keep repeating the unhealthy
habits and conditions that prompted the sickness in the first place. Desire, then, means the willingness to change, to transform those patterns
that led to our illness and not to repeat or revert to unhealthy physical
processes. We make a commitment, then, to reorient our desires, our
purposes, and our ideals toward a oneness with the Spirit within so that
we can be better channels of service for others. Here are several examples of such concepts from the readings:

Know, deep within self, that no healing comes to any save
from the divine within. Hence hold the attitude of making
self useful *for* something; not as a gratifying of self's desires
only, but as a channel to be of blessings, of help to all needing a knowledge of God.   2564-1

As should be remembered by all, though one may maintain a physical body near to normal, unless it is for a purpose other than for self-aggrandizement, how little has the soul gained?   1190-1

Don't become so overanxious as to rely upon either the mechanical adjustments or the general reactionary forces from specific exercises; but be rather the master of self in the determining to keep fit. But keep fit for a *purpose!*
                                                                                   633-10

Oftentimes the readings presented individuals with questions that demanded a fresh perspective from the recipients, challenging them to look more closely at themselves because "it is self ye are meeting; not someone else." (1056–2) One such individual was a thirty–nine–year–old locomotive engineer who was suffering from "intense agonizing pains in the right forehead and just back of the right eye." He also indicated that he had bronchial trouble and asthma, and, in addition to finding relief and learning the cause of the pain, asked, "Am I in the wrong sort of work?" (3400–1, B–1) His doctor wondered whether the condition was migraine headaches or tic douloureaux. In his first reading from Cayce on December 9, 1943, this response was given:

. . . in the life purpose—be serious with self. Are you living the purposeful life that you would have others to see? This is not a questioning of you. The question is in self! For each soul gives account for the deeds done in the body . . .
    To whom do they account? The divine within their own selves!
    And then do you wonder that you have aches and pains, troubles and worries? You are meeting your own self.
                                                                                   3400-1

In [3400]'s check reading on January 23, 1944, Cayce advised him to follow the recommended treatments in order to get at the seat of the trouble and offered explanations for the causes of migraines and allergies:

Here we find some complications—the effects of or the be-

ginning of migraine headaches. Most of these, as in this case, begin from congestions in the colon. These cause toxic conditions to make pressures on the sympathetic nerve centers and on the cerebrospinal system. And these pressures cause the violent headaches, and almost irrational activities at times.

These, as we find, should respond to colonic irrigations. But first, we would x-ray the colon, and we will find areas in the ascending colon and a portion of the transverse colon where there are fecal forces that are as cakes.   **3400-2**

According to the concept of reflexology, reflex points in the feet, hands, and ears correspond to various organs, glands, and areas in the body. Not generally known nor well understood are the reflex points in the colon. Not surprisingly, the ascending colon on the right side of the abdomen corresponds to conditions in the head and throat, such as sinus, hay fever, asthma, and nasal catarrh. Though not scientifically verified, a number of migraine sufferers have received relief after paying more careful attention to diet and receiving a series of colonics.

From a different standpoint are allergy sufferers. When [3400] asked if any of his trouble was due to an allergy, the reading stated: "Some of it is due to allergy, but what is allergy? These are the effects of the imagination upon any influences that may react upon the olfactory or the sympathetic nerves." (3400-2) Recall the case of the man mentioned earlier in this chapter who was allergic to freshly cut grass. His harsh encounter with his father impressed itself upon his consciousness, correlating that experience with the scent of newly mowed grass, and precipitated his allergic reaction to that substance.

Wanting to be healed, desiring a cure, believing in one's ability to heal physically are all powerful influences arising from deep within an individual. As summarized in one reading, "the body must determine from within itself that it will, through the help of the Divine from within, make all at a oneness with the Divine forces, and through this bring the better spiritual, physical and mental attributes to this body." (4358-1) Though this may be helped by "taking certain physics" or medicinal treatments, which allow a physical reaction to be produced in the body, "yet without this awakening in self, without this help coming from within, any outside influence would only be of a very temporary nature, but with the awakened spiritual forces from within, acting in accordance with the spiritual forces in self, the body can throw off these conditions and bring, give, manifest, much good in the physical and in its relations to others." (4358–1) Notice Cayce's use of the word *awakening* as a description of this process, as if a part of ourselves "wakes up" to a particular reality, to what is *really real* (as one of my philosophy professors used to say). Notice, too, the relationship of service to others when this effect is achieved.

Later, the reading continued the theme of wholeness, stressing the necessity of "presenting, keeping, the whole mental, moral, physical body Holy and acceptable before Him, for without this first brought into self and made a part of self there will be no permanent healing through these properties given. With this the body can give much to others." (4358–1)

The spiritual constellation of will, intent, and purpose plays a part in unifying our desires, creating a unity within ourselves as we struggle to bring a healing force to our physical bodies. The ideal helps to anchor this process:

> **Is the will, is the intent, is the purpose of the individual . . . grounded in a living ideal? rather than of an ideal of self-aggrandizement in the influences of secular things in life, or in the gratification of desires of the flesh? These, then, will enable *those* influences, those characterizations and character buildings in the life, to make for a *purposeful* life; not only being used for something but *good* for something, and will bring more satisfaction, more gratification of that of the spiritual influences as are ever present with every *thinking* individual . . . and those influences being of a spiritual creative energy, then that as is builded in the individual will be of a developing nature.   5528-1**

Spiritual Intent: We really want to be whole, to be complete, to follow through with our soul's purpose, to grow, and to develop. Practically speaking, how is this accomplished? Using the ideal, especially in

our meditation periods, can bring us closer to that oneness for which
our soul yearns and seeks. Affirmations, short prayers that one uses as a
focus for meditation, are meant to contain the essence of what we hope
to achieve; thus, they can assist us in building that spiritual force within
us that will strengthen our physical bodies. A number of individuals,
such as this person, asked Cayce for a specific affirmation for "this body–
physical." The reading first enlarged the scope of "physical," then presented the affirmation:

> **The physical should be the result of spiritual intent and
> purpose, and [one should] not . . . make affirmations for
> [the] physical without respect or relationship to the mental
> and spiritual.**
> *O Lord, let me in body, in mind and in purpose keep Thy
> ways, in such a manner as to be a channel of blessings ever to
> others—in His name.*   **1710-10**

Another individual asked if there was a meditation she could use
"for building the body and keeping it in good condition" and, if so, how
could she accomplish this. The reading responded:

> **Just as the suggestions may be used that have been made to
> the body through some of the treatments outlined—the
> *mind* acts upon the resuscitating forces of the physical be-
> ing, by and through suggestion. Just so there may be the
> realization that spiritual forces are a part of the whole physi-
> cal being. For, the *real* being is the spiritual import, intent
> and purpose, see? Thus a meditation, a centralizing, a local-
> izing of the mind upon those portions of the system af-
> fected, or upon the activities needed for the physical being,
> *influences*, directs the principal forces of the system. And it
> does resuscitate, if kept in sincerity; not merely said as rote,
> but that said being put into practical application through
> the experiences and associations with others . . .**
>
> **In the meditations, then, *open* the mind, the being, to the
> influences about same; surrounding self with the conscious-
> ness of the healing that is in the Christ Consciousness, the
> Christ-awareness.**

Thus:

Lord, use Thou me—my body, my mind—in such a way and
manner that I, as Thy servant, may fill those lives and hearts
and minds I meet—day by day—with such hope and faith and
power in Thy might, that it may bring the awareness of Thy
presence into the experience of others as well as myself.

Such as these will bring those forces and influences for
helpful experiences for the body.   **1992-3**

In considering the points made in this reading, the process we use
when we are applying a particular remedy or following a recommended
treatment is similar to how our mind through the power of suggestion
(hypnosis or self-hypnosis) is also engaged, active, and in motion. Any
positive thoughts or helpful, uplifting attitudes we possess—hope, joy,
appreciation—supply a healing, healthful diet to our body and help to
awaken "the resuscitating forces of the physical being." There is a pattern within each of us to be whole and to function in a fully normal and
healthy manner, and this pattern can be awakened by the imaginative
forces of the mind. Of course, the spiritual being must also be involved.
Healing, as discussed earlier, is not the result of just external applications or internal medications, but rather of our attuning to the Spirit
within. The term *spiritual* implies a number of considerations, including
purpose, intent, desire, and ideals. Adding this spiritual focus—meditation—helps direct the mind to those areas of our bodies needing attention and care. This concentration and focusing, done with sincere—not
automatic—effort, makes for resuscitation: revitalizing, reviving, "bringing back to life" those diseased areas. All this, of course, takes effort and
a willingness to involve all aspects of ourselves—body, mind, and spirit.
Since the physical is the *result* of these efforts, spirit and mind are naturally included and incorporated, making our bodies a clear channel
through which life energy can flow.

Another aspect of this healing focus of meditation is described in a
reading for a woman who simply asked for additional "spiritual advice
for this body." She was told:

The body is spiritual in its aspects and in its reaction. If the
body will aid self in those applications as may be made for

> same, *see* self—in the periods when the body enters into the
> quiet—*healed* as it, the body, *would* be healed. *Vision* self
> *being* aided by those applications. Know what each applica-
> tion is for, *seeing* that *doing* that within self.   326-1

This type of healing method, visualization, is mentioned by Cayce in
other readings with a similar suggestion to *see* with the mind whatever
the person desires to be accomplished, to visualize the healing taking
place. This was to be done with attitudes of expectancy and hope. However, the readings also cautioned against using visualization in regard
to specific organs; in other words, locating the diseased organ and directing the energy to that organ. Herbert Puryear summarizes the readings' caution on this technique: "The readings say that we should not
attempt to use centers, segments, or structural portions unless we consider also that the *whole* physical, mental, and spiritual structure must
be understood. Why? Because you are applying healing energy to a
symptom without necessarily affecting the *origin* of the disease." (*Covenant,*
Vol. 2, No. 12, p. 4) But utilized in a more general way, visualization is a
safe and effective technique, one of a number of different modes of
therapy to use.

Physical Applications and Attitudes

Learning about ourselves—not only what is the possible cause of our
illness, but what are our real desires and motivations, what do we truly
want out of life—helps us get to our divine roots. It may also enable us
in our hearts to answer this question posed often in the readings (from
Psalm 103): "Who healeth all thy diseases?" We do desire healing, as did
the people who received physical readings from Cayce. But the readings
contain more than just the process of getting people well. As Harmon
Bro in his article asserts: "But well for what? You may apply, inhale, eat,
relax, sweat, and be adjusted all you wish, but unless you want to get
well for a good purpose, you may as well stay sick." (3901-1, R-7) The
variety of applications to be made can assist us in the changing to a
more purposeful attitude, as stated in the following excerpt:

Do use the periods [of treatments] for prayer and meditation. Do keep the attitude in body-mind for those of better
creative influences.

Not only be good—be good for something! Do think
of others—not altogether *of* self, but as to how the
body may contribute most to that—not merely of pleasure—
but of creative forces and influences in the lives of others,
also!

This will change the general attitude, and if the applications are made—we will find better accord and better coordination for the body.   1807-6

The "why" of one's return to health was already briefly discussed
earlier in this chapter. Equally important is the "how" of making the
applications. One woman, who in her second reading simply asked for
further advice, was told:

Be consistent, but be persistent with those applications as
suggested. Not as mere rote to be gotten through with, either in the breathing exercises or the massages that are to be
given, but rather *seeing* that these are to accomplish that
within the physical reactions for the body. For each activity
has its own reaction, whether in the mental or the material
world. By the proper attitude they may be accorded one
with another, as cooperative influences; but if one is thinking one thing and doing another, then they must be com-
bative one with another. Be not double-minded.   850-2

This excerpt concisely summarizes the elements of the manner of
doing the recommended treatments. It implies, too, that we need to do
our "homework" by becoming informed of the benefits and effects of
the modalities we are using. This action means that we are taking responsibility for ourselves, making choices about the modalities to use,
and becoming acquainted with their effects. One of the most frequently
asked questions by clients at the A.R.E. Health and Rejuvenation Center
is "What is this good for?" It is helpful to know what the modality will
accomplish. Then, according to the readings, the recipient can *see* the
reaction taking place while undergoing the treatment. Holding to this

mental framework will also prevent the automatic, "rote" execution of the activity as well as enhance the aspect of oneness that we instinctively are trying to achieve in healing. As one reading advised:

> . . . keep the whole of the purposes, the attitudes, the activities *one*, and we will find cooperation, coordination in the physical forces of the body.
>
> These made to be warring one with another, will produce disturbing conditions and are the basis for much of that which becomes—as is termed in materia medica—*incurable* conditions. 263-7

In a number of readings Cayce described this "warring" of conditions taking place, noting them as conflicts between body and mind or flesh and spirit. Some of these disturbances were due to a glandular imbalance, improper blood circulation, constant irritations, or taking relief measures that did not agree with one's body. The results of such disturbances? Restlessness, a feeling of incompleteness, weight loss, nervousness, inability to rest, loss of appetite, even nightmares. How were these conditions to be corrected? Holding to one's ideal, doing what you know is correct, balancing the glands, attuning to the Divine, receiving loving care and attention from others, acting and speaking from a spirit of truth, maintaining a constructive attitude. Often in striving for a balance to meet the needs of our physical body or when our bodily systems are trying to rectify themselves, conflicts occur. Yet these are not permanent conditions, as one reading states:

> . . . these must pass away. But the hopes, the desires, the purposes may change not. And the law is perfect—that ye sow, ye reap. If ye sow it to the flesh, in the flesh, ye must reap. If ye sow it in the mind, to the mind it must be made straight. For it depends upon what spirit ye entertain. For it is only with the spirit of truth as manifested in that light, that knowledge of God deep within self, that ye may make thy paths straight. See, hear, know, act—and the world is thine. For He withholds no good thing from those who seek and love His coming. 3660-1

So we attempt, then, to set priorities or, as the readings often state, "Do the first things first." We might have a treatment plan to follow because we've already been advised what to do to get well; however, the readings sometimes recommend first setting one's house in order, getting the ideals straight, and affirming one's beliefs. For a twenty–five–year–old young man, who, according to his mother who was present for the reading, "has had chronic eczema, asthma, and hay fever since he was six months old" (3359–1, B–1), this information was presented:

> **Begin with the spiritual attitude. First know in self what ye believe about spiritual things. Know who is the author of thy faith. As was given by the lawgiver, don't look somewhere else. Neither call on heaven, until you have set your own heart and mind aright. For lo, thy redeemer liveth in thy own activity. As ye find in self the manner in which ye would treat others, ye will find in self help physically and mentally. This will change thy whole outlook on the purpose of life . . .**
>
> **Find that, and ye will begin then with the correct attitude . . .**
>
> **Don't commence taking these medicines we suggest first. If it takes six months or a year to get yourself spiritually correct, don't take a dose of the medicine until you are spiritually correct—it'll do more harm that it will do good.**
>
> **3359-1**

Another man, thirty–seven years old, wrote to Cayce on November 26, 1943, requesting a reading on his condition:

> . . . I have lost complete use of both arms due to a progressive muscular atrophy. This condition first became apparent in 1935. Though temporarily checked, it seems to be getting worse. That is why I requested the reading as soon as possible.
>
> I am very much impressed by your wonderful work and I am more than willing to cooperate in every way possible. Incidentally, I have seen many neurologists including those at the Mayo Clinic. None really seem to know what is the

cause of my affliction or how it can be cured. However, I
am positive that somewhere there is someone who can help
me.   3682-1, B-1

His reading on February 18, 1944, recommended the Wet–Cell Appliance using gold and gave directions for its series of use, along with
massages. The massage therapist received this admonition: "Take the
time to give this massage. Don't hurry through with it." (3682-1) He was
to follow these suggestions for sixty days, then request a check reading.
However, he was also advised:

> Do begin with the first things first. Don't say in self, "Well,
> I believe this and I'll give it a try." Begin first by reading
> Exodus 19:5, Deuteronomy 30, then the 23rd Psalm. Then
> begin with the 14th, 15th, 16th chapters of St. John. Learn
> each of these passages so that they may be repeated.
> Then begin to apply them with the people you meet, or
> the people who meet you; not merely as sayings. But you
> want to be a little bit happier, a little bit more optimistic, if
> you would have the Lord on your side.
> Then, when you have done this, you may begin with the
> mechanical part of the applications [Wet Cell Appliance].
> Do these and we will find changes for the better.
>   3682-1

He also asked whether any particular climate would be helpful for
his condition and was told: "Wherever the body finds it most pleasant
for its environs. It isn't the climate, it is the attitude ye need first." (3682-
1)

Unfortunately there were no follow–up reports and no check reading
was requested. Certainly a change of attitude backed up by scripture
might take time, we can surmise. But a positive, hopeful outcome was
predicted if the recommendations were followed.

Conclusion

Looking at our physical bodies as the result of the action of spirit and mind, we examine the origin of our illness, recognizing its causes—whether pathological, karmic, or error based. But we also recognize the profound depth of our own subconscious minds, where a great amount of knowledge about ourselves is stored. This knowledge can be tapped through meditation, setting ideals, the intention to live a purposeful life, and the sincere desire to *want* to be healed. Setting priorities, putting first things first, we recheck our spiritual attitudes so that we can follow through with the treatments we've chosen to apply. Now we are ready to reap the benefits of our efforts and applications as we continue on our journey toward health.

Reaping the Harvest:
The Fruits of Our Choices

. . . thy life is an expression of the divine, thy health is an expression of thy faith and thy hope in that divine power within thine own self. 2545-1

. . . there is within each organ that ability to take from the system that necessary for the rebuilding of itself, the continuous reproduction of itself. 1158-31

. . . consider the mental and physical body, for through these the spiritual may manifest, and the soul develop. 5497-1

Characteristics of Physical Applications

WE ARE SPIRITUAL beings inhabiting a physical body. Most of the time, however, in our beliefs, we reverse this statement, seeing ourselves largely as physical bodies with an inner spiritual component. In our struggles to live in this three–dimensional plane, we become subject to the laws that govern our spiritual, mental, and physical bodies. Oftentimes our illnesses, diseases, or distresses cause us to take stock of the concept we have of ourselves and where we may have strayed from the proper path. Perhaps we see a pattern that is really not healthy nor life–sustaining. We may have established a frequent dietary habit of eating steak and potatoes, and the resultant physical reaction—an upset stomach or constipation—reminds us of this unhealthy pattern. The ef-fect is first felt physically, and so we begin to take measures to correct this disturbance, maybe drinking some herbal teas or getting colonics to soothe our digestive system. We could also become aware of our state of mind. We may be agitated, worried, or upset while eating or in a hurry to finish the meal. Over time these mental states can lead to an imbalance, causing indigestion or other problems. Praying for guidance and assistance with our illness will help us reconnect with our divine source to obtain the health and healing we seek.

Gina, a student at the time at the Cayce/Reilly School of Masso-therapy, was in a car accident several years prior to her attendance at the school. While largely recovered, she still had what she referred to as a "kink" in her lower back, left side. It was a tight area that bothered her from time to time. When she began massage school, she decided to get to work on that area, to heal it, and began trying a series of chiropractic adjustments. In hydrotherapy lab class, the students were practicing ice massage on one another, taking an insulated cup of ice and applying the ice in circular movements directly on the skin to numb it—five min-utes on, five minutes off, five minutes on, then massage for a few min-utes until the numbness returns. The area of the body being iced would be some chronic—not acute or fresh—injury that still needed some work, that was still a sore spot. Gina had her fellow student apply the ice to her lower back. After the procedure, she was amazed. The "kink" was no longer present; the tightness had released and now the area was soft and pliable and pain free. She was ecstatic and reported to her chiro-practor, "I've been coming to you for several months now getting my back adjusted, but just one application of ice massage released the kink." Of course, her fellow students were quick to point out that perhaps the adjustments had prepared her lower back little by little to finally accept the healing application of the ice massage. Often when healing takes place in such an instantaneous manner—whether during a massage, an adjustment, or a hot/cold pack—we tend to canonize the treatment it-self, declaring it to be *the* authentic, ultimate healing modality, forget-ting that a number of factors probably came together at that precise moment, making the healing seem to occur "instantaneously."

In another story the application seemed incidental to the healing.

Diane, a member of a Search for God Study Group, had been bothered off and on throughout her life with constipation. Another woman in her study group recommended her taking senna tea for relief, stating that it had helped her, although others found the tea a bit strong and harsh for their systems. So Diane was told to go slowly, maybe one serving daily in the beginning. At the local health food store she purchased a small box of the dried tea leaves, boiled them in a teaball, then drank it. It worked, and Diane was pleased. Whenever an episode of constipation occurred, she made another serving of the senna tea, drank it, and got results. Finally the box was empty, another episode hit her, but Diane kept forgetting to buy the tea. One day went by, then two, then three. She was still constipated on the fourth and fifth days, until finally she remembered to stop at the health food store and buy another box. Feeling almost desperate by now, she immediately began boiling the water for the tea when she arrived home. While the water was heating up and before it had come to a complete boil, she had to use the restroom where she had a bowel movement. She laughed as she told this story, remarking how she didn't even get the chance to drink the tea. All she had to do was boil water *with the intention* of drinking the tea, and her physical system responded and released. Perhaps her body, anticipating the absorption of the remedy, began to prepare itself, much like the digestive juices in our stomachs ready themselves to receive the food when we begin merely to *think* about our next meal, what foods we'd like to eat, or at what restaurant we plan to eat. Our physical bodies respond to these cues from our mind's imaginative forces.

Of course, applications in the majority of cases are necessary and important and useful—so much so that a number of times the readings advised not even starting the protocol unless you were willing to carry out the complete treatment. Some series were quite lengthy and complicated, the treatments taken in certain sequences so that one's body would have time to adjust and readjust. One person was told to take fume baths, Glyco–Thymoline packs, massages, and osteopathic manipulations, as well as gold administered vibratorially through use of the Wet–Cell Appliance. After describing these treatments, the reading stated: "Unless all will be done, don't begin any of it." (3433–1) Maintaining consistency and being persistent in following through with the applications were stressed over and over in the readings. (These characteristics were also mentioned briefly in chapter 4.) It takes time for the body to acclimate itself to the medicinal remedies and to return to a proper balance. It may happen, too, as noted in chapter 1, that conditions might worsen and the body has to pass through this state, referred to as a "healing crisis," before it begins to feel better. So stopping the treatments at this crucial juncture would prohibit the total healing or relief from occurring, as mentioned in these readings:

> **If this is not to be carried all the way through, don't begin. For, there will be periods when there will be a great deal of distress, even in certain periods of the treatments. Yet these will bring relief, with the application consistently given.**
>
> **3244-1**

> **Do not give up too easily, and do not overindulge because you feel a great deal better. Be consistent and persistent, and we will find greater relief coming for this body.**
>
> **1512-2**

> **Now, as we find, the disturbances that prevent the better physical functioning of the body have in a great part been misunderstood. For the effects rather than the causes have been considered. Hence with applications there has come at times relief momentarily, or at others a greater period of activity and then rather the return. For many are the disturbing factors. Yet the basis of these, as we find, with consistency and persistency, may be eliminated so as to make for a much nearer normal condition and produce for the body a much more perfect physical and mental functioning.**
>
> **741-1**

As shown, the words *consistent* and *persistent* are often paired close together in the Cayce readings. *Consistent* has to do with a certain harmony or agreement, but it also means "holding always to the same principles or practice," as in a consistent behavior. *Persistent* has the quality of stubbornness or tenacity, "refusing to relent; continuing, especially in the face of opposition, interference, etc." The determination and stick-to-itiveness required for these attitudes presupposes a deep-seated willingness on the part of the recipient to work with healing principles and to explore causes rather than symptoms of illness. Making the applications "in a consistent and persistent manner," one reading promised, will "work not only towards the correcting and eliminating of the disturbances, but toward the eradicating of the causes also." (2078-1) The reading continued to explain:

> . . . while it may require a comparatively long period of consistent and practical and personal applications, these conditions may be eliminated—if there is the consistent and persistent use of the applications as may be suggested here.
>
> Do not break over from the activities once begun, or in the administrations as to diets, nor in the consistency of taking all of the things suggested; else we may find relapses that would produce other disturbances, by the very compound or complex conditions which exist.   2078-1

Mrs. [2078], a fifty-four-year-old woman who obtained this reading on January 15, 1940, wrote to Cayce three weeks later to report on her progress:

> My general condition is much better, although each week I have been spending the greater part of one day in bed with nausea and light migraine attack. Last week I increased the number of castor oil packs from two to three and this week I am doing the same. The day after I use the packs, I feel pretty punk and my mouth tastes like I had eaten up all of the bill-goat's tin cans. However, today the taste has been more "brassy" than "tinny"! So I judge from that, that the packs have done quite a bit of stirring up the poisons. High colonics (at home) have given me a great deal of comfort.
>
> 2078-1, R-3

She also began treatments with a chiropractor, Dr. Florence Wynkoop, who agreed to follow the instructions from the reading. Two days after receiving [2078]'s letter, Cayce wrote:

> . . . glad to hear you are feeling even the least better, for as
> you know your condition is deep seated and you will have
> to keep after it even when you are feeling a whole lot better
> . . . take at least two [tablespoonfuls] of olive oil after the
> packs. And the colonics will remove a great deal of the poi-
> sons—and relieve that bad taste.   2078-1, R-4

One month later, on March 19, 1940, still following the recommendations, she wrote:

> I am *greatly* improved. Have had not more than two—one
> of them quite severe—headaches and vomiting attacks since
> I started the combination of Castor Oil packs and chiro-
> practic treatments. The severe attack followed a *severe* treat-
> ment from Dr. Wynkoop, and I surely got rid of enough
> poisons for a dozen or more persons, it seemed to me. I
> both vomited and expelled from the bowels pints of green
> liquid or fluid. The green bowel passages continue, particu-
> larly after the packs and high colonics, but the color is not
> so vicious looking. Dr. Wynkoop told me last week that my
> liver was beginning to soften up . . . The entire region of the
> liver, gall bladder and duct is very tender still . . . [Her
> complexion also began to clear up, and that pleased her very
> much.] I am continuing to be careful of my diet and take
> two Castor Oil packs each week and, of course, the chiro-
> practic twice a week. I've had a few delightful periods of
> relief when I felt as though I had had a rebirth, but I find
> that I tire quite easily. Writing a letter, for instance, uses
> much of my strength. Of course, I may overdo when I feel
> improved; there are so *many* things I want to be about, but
> I suppose I shall have to continue to discipline myself in the
> virtue of patience for a time.   2078-1, R-5

In a follow-up report a week later, she had experienced a crisis, suffering from swollen hands and feet, joint pain, sore throat, a cold, odor-
ous perspiration and urine, and pains similar to ptomaine poisoning. A

few days later, however, she was feeling weaker, but better. She concluded her report: "So I feel that in a very short space of time there, I threw off and out an enormous amount of poison. Naturally, I am *greatly* encouraged about myself. And for all of this, I am deeply indebted to your generous help." (2078-1, R-7) Though there were no additional follow-up letters or reports, [2078] had evidently been making steady progress in relieving her headache symptoms by maintaining a consistent and persistent application.

Another example of these qualities being present in regard to physical applications is the case of Jonathan, who participated in the beginner's five-day massage workshop sponsored in late December by the Cayce/Reilly School of Massotherapy. On the first day of class he told the participants that he was taking this workshop to help his elderly mother, who had become more listless and debilitated, to the extent that she eventually was unable to care for herself. Though not too seriously ill, she had a number of discomforts plus losing interest in activities around her. Jonathan just *knew* that massage would be good for her and he wanted to help her. After the workshop he gave his mother daily massages, following the basic, abbreviated Cayce/Reilly routine he'd learned over the five days. After one month of massages the edema in her legs cleared up completely. Jonathan had incorporated Dr. Reilly's suggestion in his book to petrissage (knead) the legs up and down to alleviate swelling. He continued the daily massages for several months, and the improvement in her condition was remarkable. His mother had more energy, felt better, took more of an interest in life, and was back to living on her own again. Although Jonathan was encouraging her to also do castor oil packs and take some herbs, she credited the daily massages to her improvement in health and began raving about the benefits of massage to anyone who'd listen. She was indeed a changed person.

Jonathan visited Virginia Beach for a short time six months later and reported on his mother's good progress. Though just at the beginner's level of massage training, he still achieved such excellent results. "It was through being persistent and consistent," he said of his accomplishment.

Belief in the Physical Applications

When either the practitioner or the client is assured of the success of a particular modality, the results often produce a positive outcome. Being a firm believer in, for example, castor oil packs—what Dr. Bill McGarey of the A.R.E. Clinic in Phoenix, Arizona, calls "having a castor oil consciousness"—seems to help create the desired effect. A series of successful occurrences with that treatment, no doubt, builds more confidence within us in the application of that modality, inclining us to spread the word of its successful results to others. Belief in one's talents, abilities, and powers is a strong component in the healing process, as shown in the above example of Jonathan, the massage workshop participant.

Another aspect of this characteristic of belief is demonstrated in the second movie feature of the *Star Wars* series, *The Empire Strikes Back*, in which the wise wizard Yoda is introduced. After Luke Skywalker, the protagonist in the film, crash-lands his spaceship in a swamp, he watches in amazement as Yoda with his strong mystical powers levitates the ship out of the murky swamp. "I don't believe it!" Luke remarks. "That's your problem!" replies Yoda. So not believing in the possibility of an outcome *can* be a problem for us, especially when we're rigidly set in a certain frame of mind and refuse to enlarge our scope a bit. Having successful and beneficial results ourselves or hearing about or listening to the achievements of others can help us reverse our negative, unproductive thinking and focus on more positive outcomes.

One example of the power of persistent, consistent thinking was Sheila, who came to the A.R.E. Health and Rejuvenation Center to experience some of the modalities offered. She related how some time ago she had gone through a rather rough period, became very depressed, and prayed every night that she would die. How she envisioned her eventual death was that her heart would become weaker and weaker. Later, now beyond this difficult, stressful time, she discovered that she had developed cardiomyopathy, one of a variety of diseases which weakens the heart muscles. She is well aware now how important consistent thinking is, that mind is indeed the builder, and that "thoughts are things." Her massage therapist reminded her that, as she had built this weakened heart tissue, she could also reverse the process and create healthy heart muscles with her consistent thoughts of healing. This was a lesson that she felt she was meant to learn, making her more careful about what she was thinking and pondering. "We really do need to watch what we think," she remarked.

Patricia, though living in the Midwest, is also a regular visitor to the A.R.E. Health and Rejuvenation Center. She jokingly refers to herself as "the colonic lady" because of her successful, healing application of that modality. When she was much younger, she developed an infection which caused both her legs to swell up. The condition became quite serious. Her physician said she'd eventually be in a wheelchair and probably dead in ten years. Yet Patricia believed in the value of colonics and felt that they would benefit her condition. Being acquainted with a colon therapist in her area, she embarked upon a rigorous regimen, receiving a total of forty colonics before she was completely healed. She started with three a week, then eventually two a week, finally one a week, as the edema gradually diminished. She is now an avid promoter of colonics and tries to encourage others to receive them for whatever ailment they are encountering or simply as a preventative measure to maintain good health. "They really work!" she exclaims.

In one reading a twelve-year-old young man asked Cayce what weaknesses he should overcome. The reading advised him not to become "too easily discouraged at times and too enthusiastic at others." He was told to evaluate his "associations in *every* walk of life, and their relationships as one to another." The information continued:

> **For, as the physical body is but a temple, each portion must coordinate one with another for a perfect union or perfect unison of service or activity, so must the mental mind, the physical mind, the spiritual mind, coordinate as one with another. But learn their evaluations in thy experience.**
>
> **1123-1**

So, along with mental and spiritual activity initiated by the person, the physical, being the result, is seeking to balance all these elements, attempting to rectify and use whatever is at hand—the adjustments, packs, or colonics—as well as one's belief in the treatments to achieve the welcomed healing effects. This process was further elaborated upon in a reading for a forty-year-old woman who asked for mental and spiritual advice. She was told:

> **Let the mental forces know, not only that there may be help by following these things suggested but that the source of all healing comes from within. These are not curatives that are indicated; they are to *prepare* the body that the cure may be produced *by* the activity of the system itself! For it is in its very nature *creative*! Give it the opportunity to create, to reproduce *constructive* forces; physically, mentally. These arise from the spiritual forces within the body itself.**
>
> **1082-2**

One unusual story concerning this creative aspect—namely, a patient's belief in the efficacy of a treatment as well as his own attitude of hope—is narrated in Dr. Bernie Siegel's book *Love, Medicine, and Miracles* (Harper & Row, Publishers, Inc., New York, N.Y., 1986) In 1957 the patient, a Mr. Wright, had advanced lymphosarcoma, with neck tumors the size of oranges and an enlarged spleen and liver. Treatments were ineffective, yet he had hope despite his condition. A new drug was being tested and he begged to be included in the study. Even though he didn't qualify because he was considered very near death, the doctors at his insistence gave him the drug anyway, expecting him to be dead in a few days. But he perked up considerably, the tumors were half their original size—a more rapid regression than could have been achieved with heavy X-ray doses. Within ten days he was discharged from his "deathbed."

About two months later news reports carried conflicting stories about the usefulness of the drug, and Mr. Wright, very logical and scientific in his thinking, experienced a relapse. However, his doctor, seeking to explore what was really going on, explained that the early shipments of the drug had deteriorated rapidly in their bottling, but a newer, more potent strain was available, and gave his patient injections of this more recent preparation. But it was really only fresh water. Yet, the results were astounding, even more dramatic than his first near-terminal state.

Again the tumors decreased in size and he appeared to be the picture of health. Continuing to receive the water injections, he remained symptom free for more than two months.

Then the American Medical Association announced that the drug was indeed worthless and ineffective in the treatment of cancer. A few days later Mr. Wright was readmitted to the hospital, his faith and hope shattered, and in less than two days he was dead.

It has been estimated that about one-fourth to one-third of those who merely believe that the applications they are receiving or, in Mr. Wright's case, the medicine they are taking is beneficial and effective will show improvement; this so-called "placebo effect" (also mentioned earlier in chapter 4) is now accepted as genuine by most health professionals. As to why certain substances may "have different effects under different conditions," one reading states: "It is the *consciousness* of the *individual body!* Give one a dose of clear *water*, with the impression that it will act as salts—how often will it act in that manner?" (341-31) The context of this statement was in relation to eating, that people should *see* the food doing to the body what they desired it to do. After reminding us that "each cell of the blood stream, each corpuscle, is a whole *universe* in itself," the reading continued to expound on how this consciousness is built:

> One that fills the mind, the very being, with an expectancy of God will see His movement, His manifestation, in the wind, the sun, the earth, the flowers, the inhabitant *of* the earth; and so as is builded in the body, is it to gratify *just* an appetite, or is it taken to fulfill an office that *will* the better make, the better magnify, that the body, the mind, the soul, *has* chosen to stand *for?* and it will not matter so much what, where, or *when*—but knowing *that* it is consistent with that—that is desired to be accomplished *through* that body!
>
> **341-31**

Is the cup half full or half empty? The way we answer that question says a lot about our disposition, our attitude, what we choose to focus on, to believe. What do we really want to happen? Why do we want to get well? Since "the mental attitude has much to do with the general physical forces" (2823–2), we can build up our faith and belief through prayer, consistent application, and "the full trust put in the *sources* of light, life and *good* . . . " (1705–1) These elements will help establish for us the balance that we need to create the foundation for healing to occur, if this is what we truly wish for and desire.

Healing Forces

The exact process of healing will perhaps continue to remain a mystery, but that doesn't stop us from wondering about or exploring its intricacies. Just how healing happens may make for an interesting subject of speculative discussion, yet something deep within us pushes us to seek to resolve this mystery. The Cayce readings offer us a number of clues, presenting us with such concepts as attunement, specific attitudes, the setting of ideals, and self–analysis, to assist us on this healing path. There is also a consistent message presented to each individual: follow these applications and you will obtain relief. Health is promised, but the effort must be made, as mentioned in the advice presented to this nineteen–year–old woman suffering from epilepsy:

> We can only do things by *doing* them! Thinking them will not accomplish, unless put in action! Activity brings strength. Over activity may weaken the very thing attempted to be strengthened. Moderation in *all* things—let *that* be for self and for others. Keep the mind in that atmosphere and channel as holds ever before same the image of that desired. *That* is Truth!   1916-3

So following a plan of action, applying what we know our body needs, keeping a balance ("moderation"), and holding in mind the image of healing that we want can all be part of our therapy regimen. This straightforward advice is also reflected in another reading, indicating the need for a willingness on the recipient's part to do something about what he or she has learned. A forty–one–year–old man, suffering from multiple sclerosis and tuberculosis of the spine, in his fifth reading on January 10, 1944, was told:

> **The information will not do it for you. Did the Lord pre-
> vent Abel from being slain? Did He prevent Cain from slay-
> ing? Did He not say, "It is in thine own self to do"? So it is
> with individuals who may be warned or directed. It is within
> yourself to do or not to do.**   **2828-5**

The decision we make on where we might seek for help and advice
and whether we should follow it or not is an important one. For one
individual who was evidently being persuaded by others not to follow
the recommendations in his reading, that it would be futile to do so,
was told that he would have had better results if allowed to carry out
the suggestions. Cayce called it "a pity" that such a situation had been
allowed to develop and reminded the person where the true source of
strength lies: "The body should learn that in self is the force and power
through which healing may come . . . " (1308–3)

Even with conditions that appear to be difficult to cure or that do not
respond to treatment it is hard not to be swayed by the influence of
others. A sixty–one–year–old woman stated that, as far as she knew, she
had followed all the advice in her former readings "and would therefore
be grateful to be told why I received no help through the information."
She wanted in the present to "correct the cause of former failures in
order to make . . . the advice [offered in her next reading] more effective." Given on April 11, 1942, her follow–up reading explained that it
was not always her fault, that others "didn't do what was indicated to
be done . . . Mostly it was because of the manner in which administrations were made by others." (Chapter 7 covers caregivers' influence in
more detail.) The explanation continued:

> **It is not meant that information given through this channel
> should be interpreted as being infallible . . .**
>   **The interpreting of the information in the minds of oth-
> ers, as well as the manner in which the individual entity is
> influenced by others—by their material or physical knowl-
> edge, does not imply that the information given is incor-
> rect. But it does imply that if these are met under certain
> other administrations, and done in the same manner and
> attitude that the information may be given, there may be**

produced a oneness—and response in its own kind.
1472-14

Her main physical complaint, nasal catarrh, was then briefly ad-dressed. Because of disturbances in her lymph circulation, especially in her face and head, infection had occurred. Arising from many sources and of long standing, these conditions had "begun to be of a constitu-tional nature." Yet, the reading went on to explain:

> This does not imply, then, that these are incurable; but, as is the influence in *all* healing, whether the administration be purely suggestive, of a vibratory nature, from the laying on of hands, or by the spoken word, the administration of medicinal properties or even the use of means to remove diseased tissue, we find that the same source of individual-ity in the cause must be attained. That is, that which has been dissenting in its nature through the physical forces of the body must be so attuned to spiritual forces in itself as to become revitalized.
> This then, as we have indicated, does not mean that *no* condition cannot be improved, or that no condition cannot be healed. 1472-14

The reading then addressed specifically the primary ingredient for healing:

> As to what is that necessary influence to bring about cura-tive or healing or life giving forces for that individuality and personality of the individual with same, as related to the spiritual forces, may be answered only within the indi-vidual itself. For, no source passes judgment. For, the spiri-tuality, the individuality of the God-force in each entity's combined forces, must be its judge. 1472-14

What is the real source or cause of our illness or disease? Where is the "dissenting" element in our physical body? Where did we "miss the mark"? Another way of stating the question might be: "What are the urges that have brought about that material, mental and spiritual outlook that is mine today?" (2545-1) The answers to these rather personal questions lie within us, and each person must seek them on an individual basis. No one else can answer for us; in other words, as the readings state: " . . . you cannot hire someone to suffer for you nor someone to meet your own shortcomings." (3375-2) "Each soul pays for his *own* shortcomings, not someone else's!" (1056-2)

Returning to the source or "first cause" of the diseased condition was also described in another reading, part of a series on various metaphysical subjects. The question was asked: "Is it possible to give information through Psychic Readings that will lead to the cure of diseases now known as incurable?" The answer:

> It is. That which *is* was produced from some force. Nothing is greater than the force producing it. *That* may be counteracted. The condition that exists in the physical bodies we find all produced by conditions that may be met. There are in truth no incurable conditions, though the condition may be changed, or the mode of the plane's existence changed. That which exists is and was produced from a first cause, and may be met or counteracted, or changed, for the condition is the breaking of a law, and the healing forces will of necessity become the compliance with other laws that meet the needs of the condition. The healing depends upon the individual, and the attitude taken toward conditions from all manner of ways, or of the perception or consciousness of force that may be manifested through the individual.
>
> **3744-2**

Though psychic readings can point out the conditions surrounding the onset of disease and offer suggestions on how to restore the balance lost, the responsibility of compliance with the law rests ultimately with the person. The reading, however, can help the ill person understand the law that needs "to be met or complied with," for, as the information concluded, "The evasion of a law only puts conditions off, and must eventually be met." (3744-2)

A simple example would be dietary laws. One reading stated: "Do not feel or think that the body can . . . take too much meats or too much strong drink, too much of any of those that produce irritations, and not suffer the results or consequences of same!" (433-4) We are the results of our choices, or as another often-quoted excerpt states, " . . . what we think and what we eat—combined together—*make* what we *are*; physically and mentally." (288-38)

In the course, then, of analyzing ourselves, of exploring the origin of our illness, what created the disturbance in the first place, even within the process of carrying out the applications we've chosen to help heal us, we come face to face in an honest and, it is hoped, a guilt-free manner with the very thing that is preventing us from being whole. This insight and this process, then, can create for us the healing force springing up from our spiritual selves. The efforts we make, flowing through with consistency and persistence, will bring beneficial results. In a decision at a deeper level we've made a course-correction, a change in direction, and have begun to obey with a more positive attitude another law which is life-giving and healthful. The results were summarized in another reading:

> Then, as that *is* applied, as *that* is understood, there is *given* the knowledge, the understanding as to the bigger things, the greater things . . . so make then out of thine own self a whole, well-rounded individual, one seeking, one applying that that is *known*, and as *that* is applied, so is strength, grace, knowledge, understanding given as to *how* the *greater* things that are visioned by the soul from one experience to another is, and may be accomplished.   99-8

The next several sections of this chapter may help us delve further into this mysterious force that is known as healing and wholeness.

Healing Forces: Nature

One well-known aspect of the Cayce health philosophy is the holistic approach that the physical readings undertake to provide help for the seeker. In other words, in attempting to give advice for the relief or cure of an illness, a rather comprehensive, all-inclusive model was used in diagnosing and prescribing for an ailment. Yet opinions vary as to what exactly is included in the term *holistic*. *Webster's New World Dictionary* defines it as "of, concerned with, or dealing with wholes or integrated systems rather than with their parts." Holistic healing, then, according to Herbert Puryear in the *Covenant* series (Vol. 2, No. 2, p. 3), is defined as "awakening the desire to be one with the Whole." The "Whole" in this case refers to the God-force, or Higher Power, which resides within. Reflecting the concept of holism, this type of healing comprises the process of "inviting the Spirit to flow through us in accord with a high ideal, or motivating purpose, [dwelling] upon that ideal with the imaginative forces of the mind; [giving] the body proper attitudinal and suggestive instructions; and . . . physically [providing] the opportunity for balancing the atoms of the body [by] the coordination of the nervous systems and the proper circulation of the blood."

In some people's minds, though, a "holistic" approach would exclude the use of drugs or surgery, harsh interventions that might be considered too invasive to the body. Yet Cayce himself was not adverse to recommending these. However, one element that is universally agreed upon is the use of natural products to produce healing. In the readings one's own physical body is often referred to as "nature's storehouse"; hence, it "may be induced to create every influence necessary for bringing greater and better and nearer normal conditions, if the hindrances are removed." (1309-1) Relying on nature or natural elements that are stored in our bodies as our source for healing is both wise and beneficial. Nature is alive and living; it is healing. It is this natural element that helps to create our attunement to the Divine.

> **For no medicine, no appliance, cures. It only attunes the body for the activity of the living forces and living vibrations within the human system. For every element that is necessary for the sustaining of health and of the coordination of same may be created within the body if each portion is coordinating one with another.**   **1151-5**

So our body already contains the ingredients necessary for health, if the systems are maintained in a good working condition; and medicines or appliances, though not curatives, yet have a very specific role to play in the healing process. This individual was advised to "see them as they are being taken, or as they are being administered, creating—an attunement with the Divine within." (1151-5) In another reading a woman was told that "curative measures . . . are merely to assist the body to *meet* the needs in the system so that *nature's* activities may heal! *All* healing is of the mental and spiritual, *not* merely physical!" (1158-27)

Natural forces, by definition, are not made by humans. They are "rather the gift of the Creator to man to meet in the emergencies of his own experience that entanglement of flesh and matter *in* spirit association!" (1152-5) In the Cayce cosmology our souls, created by God in the beginning, gradually and eventually became entrapped in materiality, and we are making our way back in various incarnations, by choice, to our original Source, our Creator. (The "Philosophy" chapter in *There Is a River*, a biography of Cayce by Thomas Sugrue, contains a good description of this progression of events.) Could it be that somehow nature or the use of natural remedies reminds us of our true heritage, our true home, and that we are indeed spiritual beings?

> For Life is divine, and each atom in a body that becomes cut off by disease, distrust or an injury, then only needs awakening to its necessity of coordination, cooperation with the other portions that are divine, to *fulfill* the purpose for which the body, the soul, came into being.   1173-7

> For as the body is the storehouse of all influences and forces from without, it has the abilities for the creating—with the correct firing or fuel for the body—that which is able to sustain, not only sustain but to recuperate and to rebuild, revitalize, regenerate the activities of the body.   1334-1

Would natural remedies provide "the correct firing or fuel for the body"? What about non-natural products? One reading presented this information for consideration:

> If there is the constant dosing or constant application of synthetic influences, these become at times hindrances to the body. But if there are those activities from nature's storehouse, then we find these work with the Creative Energies

and impulses of an organism to create and to bring about coordinating influences in the system. **1173-8**

Later, a description of how the healing occurs was presented:

For no element outside of body produces healing, but that the attunement to the coordinating and cooperative forces of life-force as it meets the various influences that have been brought about by some error or some misapplication, the awareness of the God-Force, the Life-Force working in and through the system.

These are the manners in which healing, in which enlightenment, in which knowledge comes to the applicable experience of the individual entity. **1173-8**

In working toward healing, our body is attempting to "right itself," to adjust to whatever we are using—internal or external applications, meditation and prayer—to revitalize itself and rebalance itself. Worry, a normal and sometimes frequent response to illness, can disturb and disrupt this flow. To one person Cayce advised her not to worry, that what she was experiencing was a natural result of bodily reactions to a long-term situation. She was counseled not to aggravate the condition by "mental worry, overtaxation in a physical manner (though it does worry the body to remain idle!)—but to act in the manner as will allow *nature* to *adjust* itself . . . " (2519-3) Then, almost as an afterthought, came this advice to all physicians:

. . . this would be well for all physicians of every character to remember: That they may *only* aid nature to adjust *itself*. You can't force nature to do anything! Only *aid* it in adjusting itself to meet conditions. **2519-3**

Nature has its place. Remedial treatments have their place. Another reading delineated their roles:

The less medications, *as* medicines, the better it will be for the body; provided these are not necessary to add stimulation to some depleted or defunct activity of an organ or for

the strengthening of the body in some way or manner. But
these are rather as tonics and stimulants than as medications, as we find. For nature should be the healer. 1173-5

A tonic is any medicine that strengthens or invigorates; a stimulant
is any substance "that temporarily quickens some vital process or the
functional activity of some organ or part," such as a heart stimulant.
These types, then, according to this reading, are the preferred medicines
to administer to one's body. Even if an individual simply wants to improve upon one's condition, such as through diet or exercise, the reminder was given to use natural elements:

. . . keep to those things that are of *nature's* activity, see?
making for those conditions where there is a better normal
balance kept. Not overtaxing or *overdriving* the system, but
finding the outlets through natural channels.   1158-17

Keeping one's physical body in proper balance is a key element in
maintaining health. Oftentimes to achieve this balance the readings
suggested not overtaxing or overtiring the body, potentially by resort-
ing to too much doctoring or by the eating of non-nutritious foods.
Overdoing any aspect of one's regimen can be harmful or nonconducive
to healing—even too much exercise, overdosing on vitamins, or excessive worry or fear. One thirty-five-year-old office manager, who was
present along with his wife for his reading on January 17, 1931, was
suffering from hypotension, a depressed nervous condition, some aching and stiffness in his legs, a weak memory, and a weight problem
(obesity). His reading reminded him that "the system can, and does create within itself all necessary either to cure or to sustain the virility of a
body. Only when the system becomes so unbalanced as to need outside
forces to create a different element of consciousness in the system is it
necessary for medicinal properties or medicines for the body." (331-1)

One more comment on using natural channels for healing. One
woman asked if she should have a blood transfusion. The reading stated
that if she took the advice and applied the suggestions from her earlier
reading, her "physical body [would] arouse those activities to such a

degree that that created within thine own body will have a much more *normal* vibration to thine self than from transfusion." (557-3) The reading continued to elaborate:

> **For, realize in thine experience that all power—whether it be of that we call the gas, drug, mineral or vegetable kingdom receives its spiritual essence of activity from an All-Wise Providence that has left these manifestations in a material world . . .**
>
> **For, when the earth was brought into existence or into time and space, all the elements that are *without* man may be found in the *living* human body. Hence these in coordination, as we see in nature, as we see in the air, as we see in the fire or in the earth, makes the soul, body and mind *one* coordinating factor with the universal creative energy we call God . . .**
>
> **Coordinate thyself, then, *with* God, *with* nature, *with* the environs thou art in, *through* thine inner self.   557-3**

In a nutshell—no pun intended!—we have in nature all the ingredients for a healthy body, a healthy system, to function and operate in a proper, harmonious way. Nature is the balancer, the coordinator, the spiritualizer. It puts us more fully in touch with creative influences, with our divine source. The end result would be, as stated in another reading, "that the bodies, the minds, might be a more perfect channel for the manifestations of *God*; for the forces of the Creator are in *every* force that is made manifest *in* the earth." (341-31) Any remedies used—whether physical or mechanical applications—"are only to remove hindrances in the physical forces for the greater and better activity, and for the abilities of the body in producing the healing." (1861-5) Nature, being a manifestation or a part of God, when applied to the physical body, brings the spiritual, creative element or force needed for healing to occur.

Two natural forces of healing, osteopathy and massage (the latter included sometimes as part of hydrotherapy, "healing with water"), will now be offered for consideration, since together they constitute the most frequently recommended modalities from the Cayce readings.

Osteopathy: "There is no form of physical mechano–therapy so near in accord with *nature's* measures as correctly given osteopathic adjustments. Others may say what they may, but prove it by watching those who have them regularly, and who depend upon them!" (1158–31) With this statement and others like it comes from the readings the endorsement of this type of treatment. A number of excerpts comment on the purpose and effect of osteopathic manipulations, indicating a wide scope of value in treatment. Different from a massage, these movements are more definite, oriented to specific joint manipulations and realignment of muscle tissue.

From the standpoint of the readings it would appear that osteopathy, at least during the time period that the readings were being given, was considered by the Cayce source to be superior to other methods of manipulation. Today medical doctors (in the U.S. all osteopaths are M.D.s), chiropractors, and other therapists offer a variety of different mechanical techniques, some of which even cross over former medical and professional barriers. Because of the existence of this variety of techniques, Dr. William McGarey in his book, *The Edgar Cayce Remedies*, suggests that if one has a problem that may respond to manipulations, "it would be well to recognize the abilities of the therapist as being more important than the particular method" used. (Bantam Books, New York, N.Y., 1983, pp. 74–75) The readings seem to emphasize this importance as well: " . . . just pulling or cracking here or there . . . has nothing to do with *healing* forces! They have to be scientifically or *correctly* administered for the individual or particular disturbances . . . " (1158–24)

The founder of osteopathy, Dr. Andrew Taylor ("A.T.") Still, established the first osteopathic school, the American School of Osteopathy, in Kirksville, Missouri, in 1892, after becoming disillusioned with conventional medicine following the deaths of three family members from spinal meningitis. Rooted in Still's deeply spiritual and holistic vision, osteopathy aims to restore a working function and movement to parts of the body that become "stuck," such as the back. Considered by some practitioners more a philosophy of mind and movement than a technique, it addresses areas of the body wherever "there is stagnation of movement—whether of a joint, a body fluid, or an attitude," since "the potential for disease itself" lies in those areas, according to Helena

Bridge, a massage therapist and osteopath in England. (*The Natural Way with Back Pain: A Comprehensive Guide to Effective Treatment*, Element Books Limited, Shaftesbury, Dorset, Great Britain, 1995, p. 95) She mentions the varieties of techniques used, from soft tissue manipulation to "using 'levers' within the body to stretch a joint until it frees . . . " The difference between chiropractors and osteopaths, she points out, is that the former manipulate the facet joints of the spine usually by sharp, quick thrusts directly on the stuck joints, while the latter emphasize more the soft tissue areas. Throughout the U.S. osteopathic medicine is now widely recognized. The former governor of New York, Nelson A. Rockefeller, and former U.S. president, Richard Nixon, received regular treatments from a noted osteopath, who even accompanied Nixon on his visits to China and the Soviet Union.

In one reading Cayce explained his preference for osteopathy.

> **Let this be considered in relationship to osteopathy:**
> **As a *system* of treating human ills, osteopathy . . . is more beneficial than most measures that may be given. Why? In any preventive or curative measure, that condition to be produced is to assist the system to gain its normal equilibrium. It is known that each organ receives impulses from other portions of the system by the suggestive forces (sympathetic nervous system) and by circulatory forces (the cerebrospinal system and the blood supply itself). These course through the system in very close parallel activity in *every* single portion of the body.**
> **Hence stimulating ganglia from which impulses arise— either sympathetically or functionally—must then be helpful in the body gaining an equilibrium.   902-1**

Earlier this same reading pointed out how the body as a unit functions. Getting your feet wet, for example, could create a cold in your head. Yet getting your head wet could also create a cold in your head. This result is due, of course, to the circulatory system, which "carries the body forces in same, in the corpuscles, the elements or vitamins needed for assimilation in every organ." The description continued, ending with a humorous comment:

> For, each organ has within itself that ability to take from
> that assimilated that necessary to build itself. One wouldn't
> want a kidney built in a lung; neither would one want a
> heart even in the head (yet it is necessary to function men-
> tally that way often!).   902-1

It is interesting to note that this particular reading, 902–1, given on
February 17, 1941, with its succinct statements on the "why" of osteopathy, was not addressed to an individual, but to a particular topic: the
common cold. Yet in it we learn the reason for the preference for osteopathy. In fact, the statements were given in response to the question:
"Are osteopathic treatments of particular value in the case of a cold?"
The immediate answer was:

> It depends upon what they are for, and at what stage given.
> If there is tautness by draft upon portions of the body, ei-
> ther from exposure at time of sleeping or at time of general
> activity, the relaxing of the body through osteopathic treat-
> ments is *most* beneficial as a preventative measure.   902-1

In one of the first A.R.E. lectures I heard after moving to Virginia
Beach, Meredith Puryear, longtime supporter of the Cayce work and
member of the Glad Helpers Healing Group, related that her son Bruce
had developed a sore throat and she suggested to him that he get an
adjustment. I thought that was the most ridiculous thing I'd ever heard!
A sore throat needs some soothing medicine to swallow, not a cracking
of the neck. Little did I understand the relationship of the spine to bodily
areas and organs. According to one reading, osteopathy is "the method
by which coordination is made between various centers along the [cere-
brospinal] system." (628–2) To elaborate, the reading explained:

> This is the variation between the different schools in adjust-
> ment or massage. Some schools of adjustment work on the
> theory that if you relieve the pressure in one area the other
> naturally adjusts itself! But the osteopathic method makes
> the coordination.   628-2

Another reading gave an anatomy lesson as well as pointed out what constitutes true osteopathy. In answer to the question, "Should other glands be stimulated which have not been?" the reading responded:

> . . . these should be stimulated—but from the centers from which the *impulse* for their activity emanates!
>
> Let's describe this for a second, that the entity or body here may understand, as well as the one making the stimulation:
>
> Along the cerebrospinal system [the brain and spinal cord] we find segments. These are cushioned. Not that the segment itself is awry, but through each segment there arises an impulse or a nerve connection between it and the sympathetic system—or the nerves running parallel with same. Through the sympathetic system (as it is called, or those centers not encased in cerebrospinal system) are the connections with the cerebrospinal system.
>
> Then, in each center—that is, of the segment where these connect—there are tiny bursa, or a plasm of nerve reaction. This becomes congested, or slow in its activity to each portion of the system. For, each organ, each gland of the system, receives impulses through this manner for its activity.
>
> Hence we find there are reactions to every portion of the system by suggestion, mentally, and by the environment and surroundings.
>
> Also we find that a reaction may be stimulated *internally* to the organs of the body, by injection of properties or foods, or by activities of same.
>
> We also find the reflex from these internally to the brain centers.
>
> Then, the *science* of osteopathy is not merely the punching in a certain segment or the cracking of the bones, but it is the keeping of a *balance*—by the touch—between the sympathetic and the cerebrospinal system! *That* is real osteopathy!
>
> With the adjustments made in this way and manner, we will find not only helpful influences but healing and an aid to any condition that may exist in the body—unless there is a broken bone or the like!   **1158-24**

Coordination of bodily activities, balance of energy, and setting up
an equilibrium can all be achieved through osteopathic manipulations.
One reading included these elements as well as the reminder that just
as with medicine or any other application, the adjustments were only
corrective or stimulatory, to help the body heal itself.

> In the manipulations, there would not be so great an
> amount of adjustments as there would be the stimulating of
> those centers that keep for—and make for—the keeping of
> the proper balance, with the proper drainages to all por-
> tions of the system that have been affected—and that need
> the stimulation as the conditions are going about to adjust
> themselves.
>
> For, in *any* application that may be made of *any* nature
> for healing to a body, it is only to supply that means, that
> channel through which life energies in a body may find the
> better channel for manifestation. *Healing* is done by the
> body. Those applications to same only prepare the way for
> same to be accomplished.   632-6

How often and how long an individual should receive osteopathic
treatments, of course, varies from person to person. The readings usually recommended a series of adjustments followed by a rest period,
then resume the series. For example, to one woman the reading suggested twice a week for two to three weeks, rest a week or two, then
repeat the series. "This is the much preferable manner of taking mechanical (osteopathic) adjustments. The body responds better, and the
reactions from same are better." Her reading also stated that it would
"depend upon how well they are administered and how the body responds to same." (1158-27)

Another woman asked if once a week would be sufficient for her
son's osteopathic treatments. Again, if done properly, this frequency
would be sufficient, the reading stated. But after three to six weeks it
was to be left off for two to three weeks, then begun again. She was
reminded that the applications were not curative, but merely help attune the body "to produce proper distribution of assimilations and coordination of every reflex condition." Then this point was made: "Unless

administrations of whatever nature they may be, produce such—they are as naught." (1192-7)

As to how long to continue the series, one man was told that it would be necessary to continue the series with a few days of rest in between, that the adjustments were attuning "the centers of the body with the coordinating forces of cerebrospinal and sympathetic system." The reading pointed out, then, the two forces of healing: "Thus the body is purified or attuned so that it in itself and nature does the healing." Then, as if to answer the question, Cayce added: "As to how soon you may leave off the treatments depends upon how soon you can trust in your spiritual self, your mental self, to direct your physical being." (3384-2)

Proceeding with patience, persistence, consistency, meditation, and prayer is a requirement for achieving therapeutic results. It takes time for change to occur, for the body to be returned to a balance, for the cells to regenerate. (The next section of this chapter discusses the topic of rejuvenation.) Keeping in mind and reminding ourselves of what we wish to accomplish with our healthy body may help us waylay the feelings of failure and frustration that often arise. As one reading pointed out:

> . . . *do not* **fool self into thinking that this can be partially done and some left out and expect to find results. Do not enter in unless ye indeed intend to become, to do, to be, that which may be made as a manifestation of thy body-physical, thy body-mental. Remember ever that thy body is a temple of the living God.** *Present* **the whole body holy, acceptable unto Him whom thou dost set in thy mind as thy ideal.** 867-1

One additional remark regarding the availability of treatments. It has been noted that present–day osteopaths often do not emphasize adjustments as part of their practice, since less and less time in their education is being devoted to such manipulations. The training, however, was different in Cayce's day. Now the slack, as it were, is more and more being taken up by chiropractors. The readings on occasion recommended chiropractic care, as illustrated here:

> . . . for this particular body we would continue with the
> present chiropractor. We would ordinarily give that oste-
> opathy is more vital, but there are chiropractors and there
> are chiropractors. This is a very good one; don't lose him!
> He understands this body. These administrations will aid . . .
>   5211-1

The importance of who gives our treatments will be covered in chapter 7.

In closing this section, we should note that osteopathy was not always recommended initially in a person's treatment. Sometimes, due to
a weakened, toxic condition a series of elimination procedures was necessary to relieve the wastes and strengthen the body. There were also
instances when manipulations were not mentioned at all. For guidance
study the protocols for your specific health condition to determine
whether or not adjustments would be beneficial.

Dr. McGarey neatly sums up the effects of this type of therapy: "Osteopathic treatments stimulate the fluids, the organs, the cells—even the
atoms—of the body, to function correctly, in coordination with other
parts of the system, in a balance, a harmony of action, of life itself." (*The
Edgar Cayce Remedies*, p. 75)

Massage: One of the most frequently recommended forms of therapy
in the Cayce readings, massage involves the manipulation of soft tissue
in a therapeutic way either by hand or with the use of a mechanical or
an electrical appliance. It can be both stimulating and relaxing, affecting every part of the body—organs, glands, nerves, muscles, and blood.
Its benefits include enhanced function of joints and muscles, improved
blood and lymph circulation and general body tone, and relief from
mental and physical fatigue. With a massage literally millions of impulses are sent throughout the body along the neurological pathways,
improving nerve communication and balancing the nervous system.

Increase in circulation is a key benefit in massage therapy. Dr. Harold
Reilly reminded his massage students that whenever one could get
blood flowing to an area, the fresh blood would carry needed nutrients
and oxygen to that part and drain off wastes and toxins. A regular client

of his discovered a growth in his abdomen and mentioned it to Dr. Reilly. The client was reluctant to have a biopsy to determine the nature of it, so Dr. Reilly, when massaging the abdomen, did not massage directly on the growth—so as not to spread or enlarge it—but around it, making strokes or movements to bring more circulation to and through that area, while draining off waste products. Over a period of time the growth got smaller and smaller and finally disappeared altogether. Dr. Reilly stated that they still didn't know what it was, but the increased circulation to that area certainly helped reduce the size of the growth, eventually causing its disappearance.

Reflecting these results, one reading for a New York businessman gave this summary of the effects of massage and hydrotherapy (water therapy):

> **For the hydrotherapy and massage are preventive as well as curative measures. For the cleansing of the system allows the body-forces themselves to function normally, and thus eliminate poisons, congestions and conditions that would become acute through the body.   257-254**

In one reading, however, Cayce, after noting several hydrotherapy applications to be done by the recipient, included massage as part of the "water therapy":

> **We would have the general hydrotherapy treatments; including, first, a general cabinet sweat, the sitz baths, the thorough rubdown and massage, with special reference in the massage to the lumbar and sacral axis. Also include the superficial activity over the limbs, the knees, the feet especially . . . to stimulate coordinating activity of the cerebrospinal and sympathetic nerve systems, as well as impulses of blood supply in these areas specifically.   1772-2**

Frequently massage was used in conjunction with other modalities: steams, baths, exercise, manipulations, or dietary regimen. It affects one's physical, emotional, and mental health. For people who because of injury, illness, or age are forced to remain inactive, massage is passive

exercise, compensating partly for lack of exercise and muscular contraction. It helps return venous blood back to the heart and so eases the
strain on this vital organ.

As in osteopathy, the readings present the "why" of massage therapy
in the following excerpt, describing one of its many functions:

> **The massage is very well, but we would do this the more
> often, see? As long as there is an opportunity of it produc-
> ing the effect to all areas of the better activity to the organs
> of the body. The "why" of the massage should be consid-
> ered: Inactivity causes many of those portions along the
> spine from which impulses are received to the various or-
> gans to be lax, or taut, or to allow some to receive greater
> impulse than others. The massage aids the ganglia to receive
> impulse from nerve forces as it aids circulation through the
> various portions of the organism.   2456-4**

To apply the massage a number of mixtures were suggested in the
readings, but the most frequently mentioned lubricant was pure peanut oil, especially good for joint problems. One frequently quoted excerpt states that "Those who would take a peanut oil rub each week
need never fear arthritis." (1158-31) Elsewhere is given: "And [with] the
[peanut] oil rubs once a week, ye will never have rheumatism nor those
concurrent conditions from stalemate in liver and kidney activities."
(1206-13) It is the only oil that does not turn rancid on the skin, according to several readings, supplying nutrients to the skin, the ganglia,
muscles, nerves, and tissues as well as "elasticity and activity to the
cerebrospinal system." (2642-1) To one woman Cayce mentioned additional benefits:

> **Massage with Peanut Oil—yes, the lowly Peanut Oil has in
> its combination that which will aid in creating in the super-
> ficial circulation, and in the superficial structural forces, as
> well as in the skin and blood, those influences that make more
> pliable the skin, muscles, nerves and tendons, that go to make
> up the assistance to structural portions of the body. Its ab-
> sorption and its radiation through the body will also**

strengthen the activities of the structural body itself. 2968-1

Pure, cold-pressed peanut oil can usually be obtained in most health food stores. Olive oil was also frequently mentioned, sometimes in combination with other oils. Though Cayce did not always explain the reasoning for selecting a particular oil or combination of oils, when such was given there was a therapeutic value or benefit to it. Regarding olive oil, for example, one reading gave this explanation: " . . . as known and held by the ancients more than the present modes of medication, olive oil—properly prepared (hence pure olive oil should always be used)—is one of the most effective agents for stimulating muscular activity, or mucus-membrane activity, that may be applied to a body." (440-3) Several mixtures, formulated from the readings and recommended for sprains, strains, bruises, scars, tired legs and feet, or for a better complexion, are also available on the market today.

Regarding the frequency of massage treatments, Dr. Reilly used to say, "Get them as often as you can afford them!" Unless there are contraindications (such as fever, a fresh injury, acute infectious disease, or inflammation), massage is safe and healthful for everyone. Betty Billings, Dr. Reilly's assistant and later his wife, said that Dr. Reilly had seen virtual miracles in people who had received his treatment alone, so he was highly confident of its value and beneficial effects.

Now referred to as the Cayce/Reilly technique, this style of massage differs in several ways from Swedish; for example, it provides relaxation, whereas Swedish tends to be more stimulating. Swedish starts at the head or back, while Cayce/Reilly starts on the left arm. In Swedish the extremities are worked distal to proximal (fingers to shoulder, toes to hip), while Cayce/Reilly works proximal to distal, down the arm and leg, but always with pressure directed upward toward the heart. At the A.R.E. Health and Rejuvenation Center people who have had massages all over the world declare that this type of massage is very different from any they have received elsewhere; there is a uniqueness and specialness about it that draws accolades from these experienced recipients. Because of its blend of three different massage techniques—Swedish, osteopathic, and neuropathic augmented with special hand movements, stretches, and joint manipulations—Cayce/Reilly stands

alone among other methods. These movements and techniques are carefully and gently incorporated into the overall procedure, providing deep
relaxation and reduction of stress and anxiety to the recipient.

One of its unique characteristics is the spinal pattern movements. In
the Cayce readings four different patterns are mentioned, the most common one beginning at the first cervical vertebra and continuing all the
way down the spine. This method was adopted into the routine. It involves a series of small, close, circular movements on either side of the
spine—not on the muscles but in the groove alongside the spine, where
the cerebrospinal and autonomic nervous systems are located. Massaging this area helps to balance and coordinate these two nervous systems, the result of which affects all the systems of the body, producing
an overall healthful effect.

Massaging the abdomen with vibratory movements to the liver, gall
bladder, spleen, and pancreas as well as strokes to enhance the direction of the natural flow of the colon all help to improve organ function
and eliminate toxic wastes from the body. The importance in the Cayce
readings of proper elimination is the basis for his endorsement of ma-
nipulative therapy and massage, as shown in this question and answer:

> **(Q) Regarding health: What is the state of my health and
> what measures should I take to improve it?**
> **(A) . . . Clear the body as you do the mind of those things
> that have been hindered. The things that hinder physically
> are the poor eliminations. Set up better eliminations in the
> body. This is why osteopathy and hydrotherapy [including
> massage] come nearer to being the basis of all needed treat-
> ments for physical disabilities.   2524-5**

There are, of course, other natural healing forces mentioned in the
readings, such as herbs, various appliances, packs and poultices, and
homeopathy. As a side comment, one reading, given on May 1, 1933, for
a fifteen–year–old girl who asked about taking cod liver oil, gave this
information along with an endorsement of homeopathy:

> **Cod liver oil, of course, is an addition to a developing body
> in making for not only the structural activity, but through-**

out the lymph and all that necessary to supply the vitamins needed.

As we find, the preferable manner is to take White's Cod Liver Oil tablets; two after meals (only twice a day) would be beneficial. Take them, though, not *continuously*; but periods of three to five days, then rest for periods of an equal length of time. But take sufficient to have the desired effect.

Give the stimuli to *secrete* the necessary elements; this is much better than giving the physical body impulse and stimuli, rather than *creating* for *it* the active forces in the body!

Hence, more *often* it will be found that the activity from what is known as the [homeopathic] doses is the better; even of [allopathic] medicine!   276-5

Osteopathy and massage, however, were singled out for discussion because of their extensive occurrences throughout the readings.

Healing Forces: Rejuvenation

We have been discussing in this chapter the characteristics and benefits of physical applications. In a number of readings quoted throughout this book, another aspect is sometimes mentioned, as described by the words *resuscitate, renew, reproduce, rebuild,* or *rejuvenate.* Most of us are familiar with the concept of our body's seven–year cycle; that is, that in the course of seven years the cells in one's body have all reproduced entirely. Of course, this does not happen at once. The renewal is gradual, but constant. Normal cell division helps the body to constantly rebuild itself as well as restore areas that have lost their viability. Each cell, each molecule, each atom has a job to do, knows what it is supposed to do, and does it; this process is described in the readings as the cell, molecule, or atom having consciousness or awareness. When we are presented with such information, how do we respond?

In *Edgar Cayce on Rejuvenation of the Body,* author John Van Auken states: "I have consciously gone through four seven–year cycles using Cayce's concepts, diet, and practices. I can attest to its powerful influence on transforming bodily, attitudinal, and emotional habits and conditions into new, healthier states of being." (A.R.E. Press, Virginia Beach, Va., 1996, p. 15) The process can, of course, continue over the next cycle. "Therefore," he concludes, "if every cell is changed every seven years, then·everything and anything can be changed!"

Previously the belief was that certain tissues, such as brain cells, could not regenerate. Now medical science has evidence that the earlier regarded static brain is actually a dynamic master organ, capable of repairing damaged cells and growing new pathways.

One reading even suggests that both the recipient of the treatment *and* the practitioner understand that "there is every force in the body to [re-create] its own self—if the various portions of the system are coordinating and cooperating one with another." (1158-11) Evidently it would be helpful and healing if this concept were kept in mind by both parties. Mind, the builder, reinforces the image of health, and this consistent reminder helps restore whatever is needed by the body for healing.

Physical applications, according to another reading, "enable each organ to reproduce itself in a consistent way and manner, and it will get rid of drosses [waste matter] with its reproduction." (257-249) The reading went on to explain that growth and change take place also in the spiritual life ("ye grow in grace, in knowledge, in understanding of the law of God") and in the mental life ("in unfoldment, in the awareness of thy associations"). How the seven-year cycle affects the body in relationship to disease is also noted:

> **No need for anyone, then, to have *any* disturbance over that length of period [seven years], if—by common sense—there would be the care taken. But if your mind holds to it, and you've got a stumped toe, if will stay stumped! If you've got a bad condition in your gizzard, or liver, you'll keep it—if you think so [!]**
> **But the body—the physical, the mental and spiritual— will remove same, if ye will *let* it and not hold to the disturbance!**   **257-249**

This is hopeful news for anyone suffering from a long-term, debilitating illness. Injured tissue can be replaced. The renewal happens at the cellular level, where each atom is a universe unto itself. A healthy cell will reproduce or replicate a healthy cell. But how is this whole process orchestrated? " . . . the mind of each atom, as it is builded, [is] supervised by the whole mental mind of the body, varied by its different phases and attributes . . . " (137–81) The attitude thus is all important to the rebuilding of the body, and healing comes through the creating of an "incentive *in* that same atomic force . . . to bring about the better physical conditions in the system." (137–81) Another reading described the process in this way:

> . . . **while healing of any nature must be from within, it depends upon the attitude taken toward all elements and influences within the experience as to a manifestation of life in the material plane. In the physical body . . . each atom is a whole universe in itself . . . When there is coordination within self, in the *inner* self—when the inner shrine receives the impulse, then healing is complete; yet each atomic influence receives an impulse from various forms of application to a material body, or to a material demonstration or manifestation of a spiritual influence animating *through* a material body.** 275-32

The foods we ingest, the vitamin tablets we swallow, the massages and adjustments we receive, the positive attitudes we hold have an influence on the atoms of our body. Coordination and balance within the systems are required, as has been noted previously.

To one individual, a stock broker who was also a close associate of Cayce's and received a total of 468 readings, the information was given that he had the ability, by concentration, "to overcome conditions [that] bring distress or distraughtness to the physical body." (900–465) Earlier he had been advised to study anatomy not only to enhance this ability but to understand how the body operates and what exactly is taking place during sickness and health; in other words, he could *"become aware within self of* the body's complying with that being wrought *in* the system when distresses arise." His reading continued:

> **Hence, as has been seen through the various information as has been given regarding physical conditions in individuals,**

that, that necessary to awaken the consciousness from within an individual is necessary in its application to the physical forces *of* the body to bring recuperative and resuscitative influences in the body. *This* the process as *must* come for *every* living organism, as illness or disease is caused in a human body. The body being made up of *all* there is *without* the body in its whole anatomical force, and its essence being that of all from without; hence all from *without* corresponds to a *vibration* created from within. The sensation *of* its activity brought into consciousness by the Spirit Force, or Life within the individual, and is of a cosmic or a universal influence.   900-465

He was encouraged to continue the suggested treatments as well as the periods of silence, "seeing that as is necessary to be rebuilt within the system . . . *through* this *may* one keep themselves young; may one *rebuild within* themselves and prolong the *physical* forces as is desired *in* self!" (900–465)

Rejuvenation can ultimately lead to longevity, provided we maintain a high level of health and wellness.

One concluding comment on renewal and longevity shows how carefully the information from the readings weaves in interesting and fascinating material. The question regarded the origin of tight hamstrings. In reply Cayce points out the importance of circulation as well as makes a play on the word *hamstring*.

(Q) What makes the hamstring leaders [tendons] in the legs draw so?
(A) Poisons from those accumulations in the system, and the tendencies for the contraction of these. Keep these massaged, and we will find this will be overcome as the poisons are eliminated and a fresh blood supply is made. For the blood supply is added to three times each day if meals are taken, else we would never recuperate or change a whole body every seven years; it is a *constant* growth. No condition of a physical nature should be *remaining* unless it has been hamstrung by operative forces or strictures or tissue that may not be absorbed; and even this may be changed if

it is taken patiently and persistently—in *any* body!   133-4

All parts of the body have this capability of regenerating cells and tissue. Perhaps what prevents this from occurring are our own limiting thought processes—we can't possibly survive long after one hundred years!—but the possibility of having a new, improved body every seven years paints indeed a staggering and welcomed picture of health and healing.

Conclusion

We can become whole or well; it is in our nature to be so. To attempt to reach this state, we apply a variety of medicinal treatments and make some lifestyle changes to better our physical beings. These applications in themselves set up vibrations that create the atmosphere we need—both inner and outer—to produce better, total health. But not to be left out of any healing equation are the caregivers and practitioners, those upon whom we rely and whose help is both necessary and important in our ongoing process toward wholeness. The special role of these providers is covered in the following chapter.

7

Being Channels of Blessing:
Advice for Caregivers and Practitioners

. . . individuals must first seek that they be of service. Service rarely seeks individuals.   254-31

. . . ye grow in grace and in knowledge and in understanding, as ye apply that ye know day by day.   969-1

To each individual soul has been given the privilege, yea the opportunity, to become a co-worker with the Lord among his brethren.   3019-1

The Value of Service

FACE-TO-FACE encounters for those doing volunteer work on a regular basis benefits one's health as well, according to a poll sponsored by *Spirituality and Health* magazine (May/June 2003). The study, conducted on the Internet by Equation Research, revealed that 58 percent of the 1,413 participants think that personal contact work is good for the health of the volunteers, producing such results as stress relief and decreased sensitivity to physical and emotional pain. From their own experience or knowledge of the research, respondents also felt that helping someone on a regular basis would make them feel good. Only 5 percent said they didn't believe there were any benefits. The poll had a 4 percent margin of error.

Seventy-seven percent of those who answered the poll stated that they engage in some form of volunteer work, but only 13 percent of the volunteers worked consistently in a personal contact situation. The latter group spent at least four hours a month helping others in a face-to-face situation, performing such services as tutoring, aiding the sick, working with the homeless as well as informal acts such as giving advice to someone or helping a neighbor.

The author of this first national study to look at the kind of helping that strengthens personal health, Allan Luks, heads Big Brother Big Sister of New York City. He also noted that the health benefits of volunteering are experienced only when people work consistently and personally with strangers, not just family members or friends. Referred to as the "helping connection," this type of behavior reflects the volunteerism that Americans see themselves as engaging in: close to half of all adult Americans volunteer; in 2001 it was 44 percent or 84 million people.

The main reason people cite for becoming involved is compassion for others, mentioned by 90 percent in the study. When asked about their feelings when they help people, the majority reported, "It makes me feel good." A concluding comment from this study mirrors an important concept in the Cayce readings: " . . . the key to volunteering . . . is in our bones. Just as the rush of energy from taking a walk immediately reminds us that our bodies are meant to move, the rush of good feeling from helping a stranger reminds us that we are all connected." (http://www.spiritualityhealth.com/newsh/items/article/item_5989.html; p. 6)

Some of us make the choice to be in one of the helping professions, while others by circumstance may have the opportunity thrust upon us when a family member or a friend becomes ill. In either case we may feel called upon to become what the readings term "channels of blessing" to those in need. What does this mean? What does it imply? Describing the characteristics of this phrase will be the scope of this present chapter, with special emphasis on the roles of caregiver and practitioner.

Qualities of Care and Concern

Ill people are at times no fun to be around. They can be cranky, impatient, irritable, demanding, and intolerable. Often it takes a special person with a lot of patience and love to work with someone who is not feeling well or who is suffering from a long-term sickness. Much of the advice, encouragement, suggestions, and promptings given to ill people in their Cayce readings—especially regarding attitudes and beliefs— could be applied equally as well to the caregivers and those working in any capacity with the sick person. Family members, nurses, or physicians were sometimes the ones making the request for the reading out of concern for their loved ones or their patients. Early on in Cayce's work as a psychic, many of his readings were given to doctors who were baffled by their patients' condition and wished to learn the causes and treatments for cure. In fact, those early readings were largely all health related; it wasn't until later, when the success and accuracy of these were noted, that the subject matter of the readings expanded to include metaphysical topics, such as astrology, dreams, and reincarnation.

Yet of the 14,145 actual copies of the readings contained in the A.R.E. Library, the largest category is the physical readings: 9,541 or about 67 percent of the total. The life readings—1,947 or about 16 percent—is the next highest category. The "categories" are based on the suggestions given to Cayce at the beginning of the reading. They do not take into account that different subjects might be mentioned in one reading of a particular category. Thus, a description of one's past lives might include references to one's physical health or those receiving the information might ask about health concerns in their life reading. So the greater bulk of the Cayce material still relates to health and healing.

If one were to take the notion that in order to reverse the disease process, in order to be healed or cured, the most important step initially would be to work with attitudes, how should the caregiver respond? Perhaps in much the same way as the person who is being cared for, observing at first one's attitude toward the process itself. One A.R.E. employee, for instance, stated how she's learned to really enjoy her colds. Whenever she feels a cold coming on, it's time to take care of herself, curl up in bed, drink a hot cup of tea, rest and relax, take some time off. Each time she sneezes or coughs or blows her nose, she thinks of how much more toxic wastes are being eliminated from her system and thus she's getting closer to being well. This positive approach works wonders for her.

One can also work with removing any doubts and fears, as suggested often in the readings. Notice the conditional phrase used in this advice given in a thirteen-year-old's reading:

> . . . if the attitudes and aptitudes are kept in accord with that indicated for those about the entity, and there are the applications of those conditions given, the body will recover entirely from these disturbances [epilepsy].
>
> Then, in counsel to those about the entity:
>
> Do not allow doubt and fear to enter in. *Know* the source of all that is good. *Know* that there is the power within the body to associate the ideas, the purposes, the desires, with the Infinite, to make it whole within; and this includes those about the body. **2153-7**

In some instances to promote healing the environment had to be changed as well; in one case, the change was needed "so that the spiritual promises may be put to active service." (1427-1) This man was advised to spend four weeks at Still-Hildreth Osteopathic Sanatorium in Macon, Missouri, in order to have manipulations ("corrections made in the cerebrospinal system to produce coordination between the sympathetic and the cerebrospinal system") and to relieve pressures and mental anxiety. He was also told to pray and study, and to work with replacing his bad habits "with the habits of doing *good*, doing right, doing justice, being merciful." The reading continued:

> These [habits] are naturally a part of the whole of the entity's self, and the harm comes to self from only anxiety, shame and inordinate desires from those about the entity.
>
> *Do not*—those, then, about the entity—*condemn;* lest a worse fate befall thee!
>
> For these conditions may be overcome with this body if the entity will turn first to the spiritual self, and seek spiri-

tual aid and guidance from within . . .   1427-1

Although the ill person is to take responsibility for his/her own heal-ing process, doing whatever it takes—a shift in attitudes, increased prayer, setting ideals, or lifestyle changes—to achieve the healing, the caregivers, practitioners, and others who come in contact with the sick individual share equal responsibilities. They are to be cognizant of their own beliefs and attitudes just as much as those who are ill. No condem-nation, no judgment, no fear, doubt, or worry are to characterize their mindset. The Golden Rule—do unto others as you would have others do unto you—is to be applied in a loving and heartfelt way.

One woman in her physical reading was reminded of the goal or purpose for getting well: "What need is there for a better body, save to serve thy fellow man the better?" (1620-1) This advice, the reading said, was not meant only for teachers, ministers, "those who wait on this, that or the other influence, but to each and every soul—and to every phase of the soul's activity in a material world!" (1620–1) Being of service to others or being channels of blessing was often cited as the paramount reason to attain health. After suggesting that she purify and cleanse both mind and body, her reading concluded:

> *Practice* then in thy daily experience, and thy associations with thy fellow man, charity to all, love to all; finding fault with none; being patient with all, showing brotherly love and brotherly kindness. Against these there *is* no law! And ye who have put on and as ye put on these, by the applica-tion of them in thy dealings with thy fellow man, ye become free of the laws that are of body or of mind; for ye are then conscious of being one *with* the Creative Forces that bring into the experience and consciousness of all the love of the Father for the children of men.
>
> And it is only as ye deal with thy fellow man that ye show forth His love. For as ye do it unto the least of these, thy brethren, ye do it unto thy Maker.   1620-1

Jan, a massage therapist, had a new client Marie who was in town visiting relatives. Marie requested an acupressure treatment, stating that she recently had had surgery following months of chemotherapy for breast cancer. Jan noticed that Marie was rather abrupt and standoffish in her manner, but immediately refused to react to it, realizing that the aloofness had nothing to do with her personally. As she began the session, Jan remembered her niece who had also suffered with breast cancer. She thought about all the difficulties and emotional turmoil she'd gone through with it. The client Marie suddenly opened up and began relating how she'd hated her job, wanted to quit it, but her husband insisted she remain in it. When she developed the cancer, of course, she had to leave it, remarking that in a way she was glad to have this opportunity to at last quit a work in which she was not happy. Marie seemed to soften and appeared relieved to be able to share those feelings. What happened to create this change? Did Jan's sympathy for her niece who came to mind set up an energetic shift, a vibratory change, that elicited a response or struck a chord in Marie, causing her to recognize on some level a sympathetic, caring soul?

Along with her education as a massage therapist and acupressurist, Jan had also attended training workshops with Dr. Elisabeth Kübler-Ross, well-known expert on death and dying. One of the questions Dr. Kübler-Ross asked the participants was, "Who here is very unhappy with their job?" After some hands were raised, she ordered, "As soon as you return home, quit it!" Of course, people began to rationalize and explain how this couldn't possibly be done at this time, it just wasn't feasible, etc., etc. Yet she knew the ill health engendered in many who feel trapped or stuck in unproductive, unfulfilling work and that over a period of time these feelings could make you ill. Dr. Harold Reilly told one of his trainees, "Don't ever massage someone you don't like. It could make the person sick." When two individuals come together—one to receive help, the other to give it—there is a type of dynamic, a "union of forces" which comes into play, each one bringing to the moment a spiritual quality, an essence of the totality of who each is.

Michael's experience involved two back surgeries to repair an area worn out from overuse of lifting and bending required in his warehouse job. While recuperating from the second surgery, he noticed a paperback book that someone had tossed in the trash can. Never much of a reader, he decided since he was going to be in bed for a while, he might as well be doing something. An intern retrieved the book for him, Michael read it, and later stated, "It changed my life!" The book was *There Is a River*, the biography of Edgar Cayce by Thomas Sugrue. He began meditating and hoped one day to visit the A.R.E. in Virginia Beach. But the second surgery was "botched," in his words, and the resultant nerve damage caused constant pain, alleviated considerably with meditation.

Five years later Michael finally made it to Virginia Beach and decided to receive a Therapeutic Touch treatment at the Health and Rejuvenation Center, where he shared his story. He had given up on doctors and had turned to meditation and energy medicine, receiving some relief from various healers in his area. He wants to teach meditation to others since he derives such benefit from it. During the TT session he felt energy flowing throughout his system. At one point his whole body jolted. "What was that?" he asked. "I don't know," answered the practitioner. "Perhaps a release of energy." At the end of the session Michael reported that for the first time in five years he was pain-free. His range of motion also improved. The next day before he returned home, he visited the Center and demonstrated several times how he could bend over and touch his toes, something he'd not been able to do since the second surgery. He was ecstatic. His belief that energy medicine could help his condition as well as his desire to serve others as a meditation teacher—was this a combination, a "union of forces" within him, that created the remarkable change in his system? And did the attitude of concern on the practitioner's part add to and intensify the energy already present?

One rather poetic description from the readings, comparing two individuals to two brooks, is found in the following:

> **Two brooks in all of their beauty, in all of their freshness, seek to wend their ways upon the bosom of the earth; each enjoying the beauties that they are given. Yet as they unite they give then strength and the power and the majesty of His beings in the abilities to give to those forces and powers of many. In a way they intermingle as one and yet each enjoys those beauties, those abilities, those effacements of self in this union for the glory of the power and the might that may be manifested of that they *as* individuals worship as the one God.**   **688-4**

This reading was given for a man and a woman who were seeking "counsel and guidance as to their spiritual and mental development, and connections in past incarnations, especially in relation to working together in healing work." Thus, it describes the qualities of two individuals who unite for a common purpose.

Development of the Healer

A number of comments from the readings refer to a magnification of energy, especially prevalent when two or more people take part in the healing session or when two or more offer prayer for those requesting help or aid. While the magnification is present simply because there are more bodies taking part, the *quality* of the healing force may depend on a number of variables: how connected the individuals in the group are to one another, the attitudes of each of the group members, each one's own connection to Spirit or the God–force, and the work each has done on a personal and soul development level.

Anyone who reaches out to another—or to oneself—in a caring and loving way, from the heart, is a healer, so one doesn't necessarily have to belong to a helping profession to do healing work. Some people may feel that this is their calling or others have told them they have "healing hands," so these individuals begin to study, take courses, and educate themselves about the various concepts of healing and to acquire certain skills for doing healing work. There is also a spirit of dedication and commitment that is part of the process; for some this may require setting aside certain needs or personal projects in order to fulfill a higher goal. According to Alice Bailey in *Esoteric Healing*, "the healing art is not a vague mystical process, or wishful thinking and simple good intentions . . . it presupposes the mastering of the science of soul contact . . . the constant practice of alignment . . . " (Lucis Publishing Company, New York, N.Y., 1953, p. 557) She also maintains that in the future healers will undergo years of intensive training, much like the current medical profession, combining "orthodox study and knowledge with the art of spiritual healing." (p. 557)

A number of schools or programs offer a graduated course of study leading to certification, a diploma, or credits toward licensing or the authority to practice a particular field of study. If one wants to be a professional healer, for instance, it would be appropriate to choose an educational basis first in order to facilitate one's practice. In most areas there are licensing laws that govern who may legally touch and charge a fee, and the non–health professional would need to operate within the scope of these regulations.

Many practitioners, however, enter the field of healing with an already established basic education in a helping profession, such as nursing, chiropractic, medicine, psychotherapy, physical therapy, or massage, that require a certificate or license or is regulated by a licensing board in one's individual state. The expertise, then, of an energetic healing modality can be added to this educational preparation. For example, Therapeutic Touch, developed by Dolores Krieger, Ph.D., R.N., and Dora Kunz, is considered a nursing skill now used throughout the U.S. and Canada as part of nursing practice. Likewise, Healing Touch, an energy-based therapeutic approach to healing developed by Janet Mentgen, R.N., H.N.C., B.S.N., offers a multilevel program moving from beginner to advance practice and is used extensively in the nursing profession as well as a spiritual ministry in churches and for animals.

In addition to educational development, the healer is strongly encouraged to honor his/her needs through self-care. "Maintaining a personal state of wellness and vitality, reducing fatigue and stress is necessary for this work. The physical body needs to be in a relaxed state, the emotions calm, the mind clear of tension and worry, and the spiritual self quiet and still." (Mentgen and Bulbrook, *Healing Touch Level I Notebook,* North Carolina Center for Healing Touch, Carrboro, N.C., rev. ed. 2001, pp. 42–43) Other qualities considered traditional to the healer are compassion, care, and love for the client, setting one's ego aside, being nonjudgmental, as well as being open, curious, and flexible to the adventure that is healing work. "The healer's intent is to help another, to see that person whole, and to focus on the intention of healing." (p. 42) (More about *intent* in the next section of this chapter.)

The four-year program at the Barbara Brennan School of Healing®, headquartered in Boca Raton, Florida, offers a B.S. degree in Brennan Healing Science accredited by the Florida Department of Education. One of the requirements for attendance is that the student, while in school, engage in two private sessions a month with a psychotherapist or other qualified mental health practitioner. This practice enables the student to deal with issues that may arise through healing work, such as projection, boundaries, and transference. It is a well-known axiom that a healer cannot take the client further than the healer has gone. If the healer has the same fear, for example, as the client and has not dealt with or worked through the fear, the client will not get far along in the process either. According to some teachers at the Brennan school, those willing and open to self-work often are more receptive and quicker to learning the skills being taught and presented, having fewer blockages in their energy fields. Knowledge along with acceptance of one's issues, as well as the desire to work on them, opens the student to better receptivity energetically.

During my freshman year at the Barbara Brennan School we were practicing "chelation," as described in Brennan's *Hands of Light* (Pleiades Books, New York, N.Y., 1987). Day after day, class after class, we did "chelation." Finally one student asked, "When are we going to learn a different technique?" The teacher responded: "We can teach you all the different techniques you'd want to learn, but if you're not willing to work on yourselves, none of them would be effective."

Having the proper intention and the desire to heal and willing to make the effort are characteristics of one wishing to heal, according to the Cayce readings. In the Prayer Group series several of the Glad Helpers asked questions about their healing ability and how to develop it. One person was told to work first on understanding herself and to allow the spirit to lead her. The *Healing Touch Level I Notebook* states, "Eventually the energy itself will be your teacher." (p. 44) Here is the question–and–answer exchange from the readings:

> **(Q) How can I best develop the magnetic power for healing?**
> **(A) First understanding self; and do not become mechanical or rote in action. Rather be the growth as the spirit moves self, as the understanding comes—but *much* may be accomplished through *these* channels.   281-9**

Another person asked: "Could I become a healer? If so, what method should I use?" The reading advised: "That as seemeth to thee that channel through which an individual, or entity, may get hold of that which is being given out by self." (281-6) Then it mentioned the various types of "channels through which healing may come": individual contact, faith, laying on of hands, or what will create in the mind "that consciousness that makes for the closer contact with the universal, or the *creative* forces, in its experience." The reading ended by advising the person to use what "is nearest akin to that concept built. Use that thou hast, then, in hand." (281-6) In other words, it was to be left up to the individual which method to use—whatever seemed to fit the situation or whatever the individual felt drawn to or attracted to, *that* method was to be utilized at that moment. One individual was reminded that the Master Jesus used various methods in His healing work:

> **What were the methods used by Him . . . ? Just by speaking, just by prayer, just by fasting? No. Was there not anointing? Was there not washing? Was there not mechano-therapy? Were not even other conditions used in combination with them all? . . .**
> **Use *all!***   **1546-1**

Further information on healing methods was given to a sixty-nine-year-old physician who asked for comments on his life and work. The reading stated:

> **. . . there is good in *all* methods—and they have their place. But from whence comes the healing? Whether there is administered a drug, a correcting or an adjustment of a subluxation, or the alleviating of a strain upon the muscles, or the revivifying through electrical forces; they are *one*, and the healing comes from *within*. Not by the method does the healing come, though the consciousness of the individual *is* such that this or that method *is* the one that is more effective in the individual case in arousing the forces from within. But *methods* are *not* ideals. The *ideal* must be kept in the proper *source* . . .**   **969-1**

In light of the readings, then, the particular modality used seemed incidental to the spiritual guidance and development of the healer, as demonstrated in the answer to this question: "By what steps are developed the powers of spiritual healing?" The person who asked this question, [699], was a member of Study Group No. 9, which also obtained readings from Cayce and was given the designated number [705]. The reply was:

> **Through spiritual growth. By what powers doth a grain of corn maintain its ability to produce corn; that divine gift to the first corn? By not trying to be something else than a grain of corn! Thus may there come an understanding to any soul, to any that will say "Use me, O God, as Thou will." But not remaining idle! For, as has been given, *activity is* the key to understanding. Rather had there be a purpose or an act in error than no act. For movement is the effect of spirit. Spirit is life. But let the inner self, the divine self, the knowledge of same be directed only by Him.**
>
> **705-2**

Following one's inner guidance and acting upon it will help one develop the gift of healing. To one woman the reading also advised "the study of vibration as related to human emotion" and "studies . . . combined or compared with the teachings of the Teacher of teachers [Jesus]." (2029-1) When one of the Glad Helpers asked Cayce to define vibration in relation to healing, this succinct answer came: "Vibration is, in its simple essence or word, *raising* the Christ Consciousness in self to such an extent as it may flow *out* of self to him thou would direct it to." (281-7) So in addition to a knowledge base—which may include courses in anatomy and physiology, learning about field theory and energy concepts, as well as having a general knowledge about physical, mental, and spiritual dimensions—knowing how to meditate in order to raise the Christ Consciousness is equally important; in fact, it is essential to one's growth as a healer and is used as the basis or starting point for all healing work. Its importance was also stressed to the Glad Helpers Prayer Group and the effects were described in the following:

When a body, separate from that one ill, then, has so attuned or raised its own vibrations sufficiently, it may—by
the motion of the spoken word—awaken the activity of the
emotions to such an extent as to revivify, resuscitate or to
change the rotary force or influence or the atomic forces in
the activity of the structural portion, or the vitale forces of
a body, in such a way and manner as to set it again in motion.

Thus does spiritual or psychic influence of body upon
body bring healing to *any* individual; where another body
may raise that necessary influence in the hormone of the
circulatory forces as to take from that within itself to revivify or resuscitate diseased, disordered or distressed conditions within a body.   281-24

Meditation helps one focus and maintain a point of reference. This
focused intent or centering keeps the healer fully present, connected to
oneself, and open to another, clearing the ego and making for a balanced flow of energy exchange throughout the healing session. A moment of quiet to focus, to pray silently, to connect with one's ideal, or to
visualize a flow of healing energy—these are all techniques of centering
that healers may use when beginning their work, directing their attention momentarily inward before relating outward to the client. Ideally
the healer remains centered throughout the entire healing session.

Who can heal? The readings say that we are all healers, that in any
given moment we have the potential to be a blessing to someone. Do
we want this? Are we willing to be used in this manner? One woman
was told:

Each and every soul that seeks and that contacts consciously
spiritual forces that are constructive, is a healing force both
mentally and (if mentally) physically. Hence the body with
its will, with its desire, with its development, may raise those
influences within self as to bring healing. By touch. For, as
healing is through a physical channel, and as the various
activities of body units are raised in their vibration to send
out influences to others, there may be seen in self that while
all body units are not wholly in unison, but if these are

raised properly (which means the will, the desire to be used by Infinity or the God-force in self), it may heal self as well as others. For, in healing others the healing comes to self.

443-3

This notion of healing oneself through healing others also appears in the answer to a query from one of the Glad Helpers, [69], who asked: "Is it right to try to heal others when one has failed to accomplish healing in one's own life?" A rather thoughtful question, such a concern would naturally arise in the mind of any would-be healer. The reply was:

Healing others is healing self. For, to give out that which aids others in reaching that which creates the perfect vibration of life in their physical selves, through the mental attitudes and aptitudes of the body, brings to self better understanding.
Yes, in healing others one heals self. 281-18

So we don't necessarily have to wait until we are physically and mentally in perfect health before we begin our healing work. We can start where we are now, with raising our vibrations through meditation, with setting ideals, with working on having the proper attitudes, and setting our intent for the highest good for ourselves and for those whom we contact.

The Power of Intent

Next to centering, the motivation of the practitioner is an important quality for achieving positive results. Not only does the healer have a strong desire to help but also an understanding of how to achieve the goal, how to facilitate the intervention, and giving up attachment to the outcome. Understanding one's motives (why one wishes to help or to heal) is part of the self-learning process, making the healing act one of careful consideration and mindfulness. Much like the definition of vibration mentioned earlier, the energy raised in silence and meditation flows out in focused thought (intent) to the recipient, with the mind directing the flow of energy. How this transfer of energy occurs cannot be explained scientifically, but a possible analogy from physics has been suggested, as described by Dolores Krieger in her book *Therapeutic Touch Inner Workbook: Ventures in Transpersonal Healing:*

> . . . it is the surrounding nonphysical field that carries the charge of electrons between objects, and this transfer occurs whether or not the objects come into contact. The explanation is that electrons in the outermost orbit at the molecular level are bound very loosely and, therefore, can be easily dislodged, carrying the electrical charge with them across the intervening space without a physical bridge to convey them. (Bear & Company, Santa Fe, N.M., 1997, p. 125)

In a lecture Dr. Krieger spoke about an experiment in which she was involved to help test this energy transfer. The client was in a sealed room, with instruments set up to monitor the transfer of energy. Just when Dr. Krieger entered the room to administer the Therapeutic Touch treatment, she looked at the client. The needles on the dials began moving, as if to register that some type of transference was already taking place before she had even started her healing session. A connection had been made prior to the beginning of the actual treatment. From this experiment we can conjecture that when a client or patient calls to inquire about or make an appointment for a massage, an adjustment, or a Therapeutic Touch treatment, it can be said that the healing has already begun to take place, with the initial contact being made over the telephone. Some type of energy transfer is already occurring, setting the stage for the subsequent healing process.

In his book *Your Inner Physician and You* (North Atlantic Books, Berkeley, Cal., 1997) Dr. John Upledger relates his initial introduction to the power of intention when in the late '60s he and other physicians began using acupuncture at several free clinics in Florida. Most of the clients were active drug users, and acupuncture was inexpensive and did not involve pills. He noticed that some of the doctors had great success with the treatment, while others didn't, even on the same patients. "At first I thought it was suggestion, so we tried to control any positive or negative comments about expectation. We even went so far as to say nothing at all to the patient before, during, or after the treatment." (p. 101)

What they discovered is that a strong correlation seemed to exist in the unspoken attitude of the practitioner. Those who genuinely believed in the beneficial effects of acupuncture got better results than those who did not believe it would work. Two doctors who really thought it was all "poppycock" did not get good results at all. Sometimes Dr. Upledger would treat the same patient the following day and would get positive results immediately. The results were easy to test, for patients would have immediate relief: pain would disappear, asthmatics would breathe easier, cravings for heroine would subside, and the shingles rash would fade—all during the treatment. It became apparent that it wasn't where or how you put the needles that counted, but *who* put them there. More than just the power of suggestion, the therapist's attitude and intention seemed to greatly affect the outcome of the treatment.

Though there is room for a lot of research in this area, some initial experiments "have begun to measure the effect of attitude upon electrical resistance in a circuit between the therapist and the patient . . . higher electrical resistance correlates to negative attitude in the therapist as well as the patient." (p. 102) Evidence supporting the attitude-effect concept was so strong that therapists were advised not to work on someone if on any particular day they couldn't leave their personal problems outside the treatment room or if they had a poor attitude toward a certain patient. "The therapist's attitude (be he/she a surgeon, physician, dentist, physical therapist, Rolfer, acupuncturist, CranioSacral Therapist, or anyone else) has much to do with the success of the patient in his/her healing process." (p. 108) Those with happy, upbeat, confident dispositions simply got better results than those who were chronically angry, cynical, or depressed. The success rate seemed to reach beyond technique.

Using a few readings about the receiving of massage as an example, we can see demonstrated the importance of intention. One man was told not only to get a massage (along with a criterion for choosing a therapist), but the advice also seemed to be for the massage practitioner:

A gentle massage to quiet the body would be well, with prayer—and not by those who do not live what they pray.

> **Do not merely pray that he will be well, but well for what?**
> **Do not pray for the body to be well for what the body can**
> **do for self but for those whom he has aided and also hin-**
> **dered.** 3439-1

For another man the time during the massages was to be a "period for meditation and prayer, and for the conversation about the spiritual life to the unfolding mind and body." (5406-1) Another was told that "the spiritual, the mental, the attitudes of the associate and companion will mean much; as also will the character of the individual [in the] daily administering of the massages . . . and a good conversation during same." (2642-1) Earlier in this reading the quality of the massage was described:

> **Do not hurry through the massage. Take time to give same,**
> **and let it be done with the spirit of truth, of hope, of pur-**
> **pose, of the suggestive influence as will aid in establishing**
> **the coordinations needed for the rebuilding, the replenish-**
> **ing for this body of those conditions.** 2642-1

A response must be awakened in the body for the healing to begin. Whether done with the laying on of hands, a massage, a pack, or an adjustment, there is a force that will flow through us when we begin to apply what we know. "All methods of healing—whether of the physical, the mental, or the spiritual—simply awaken within the cells and atoms of our bodies the willingness to allow this life force to flow through us." (*Covenant*, Vol. 2, No. 12, p. 4) In achieving this awakening, we become, then, authentic channels of blessing to those for whom we care.

Role of Practitioner and Caregiver

Quite a lot, then, depends upon the mental and spiritual develop-ment of those administering healing in any way. This development would reflect not only one's attitudes but also *how* the treatments are to be done, as shown in these readings: " . . . if the treatment is given as *rote*—because it's told to be done, how much may be expected? Not a very great deal." (456-1) " . . . for these [treatments] need to be given not merely that they may be gotten through with . . . but with love and care. For, all must be kept in that attitude of a search for *His* purpose with each. And let all know that as they minister, in love, in care, for one of His children, His purpose with them—too—is for good." (2619-1) In some readings, especially those for children, the success rate seems to lie primarily upon the parents or caregivers.

For a nine-year-old boy with muscular dystrophy the reading offered this hopeful information:

> . . . we may bring help for this body, we may bring better quietude within. As to just how far these helpful forces may be obtained, much will depend upon the faith or the prayerful attitude of those about the body and those making administrations for the body . . .
>
> Whether these treatments will cause complete development of the control through brain reflexes, or partial, will depend—as indicated—on those about the body, and then the persistency with which these will be used.   3649-1

An eight-year-old boy with epilepsy was told that his condition was prenatal "and must be met by the body as well as by those responsible for the body." (3156-1) The treatments given in his protocol were not to be delegated too often to others, but rather should be administered largely by the parents. The reading promised: "We will bring help if there is persistence and if, in the lives of the mother and father, there is consistent living of that they pray for." (3156-1)

A twenty-three-year-old woman was reminded in her sixteenth reading that in her epilepsy she was meeting a past condition and that she as well as those around her were to be consistent and persistent in the treatments. This additional insight and hopeful outcome were also mentioned:

> . . . "Where two or three seek in My Name," He has given, "there will I be also." Is this consciousness to be awakened, then seek often—*all*—that would minister with the body in gaining that understanding, that the ministrations as given will bring about a more perfect accord in this material body,

and it—the cure—will come to pass.   543-16

Doing things halfway will merely achieve partial results. "If these [treatments] will be carried through, help may come. If these will be given only as partially or as not necessary for this or that, then only that much of help or aid will come." (1289-2) In this reading for an eleven-year-old boy with epilepsy additional encouragement was given to his caregivers: "If we can awaken in those who are responsible, in those who would bring help and relief, the consciousness that the Divine *may* aid . . . we may bring with the physical that of spiritual healing also, that may aid." (1289-2)

In a reading for a thirteen-year-old girl with epilepsy, the parents were cautioned about their attitudes, especially self-condemnation, and told to spiritualize their activities so that God would be in direct charge. They were also advised:

> Not [to act] as in a spasmodic reaction, blowing hot and cold, overzealous one day and then again fearful and doubtful another. For, know—the strength, the health, the financial, the whole of an individual's purpose is in Him. For He is thy health, thy wealth, thy position, thy purpose—if ye will but make Him such. Not as to become fanatical or imposing upon others any tenet that would be or cause objections, but live in thine own inner self with that awareness which is His promise to thee—"If ye will be my children, I will be thy God."
>
> *Who* may ask more?   2153-11

Being God-centered and keeping a spiritual purpose uppermost in one's heart and mind are other important attributes for those administering healing in any capacity, as described in this excerpt:

> Let those who would wait, those who minister with, those who minister for the healing of *this* body [a thirteen-year-old boy with epilepsy]—in its gaining of its coordination, in the gaining of its rightful position in the affairs and among peoples know that they labor *with* the Lord, those

who look to Him for aid; for in Him *is* the life and the light, the understanding and the healing *must* come from within.

146-3

Another reading predicted healing for the caregivers as well, harkening back to the concept mentioned earlier, that in healing others one heals oneself.

. . . there is to be a healing *also* in the minds and purposes of those upon whom the body is dependent in the present for the seeking *for* corrections in a spiritual and mental manner; that the physical expression may be the greater channel for manifestation of the spiritual laws. 2153-7

The physical environment is where the spiritual can manifest. So any help that a person provides—whether in a hands-on effort, financially, or as a part-time support person—can enable and enhance the spiritual aspect of the one who is ill. For those who may decide to make this type of service a profession, with all its attendant anxieties about adequate financial support, right business location, need for continuing education, etc., the readings offer encouragement and advice to build a work that is helpful, selfless, and in harmony with one's ideals. To one woman who was attempting to make it as a massage therapist, Cayce offered the following suggestions, which could easily be applied to any other service profession. Here is the question-and-answer exchange:

(Q) How may I make my own profession, as a licensed masseuse, more suitable for me?
(A) By applying in thy daily applications of its good offices that which is best within thee; and with the desire and purpose not merely to have a job, not merely to have a means of achieving material gains, but to do a work entrusted to thee by a divine power that enables thee to be to each soul to whom ye apply thy work, thy profession, a channel, a means of making manifest His love among thy fellow men.
Applied in such a way and manner it *cannot*, it *will not* fail. And ye will find a greater increase. Not by loud boasting,

no. But let thy prayer and thy meditation be, as ye make application to others, *"Lord, lead Thou me the way!"*   2275-1

When she asked later in the reading about how to establish a clien-
tele, this advice was given:

Let each client, each person ye serve, be that as He gave—
"He that would be the greatest among you will be and is the
servant of all."
   In that attitude, in that manner, that way of expressing
self, ye *build* that which is creative and helpful; and not only
does it bring peace and harmony but love with same . . .
                                                         2275-1

In summary we could say that being a channel of peace, harmony,
and love is the chief duty and responsibility of any caregiver or practitioner who is directly or indirectly involved in caring for another. In
aiding a body one is aiding a temple of the spirit as well, making it, as
one reading described it, "the more beautiful place for the worshipful-
ness in its every function, in its every organ, to glorify those purposes
whereunto each organ, each functioning, has been set for the glorifying
of the spirit of creative forces in a material world." (443-3) There can be
no more nobler achievement that this!

Conclusion

For those in the helping professions or who serve as supporters or
caregivers, being channels of blessing to others may be a natural outlet
for their ideals of love and service. These special folks, acting in a selfless manner, can bring light and healing where there is darkness and
disease. Recognizing their own needs for spiritual and self-development, these people through study and practice have made the effort to
strengthen their intent and to apply those spiritual principles in their
everyday lives. As a result, they become conduits of healing energy,
bringing refreshment and hope to those in need and making the earth
a better place because of their activity in it.

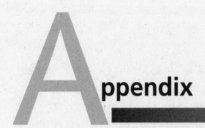

Appendix

Excerpts from the following Edgar Cayce readings are intended as supplementary material for the reader seeking a more practical application or additional help in the pursuit of health and healing. They are grouped under certain categories for easy reference. Several of the excerpts are informational, some are inspirational, while others contain advice that was considered useful for anyone to follow.

Physical

Cooking

(Q) Is food cooked in aluminum utensils bad for this system?
(A) Certain characters of food cooked in aluminum are bad for *any* system, and where a systemic condition exists—or a disturbed hepatic circulation or assimilating force, a disturbed hepatic eliminating force—they are naturally so. Cook rather in granite, or better still in Patapar Paper.   **1196-7**

Diet

Use more vegetables in the diet and less meats of any kind; though certain characters, as fowl or lamb, may be taken in moderation. The greater portion of the diet, however, should consist of the various characters of vegetables, but eat two to three of those that grow above the ground to one that grows under the ground.   **5063-1**

Take often raw vegetables and fruits, and most of the vegetables should be those grown above the ground, prepared in their own juices or cooked in Patapar paper. The salts from the green vegetables are needed; not those where preservatives have been sprayed on them for shipping, but those that are green.   **3692–1**

(Q) Can coffee and tea be used by this body without harmful effects?
(A) No one can use them without *affecting* the body. As to whether they are harmful or not depends upon the extent to which they are used. Use one or the other; don't use them both. Tea is more harmful than coffee. Coffee is a food if it is taken without cream or sugar, and especially without cream; and if taken without the caffeine—as Kaffa Hag, or the like—it's really a food for the body.   **816–5**

Have an eighty percent alkaline–producing diet to a twenty percent acid–producing diet . . . but *do not combine* cereals with the citrus fruit juices at the same meal. Do not use white potatoes and white bread at the same meal. If these are considered in the diet, the conditions will be found to be much better.   **1601–1**

For as the body knows (though do not let the attitudes produce the acids; or the resentments or disappointments or any of those factors of the mind itself), it should leave off altogether the white breads, white potatoes (unless merely the jackets are taken). Do not combine *any* of starches with any quantities of sweets. Do not take food values that cause great quantity of alcoholic reaction. This does not refer to alcohol, but sweets *and* certain starches produce a character of fermentation that is alcoholic that makes for excess of fatty portions for the body.

1125–2

Do not take citrus juices with cereals or large quantities of starches at the same meal. However, these both should be taken, but alternated— the citrus fruits one day, the cereals or starches the next, and so on. When taking orange juice, add a little lemon or lime to same. Do not add lemon or lime to grapefruit, nor to the pine apple or grape juice; but add same to the orange juice.   **1593–1**

(Q) Should I drink plenty of water, and how many glasses each day?
(A) Drink plenty of water. This as we find is most helpful to the body.

Six, eight, ten glasses a day. **1196-9**

At all times take as much water in the system as possible. Drink *more* water than has been common with the body. Take water when first arising in the morning and the last thing before retiring—no matter if same must act through the kidneys, this *needs* to be cleansed—the whole system. Water cleanses it better than purgatives. **4843-1**

. . . drink plenty of water each day—six or eight glasses. It is true that this tends to flush the kidneys, and it may at times cause some inconvenience in the evening; but they must be flushed out—and water is the better to use for same, see? **1586-1**

(Q) Am I allergic to certain foods?
(A) If you imagine it, you can be allergic to most anything, if you want to! **3268-2**

Exercise

The exercise that we would follow . . . would be the stretching much in the manner as the exercise of the cat or the panther, or that type of activity; stretching the muscular forces, not as strains but as to cause the tendons and muscles to be put into position for the formation of strength-building to the body. **4003-1**

(Q) Just how much exercise should be taken each day . . . ?
(A) If it is taken one minute today, make it a minute and fifteen seconds tomorrow! and then a minute and thirty seconds the next day! Then it may be necessary to go back to the one minute, see? Vary according to the ability, but *force* self to take a little more exercise each day if it is practical. **849-57**

(Q) What exercise, if any?
(A) Walking, and the exercise that would be of the setting-up nature morning and evening would be the better for the body. Not too strenuous, but for three to four minutes in the beginning—which may be extended. **592-1**

When body has prepared for retiring, or dressed for the exercise—begin with that of raising self on toes (barefooted) and then stooping as low as the body can; this with the body remaining on the toes. Do this for at least ten up and down movements, and then standing flat on floor, bend the body forward to where the palms or fingertips may touch the floor; this slowly, but at least ten times. Then standing flat, with the arms raised above head, stoop at least ten times. Then holding hands on hips, circulate the upper portion of body, each side, at least five times.

After same, take a thorough rub with a coarse cloth or towel along the spine, from head to central portion of the back, until the flesh is aglow. Then from the whole *length* of the spine—head to the base of spine—at least five or six such rubs, not to *irritate* the flesh, as to cause too much trouble, but to *stimulate* the circulation throughout the physical forces of the body.   **155-1**

In the exercises—naturally as these have been a part of the body's activities for retaining its present strength or vitality, they should be kept; not too strenuous but in moderation, *especially* the activities of walking, of muscular forces, of dancing or of such natures in which both arms and lower limbs are used.   **1703-1**

We would take the exercises in the open. The body should sleep light; that is, just sufficient cover to keep warm, but never heavily covered. Get plenty of fresh air. When the exercises are taken, morning and evening, the body should be then well rubbed down with cold water from the first cervical to the end of the spine, see. And then rubbed until the circulation comes to the surface, with a coarse towel, you see.
                                    4839-1

Hydrotherapy
(Q) Do you advise the use of colonics or Epsom Salts baths for the body? (A) When these are necessary, yes. For, *every* one—everybody—should take an internal bath occasionally, as well as an external one. They would all be better off if they would!   **440-2**

Nature
The *natural* things . . . are the things that make for the better physical body in normal activity. *Normalcy*, not extreme in any manner! and there

will be shown thee day by day that which will be the necessary for thine *own* development. To some certain amount of exercise, certain amounts of rest, certain amounts of various characters of breathing, of purification, of prayer, of reading—as is found necessary; but of *all* be true to that thou promiseth that source from which all health, all aid, must come! Don't fool yourself; for you *cannot* fool your Maker, and if there is fooling it is yourself—for your brother will soon find you out!

5752-2

Packs

For an hour each day, for five days in succession, apply Castor Oil Packs over the liver and gall duct. Use at least three to four thicknesses of flannel saturated with Castor Oil. Apply these directly to the body and when covered, to prevent soiling linens, apply the electric pad. Keep these sufficiently warm as to cause the radiation to be absorbed through the area.

After the first pack is taken, begin taking small doses of Olive Oil, a teaspoonful every four hours. Keep this up for the five days.

Then leave off the Packs about a week, and then have another series, and so on. **5060-1**

[*Note*: There exists quite a variety of sequences in the use of castor oil packs. The most frequent one that is often recommended by the A.R.E. is: three days of packs, followed by four days off, then repeat for three weeks; no packs the fourth week; repeat the series, if desired. Olive oil is usually taken on the third day, after the third pack was taken; dosages ranged from a few teaspoons up to half a teacup.]

Recreation/Rest/ Vacation

(Q) Should I rest daily?

(A) Each body should have rest periods, and so should this body. Have rest periods. These would preferably be *after* meals; or as the old saw goes: "After breakfast work a while, after lunch rest a while, after dinner walk a mile." This routine would be very well to be considered by most people, and would be very well for this one. **1158-11**

Then budget the time, that there may be a regular period for sustaining the physical being, also for sustaining the mental and spiritual being. As it is necessary for recreation and rest for the physical, so it is necessary that there be recreation and rest for the mental. The spirit is willing, the flesh is weak. Do not court the flesh, but do give voice and heed to keeping the body as the temple of the living God, as indeed it is. Purify it. Keep it clean—in physical, as well as in mind, that it indeed may offer that channel through which thy Maker may speak to thee.

3691-1

(Q) In the vacation season, should I seek rest and recreation in some quiet place, or would travel from place to place be preferable?
(A) The seeking of rest in one place for study, meditation, and—most of all—as thou hast naturally studied and do naturally study others—study self; not only as to what others are due thee, but what thou art due to thy fellow man. Remember ever, as He has given, the questions that must be thine own self. Remember, each soul must oft stand and watch itself pass by. It oft must meet its own self and that it has meted to its fellow man. Or, as He has given, "As ye do it unto the least of these, my brethren, ye do it unto me." Hence in thy meditation and thy rest, seek the recreations in those surroundings that are close to water and sands and hills and dales, and those things that deal with waters; for there may come an awakening that will indeed make thy experience worth while.   **816-3**

(Q) Where shall I spend vacation this summer to obtain most benefits?
(A) Where there is the sand and sea and pines, or where there is the social activity which is in keeping with the hopes and desires of the body. But, wherever these would be much better for the body, so there will be sand, sea, water, pines. A great deal of the ultra-violet rays will be well for the body, but not too much of same.   **2582-4**

In those periods when ye would enjoy a vacation with thy friend, do ye speak of the love of the Christ? Do this oft, ye will be a much greater channel of blessings to thy fellow man. Ye also will find in thine own heart, in thine own conscience, harmony, peace, not as the world knows peace, but only as comes from just being kind, just being patient, just being long-suffering with thy fellow man.   **5083-2**

(Q) Where should I go on my vacation in September?

(A) This should be a choice by self, and in the meantime if there is the use of these periods of relaxation, let that be the guide. For this *will* create forces and influences that—well, that haven't been even suspected by the body to be able to think about! **416-9**

Rejuvenation

For the body renews itself, every atom, in seven years. How have ye lived for the last seven? And then the seven before? What would ye do with thy mind and thy body if they were wholly restored to normalcy in this experience? Would these be put to the use of gratifying thine own appetites as at first? Will these be used for the magnifying of the appreciation of the love to the infinite? For who healeth all thy diseases? If ye think it is the doctor or the surgeon, who is thy doctor? Is his life different from your own? Life itself, comes from the infinite. There ye must begin if ye would have healing for this body, not merely by saying, "Yes, I believe Jesus was the Son of God—yes, I believe He died that I might have an advocate with the Father."

Yes, this also—but what are ye doing about it? Are ye living like that? Do ye treat thy brother, thy neighbor, thy friend, thy foe, as though this were true? For no matter what ye say, the manner in which ye treat thy fellow man is the answer to what ye really believe. For the manner in which ye treat thy neighbor is the manner in which ye are treating thy Maker. And be not deceived, God is not mocked; whatsoever a man soweth that must he also reap. **3684-1**

Sleep

(Q) I usually wake very early in the morning. Can anything be done to make me sleep better?

(A) This is more of habit, that arises from a nervous reaction or of such natures. If the body will use a little lemon juice just before retiring, with salt, this will materially aid the body in having better sleep.

(Q) How much sleep does this body need?

(A) Seven and a half to eight hours should be for *most* bodies. **816-1**

Weight loss

(Q) What should be done to reduce and what should be the normal weight of the body?

(A) That as desired by the body may be made the normal weight. This should be done through the exercising and dieting of the system, according to the real innate desires of the body, to bring those conditions for the system. With a corrected system, see, the *normal* conditions will ensue.   **3986–1**

Mental

Anxiety

. . . as is understood—anxiety is like fear, and is as canker to any disturbed *nervous* condition of a body, if it takes hold.

But rather do that the hands and the mind *find* to do; knowing that what is best—and that will give the greater opportunity for the self to be of greater service—will be thy lot; if that is thy purpose and if thy life is lived in that manner.   **1472–7**

Attitudes

The mental attitude has *much* to do with the general conditions; the *determination* to fight it through. These are necessary, and will include the work as well as play, as well as social activity; but don't let one interfere with the other!   **849–53**

The body, with its physical condition, would do well to remember that the giving out of the mental attitude toward others, is the same as will be received to itself, and that as these thoughts or vibrations or expressions give out to others, we receive these in return; that if we would bring the best to self and others, we should give of our best to others, see . . .

Keep the mental forces in accord with [your] own higher self, and rise above the conditions that would beset the mind, for if we would give of our best to those who depend upon us we must have bodies physically fit, and minds above the lower level. Do that!   **3991–1**

In the abilities, keep in the way in which ye judge not, if ye would not

SEEKING INFORMATION ON

holistic health, spirituality, dreams, intuition or ancient civilizations?

Call 1-800-723-1112, visit our Web site, or mail in this postage-paid card for a FREE catalog of books and membership information.

Name: _____

Address: _____

City: _____

State/Province: _____

Postal/Zip Code: _____ Country: _____

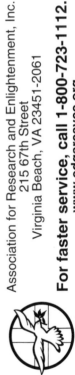

Association for Research and Enlightenment, Inc.
215 67th Street
Virginia Beach, VA 23451-2061

For faster service, call 1-800-723-1112.
www.edgarcayce.org

PBIN

BUSINESS REPLY MAIL

FIRST CLASS   PERMIT NO. 2456   VIRGINIA BEACH, VA

POSTAGE WILL BE PAID BY ADDRESSEE

ASSOCIATION FOR RESEARCH
AND ENLIGHTENMENT INC
215 67TH STREET
VIRGINIA BEACH VA · 23451-9819

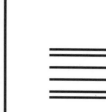

be judged. Remember, with what measure ye mete to others must eventually be meted to thee. If ye would have friends, if ye would have love,
if ye would have patience, manifest same. Each of these are the attributes of the spirit of truth and as ye apply same in thy experience, the
greater becomes thy measure of faith.

For if ye have not faith in others, how can ye have faith in God? If ye
have not faith in God, how can ye find it in thyself?

Keep sweet, keep true, keep earnest!   **5079–1**

Know first, in the spiritual attitude, as ye attempt to analyze self and
self's abilities, self's faults, self's virtues, that the nearer ye may build
thy mind to the Christ Consciousness the better may be the mental
being, and a great deal of strength may be gained in the physical being
also.   **5064–1**

Hold to that which is pure, in every form, in ever phase, and it will melt
the obstacles away before thee as ye apply same; leaving off resentments; knowing they are only seeking to express self, manifest self. But
keeping God and His purpose ever foremost, these hindrances and disturbances will lessen more and more.   **1472–10**

See in self, then, the virtues as well as the faults. Then, magnify the
virtues, minimize the faults.

Don't condemn self more than you would be condemned by thy
Maker. Don't pass over frailties of others because of strength in self, but
see thyself as thy abilities and the urges, and know that in Creative
Energies, in God, in Christ as God, ye may find strength for the application of thy ideals.   **5075–1**

Would the entity gain confidence in others, it must be first within self.
Would the entity trust others, the trust must first be within self. Would
the body find the closer relationship *with* self, the body must first *know*
self in its relation to that portion of the Whole, see?   **78–3**

Remember, there is a law—divine—with what measure ye mete to others, in thy conversation, in thy activity, it will be measured to thee again.

Take thought oft, then, to speak well or keep silent—of self, of others.
Not as an extravagancy in any sense, but the truth, ever. These have

brought discouragements. Then meet same with the optimistic abilities to attain to that oneness with the universal consciousness, which brings of itself its reward—as does virtue, as does kindness, as does patience, as does brotherly love. **2809–1**

Do continue with the mental attitude of cooperative, constructive thinking. Don't talk one way and act another. Be consistent, be persistent. Use the abilities, mentally and physically, in constructive thinking, writing and acting. And *as* these are used in helping others, it will bring help to the body. **849–61**

. . . if ye will meditate the more upon how that as He gave, love and forgiveness, faith and hope may overcome spites, fears, distrust, ye may open thy heart, ye may open thyself to the opportunities that *constantly* lie before thee in thy activities in the present. **1599–1**

Keep in that of constructive thought; because, to be sure, the thoughts of the body act upon the emotions as well as the assimilating forces. Poisons are accumulated or produced by anger or by resentment or animosity. Keep sweet! **23–3**

Do keep the attitude creative. Know from what source all healing must come. For it is not of self, it is the practical use of elements of which the individual man is made and in which the constitution is lacking. These must be added. All power, all force is one source—the Creative Force or God. Without such there is little hope. In using these there is hope.

Do these things consistently and persistently, not as something just to be hurried through with but be persistent, be consistent and we will bring better conditions for this body. **4099–1**

. . . don't become pessimistic because of those conditions arising that outwardly appear to be causing the body to become a "shut in" without the use of other than the mind. But remember, mind is the builder.

And who healeth thy diseases? From what source cometh love, mercy and grace? Know that He is the same yesterday, today and forever.

Though the body may become as though it were useless in the ability for movements, we would put more faith, more hope, more trust in Him. **3681–1**

For all that you may know of God is within yourself. What are you doing about it? What are you doing with it? Are you proud of the way you have treated some people? Would ye like for thy God to treat thee in the manner you have treated some people? Look within. For there ye may know if God is within thine own self and what ye are doing about it. Use it, don't abuse it. Use it to the glory of the Father. Then it will be to the honor of self.   **3689-1**

Beware of too much mental strain, especially when there is the digestion taking place in the body for the weaknesses, tendencies are toward those of the pressure to the hypogastrics that would cause headaches or nausea and the resultant activity of those portions that bring the distress in the lower digestive system.

These rather as warnings than as conditions that cause distress. Keep physically fit through activity of the body, physically and mentally but keep well balanced.   **165-4**

For if the individual entity thinks only of self, others will not think much of the individual. If ye would have friends, be friendly. If ye would have love, give love to others. For he [who] would save his life shall lose it. For life is the manifestation of God and to have God in thine experience, which is all love, all hope, all faith, all kindness, all gentleness, all patience, ye must manifest such in thy dealings with others.   **5032-1**

Consistency
. . . analyze self. See where your shortcomings have been. See how that you must make your life a *consistent* one!

For consistency in the experience of any is *indeed* a jewel of great value.   **1587-1**

Depression
(Q) How can I prevent myself from becoming blue and depressed at times? And how can I prevent myself from crying so easily?
(A) By not remaining alone! Be joyous! Whistle, sing, holler, anything that makes for activity! Just don't allow it to come on! Put it on someone else! Be with someone else!   **386-3**

Be not weary in well doing [Galatians 6:9]. Do not give up easily. Those conditions that bring about depressing forces to the body, as are exercised at times, naturally bring depressed feelings. Overcome these by doing for others.   **147–31**

Yet again we find, as is the experience of each soul, there are those periods of affluence and those periods of depression; that come to each and every soul in materiality. But if the trust, the hope, is put not in self, not in self's ability, but rather in Him that is the Giver, the Maker of all good and perfect gifts, it will be found that the more the reliance is put in those influences of Him—in the activities in the material world—greater will come the abilities for finding harmony, peace and understanding.   **1058–1**

Fear

If this entity, in this particular sojourn, would make advancements materially, mentally, spiritually, it must first apply in self that which will wholly cast out fear; fear of others, fear of influences, fear of what may come to pass. For if the entity comes to that consciousness which is a part of the universal consciousness, that ye abide—in body, mind and purpose—as one with the Creative Forces, ye are at peace with the world and have nothing to fear. For God will not allow any soul to be tempted beyond that it is able to bear—if the soul puts its whole trust in the Creative Forces manifested in the Christ Consciousness.   **5030–1**

Forgiveness

. . . if ye are to be forgiven, ye must in thyself be forgiving. For the manner in which ye treat others is the manner in which ye are treating thy Maker. Remember, it is yourself you have to live with the most. Others can move out of the way. You can't move, or you can't refrain from meeting thine own self.   **4028–1**

Hurts arise from misunderstandings. Thus the injunction to forgive as ye would be forgiven. As given to each soul, if you would offer praise or honor to thy God and have aught against thy brother or a brother against thee, first make thy peace with thy brother. Then thy offering, thy praise, may be other than sounding brass or a tinkling cymbal. Otherwise, it will mean nothing to anyone except to fool thine own self.   **3253–2**

Humor

. . . above all, *keep* that ability to see the humor in any experience, whether it is the most sacred, the most cherished experience, or that which comes as a trial or as a temptation from outside influence.

Keep and be able to see—keep that ability to see the ridiculous even in the most sacred thing. Not that it may be used, of course, as to hinder others, but in thine *own* life. These keep.   **2560–1**

. . . in prayer, in meditation, in longing, in hoping . . . in doing the things and being the things in thine inner self ye hope for and long for—these are the manners and the ways of approach, and of overcoming those tendencies which arise in the emotions.

Not as one to be long–faced. For, the earth is the Lord's and the fullness thereof—in *joy!* Do not see the dark side too oft. Turn it over—there's another side to every question. Cultivate in self humor, wit. Ye enjoy it in others, others enjoy it in thee. But too oft it becomes to thee foolishness. *Know* that thy Lord, thy God, *laughed*—even at the Cross. For He wept with those who wept, and rejoiced with those who rejoiced.

2995–1

Remember that a good laugh, an arousing even to what might in some be called hilariousness, is good for the body, physically, mentally, and gives the opportunity for greater mental and spiritual awakening . . .

Be *mindful* of the little things, but *do* see the humor, do see the laughable side, and not always the tears, the drab, hard sides. For, there is more than one phase of any problem, any condition, any relationship. Life *is* of the Creative Forces, and an individual uses same for weal or woe . . .

First find self. Awake to the joy in the earth, even under trial ye give expression of same. Manifest it in thy life, rather than the sorrow. This will need cultivating. But Life itself is a cultivating of the joy, of laughter, of those things that bring hope—and attempting this will not only bring those things that are of a creative influence in the experience of the entity but a joy in same.   **2647–1**

(Q) How long will it take before a return to normal health?
(A) This will depend, of course, upon the applications and the response
the body makes; and the attitude that is held. These treatments, as we
find, should make for a relief *soon*; in ten days to two weeks *some
changes*—but we need not expect there not to be those periods when
there will be bad reactions; for the weather, the temperature, the atmospheric pressures and the general surroundings will make blue days as
well as brighter days. But don't forget the recipe of making three people
laugh every day!   **798-1**

Ideals

First know in self in what thou hast believed, and then set that as the
ideal. Not in material things, not in the activities of individuals, not in
that which partakes of the earth as earthy; but those attributes of the
soul that may find activity in the earth—these make for those things
that the entity may set; for these become as experiences that may bring
for the entity that basis upon which there may come not only peace
and harmony and understanding, but make for the experience throughout this sojourn as one worth while. And when the darker days come,
and when the shadows come that would make thee afraid, turn within
and have a good time at scaring the bogies away from those that would
fear, that would doubt.   **815-2**

. . . if ye would have peace, if ye would "iron out" kinks, if ye would
know your relationships to others, set in thine inner self as to what is
thine ideal. What is thy purpose in life? Is it to *get*, through the attitude
of "Gimmee—Gimmee—Gimmee!" or is it to *give—give—give!* If it is the
latter, then there should be the knowledge and security from within as
given of old:
   "Let others do as they may, but for me—I will *know* the living
God" . . .   **815-3**

. . . if you will read the Book of Revelation with the idea of the body as
the interpretation, you will understand yourself and learn to really analyze, psychoanalyze, mentally analyze others. But you will have to learn
to apply it in self first. For the motivating force in each one of those
patterns represented, is that which the individual entity entertains as

the ideal. This is the motivating spirit, the motivating purpose. When it is out of attune, or not coordinating with the First Cause, there may not be the greater unfoldment. For, it is in self that it becomes out of attune. It loses its power or ability. It loses creative energy or its hold upon the First Cause that is the Creator or God.   **4083-1**

Let not thy judgments nor yet thy disappointments . . . cause thee to become discouraged. Indeed hardships may be a part of thy experience, and a great many disappointments come with such ideas; but if the ideals are set in spiritual sources the results will be good . . . For each and every soul must find the answer to the best that is within the entity itself. All that the entity may know of divinity or of God, or of the universal law, is to be, may be, can be, manifested within the entity itself.   **5007-1**

For, if this entity—as others—will embrace and be embraced with that thought, that idea which is the basis of faith and hope, "Have Thy way with me, O Lord! Not my will but Thine be done," and hold to same, it will be as a guiding light, as a criterion in every influence. And it may save much suffering, it may ease many a disappointment, it may bring light to the entity often out of shadows and out of the slough of doubt, and out of the casements of fear!   **1597-1**

Know that ye are in the earth as an opportunity for self, for social unfoldment . . . so live that others, all others would wish to be like [5256]. That is an ideal manner of conduct.

   What is required in this? In self knowing thine own ideals, spiritually, mentally, materially, not merely as "I think this should be it, I think that would be wonderful, that this or that" but write them down on paper and see what they look like. You'll be surprised how oft you can change them from one day to another.

   Then, knowing the ideal, practice it. Don't have an ideal and then not practice it in thy daily activities.   **5256-1**

A self-analysis of the desires and wishes, and the *fixing* of self as toward some ideal outside of self will enable the body to better meet—mentally and materially—those conditions and problems that present themselves from time to time.

These, as the body—the mental abilities—will recognize, are necessary; for one to *have* an ideal to make for the impulse and activities towards working for some conditions as outside of self.   **78-5**

Know that ye are going through a period of testing. Remain true to all that has been committed to thee, and know that each day is an opportunity, and an experience. Speak a word for thy ideal. Not as to force an issue but ever constructive. Sow the seed of truth, the seed of the spirit. God will give the increase.   **3245-1**

Joy

Be joyous. Be happy at all times, and apply in the daily experience that which is not only a desire to be of help to someone else, but *physically* help others and it will help self the more—mentally *and* physically!

386-3

Keep the heart *singing!* Keep the mind clear! Keep the face toward the *light!* the shadows then are *behind!*

Keep the way open, and be ready to meet the needs, rather than *giving up* before the work is well begun!   **39-4**

Music

Dare oftener to be yourself, but let yourself be in accord with that which is of the spiritual import or prompting; as in the beauty of music, the rhythm even in mathematics, the rhythm even in the score in music and that which answers to the high emotions of affection, companionship, activities in the associations. Yet these must be kept in a balance that never causes the entity to condemn self or to condone or condemn others.   **4028-1**

Openness

. . . open thyself more to the possibilities and the probabilities that are about thee day by day, and ye will find greater blessings may come to thee.   **3246-1**

Optimism

Each individual has its own experience to meet. Being overanxious may only bring those influences that bring their *own* development. But keep that which may commonly be called an optimistic frame of mind, seeing the best in others and in self, making those proper adjustments in the own physical experience for a greater growth and a greater preparation in body for the meeting of emergencies or of conditions that arise. In this may there be brought not only the better attitude but the better physical condition to meet all.   **819-1**

Keep optimistic and prayerful, and with a song on the lips often, if you want the body to be cheerful!   **23-11**

Patience
Learn ye patience, if ye would have an understanding, if ye would gain harmony and grace in this experience! "For in patience do ye possess your souls." It's when individuals have become impatient, and desire their own will or desire their expression or desire that they as individuals be heard, that they become less and less in that close association with the Divine—and more of that as is human and of the animal becomes manifest. This is a power, to be sure, but fraught with egotism becomes a destructive power.

And bad is only good gone wrong, or going away from God.

1201-2

Self-Expression
(Q) What is the cause of my not being able to express myself so others will understand what I mean, and how can I correct this?
(A) Practice it . . . Practice by telling it to yourself in the mirror. You can become a good speaker.   **5163-1**

Self-Confidence
(Q) What can I do to acquire self-confidence and greater mental balance?
(A) Study to show thyself approved unto thy Maker, rightly divining the words of truth, keeping self unspotted from the world. Be true to that thou knowest to do, and with thy heart, thy mind and thy body keep inviolate all pledges made to self and to thy Maker.   **1058-1**

Thankfulness

Life itself is a manifestation of that called God in the earth. Give thanks for the very fact that ye are conscious of yourself, even with the frailties of the body; that thy mind and thy purposes and thy hands may do much to show the appreciation in self of the opportunity in this experience to be a channel of blessings to others, in making known to others the love of the Christ for those who are weak in body, who are hindered from the activities of a normal physical world.   **5064-1**

Then, to *all*: As ye do in the spirit of *true* thanksgiving come to realize, as ye find in thy daily experience with thy fellow man—he that is unappreciative of opportunity, of care, of thought, of long-suffering, to thine *own* mind becomes very little.

    . . . remember, Thanksgiving is thy *opportunity* to show thy appreciation to thy friend, thy home, thy mother, thy children—yea, most of all to thy God!   **3976-21**

When the body mentally and physically takes into account the conditions, and that it has to be thankful for—the companionship, the relationships—these should bring greater spiritual awakening for the body. Not because of duty, but because of the glorious mental and spiritual opportunities that are offered.   **533-18**

. . . as ye pray, *live*, *act!* So conduct thine own life as to show thy appreciation of that which thou hast received. For he, or she, who neglects to be thankful builds that which is condemning in the own self.

                                                            254-115

Spiritual

Application

Use judgments, use discretions in the activities and in the application of those administrations indicated. There will be days, to be sure, when the body will be overly tired; there will be others when through the very necessity of change and activity the body will feel better—and this should be a part of the body's actions. *Do not* curtail social relationships or activities because of the fact that "I must hurry home to get a treatment." But rather that the treatment may be given on days to stimulate the body so that there is more of the desire for social activities for periods of this or that activity that requires the leaving off of the applications for the day; but *do not* become discouraged—for improvements are at hand. **1196-9**

As the body has experienced through many of its experiences, when you work towards a thing you do not allow little disturbing factors or a continual changing to this form or that form to interfere. Be sure you are on the right road, then go ahead—to that which will bring health, if properly applied. **1196-7**

Arts
. . . keep daily—yea, twice daily—the constant meditation or prayer for definite determining activities for harmony.

Keep about the body the colors of purple and lavender, and all things bright; music that is of harmony—as of the Spring Song, the Blue Danube and that character of music, with either the stringed instruments or the organ. These are the vibrations that will set again near normalcy—yea, normalcy, mentally and physically, may be brought to this body, if these influences will be consistently kept about this body.
2712-1

Attunement
How, you ask then, may the entity so attune self?

By looking on the beauty of a sunset, of a rose, of a lily, or any of those things in nature, and—by the very nature of the mood that these create in self—arouse or bring forth those melodies upon the instruments of the day; the piano, the organ, the reed or even the stringed instruments; to express the nature of these as they express themselves in their unfoldment.

And gradually may the entity so enter into the accord with same as to in self *attune* self to that unfoldment, that beauty, that nature to which it adapts itself for the healing forces necessary for man's awakening to his relationships to the Creative Forces. **949-12**

Healing

(Q) Approximately how long will it take to get results?
(A) If it requires time—as indicated, be consistent, be persistent. These are not questions so much as to whether results are to come tomorrow or next month or next year, but it is a case of the necessity of body, mind and purpose being one. As this is accomplished we will find that the body will grow in grace, in knowledge, in understanding. It is by the grace of the divine that healing may come. **3694-1**

(Q) Is there any hope of a cure?
(A) While there's life there's hope, but there must be persistence, consistence and faith in the divine, that the entity has a purposefulness in its experience in the earth. **4066-1**

Meditation/Prayer

[Spiritual foods] are needed by the body just as the body physical needs fuel in the diet. The body mental and spiritual needs spiritual food— prayer, meditation, thinking upon spiritual things. For thy body is indeed the temple of the living God. Treat it as such, physically and mentally. **4008-1**

(Q) Please give affirmation that would help me physically, mentally and spiritually.
(A) *Into Thy hands, O Father, I give myself; in body, in mind; that Thy forces of good, Thy influence, may be manifested to those I contact day by day.*

Not only this as rote, but as feeling and active in word and truth. **379-12**

(Q) What will help me in coming to right decisions as to my life?
(A) Prayer and meditation, to be sure. For, as He has given, "Behold I stand at the door and knock. If ye will open I will enter in."

Then, in thine own mind, decide as to whether this or that direction is right. Then pray on it, and leave it alone. Then suddenly ye will have the answer, Yes or No.

Then, with that Yes or No, take it again to Him in prayer, "Show me the way." And Yes or No will again direct thee from deep within.

That is practical direction. **3250-1**

Nature

May we indeed inculcate in the lives of others that like the rose, that like the baby breath, like every flower that blooms. For it does its best with what has been given it by man, to glorify its Maker with all its beauty, its color, with all of its love for the appreciation of spring, of the rain, the sunshine, the shadows. And so the man in like manner, with the worries, the troubles, heartaches, the disappointments, may draw closer and closer to God, knowing that this may be done as in the Son. He gave Himself that man might know that appreciation, that love, and how that in meting it to others we come to learn, to know the meaning of disappointments, of little hates, little jealousies, and of how they may grow by entertaining them, and how that the joys may grow also just by entertaining them, as do the flowers that God hath given, that man might see His face in the beautiful flowers. Consider the color, the beauty of the lily as it grows from its ugly muck, or the shrinking violet as it sends out its color, its odor to enrich even the very heart of God. Consider the rose as to how it unfolds with the color of the day, and with the opening itself to the sunshine, into the rain.   **5122–1**

Scripture reading

. . . present self in that manner of accepting that presented in St. John 14, 15, 16, 17. As the body reads, as the body meditates upon this, there will be found that need for the activities which have brought about this present conflict in a manner, within self. Then as ye apply it, let thy activities be that there is not question in self, as well as in those ye attempt to aid in bringing an at–onement with the divine within.

4001–3

Do begin with the first things first. Don't say in self, "Well, I believe this and I'll give it a try." Begin first by reading Exodus 19:5, Deuteronomy 30, then the 23rd Psalm. Then begin with the 14th, 15th, 16th chapters of St. John. Learn each of these passages so that they may be repeated.

Then begin to apply them with the people you meet, or the people who meet you; not merely as sayings. But you want to be a little bit happier, a little bit more optimistic, if you would have the Lord on your side.   **3682–1**

(Q) What would be the best metaphysical studies for me just now?
(A) Fourteenth, fifteenth, sixteenth, seventeenth of John! and put thyself
in same! Know that He is speaking to *thee!*   **1599-1**

(Q) How am I to overcome a persecution complex?
(A) Supply the mental forces with a spiritual promise. Read, apply the
30th of Deuteronomy, and the 14th, 15th, 16th and 17th of John as personal things. Not merely learn these as a routine but make practical
application of them. We will overcome this fear complex as well as the
feeling of being inefficient. And in His might and power is all strength
and all aptitude.
    Do that.   **3251-1**

Service

. . . only as an individual gives itself in service does it become aware.
For as the divine love has manifested, does become manifested, that
alone ye have given away do ye possess. That *alone* is the manner in
which the growth, the awareness, the consciousness grows to be.

1472-1

Administering to others is the best way to help self. More individuals
become so anxious about their own troubles, and yet helping others is
the best way to rid yourself of your own troubles. For what is the pattern? He gave up Heaven and entered physical being that ye might
have access to the Father. Then what are you grumbling about because
you dislike your mother? She dislikes you as much, but change this into
love. Be kind, be gentle, be patient, be long-suffering, for if thy God was
not long-suffering with thee, what chance would you have?   **5081-1**

(Q) Which of my aptitudes, active or latent, shall I follow for the greatest
success in adult life, financially?
(A) Forget the financial angle and consider rather that outlet for the
greatest contribution the entity may make to the making of the world a
better place in which to live. Let the financial gain be a result of the
abilities being used . . .   **4084-1**

. . . there is that awareness that should be in self, that the very fact ye
are conscious of thy activity in the material plane should be evidence

that thy Father-God hath need of thy service in the earth, and that through the present activity ye are given the opportunity to be a channel of blessing to someone.

For, to obtain the consciousness and awareness of coming into His presence, or as one would call to heaven, it will be as if it were leaning on the arm of someone ye have tried to help. For as ye do it unto thy brother, ye do it unto thy Maker. Know they are immutable laws. God is, and ye as a daughter, as a servant of the most high God are His handmaid. Then act like it!   **5177-1**

. . . let all so examine their hearts and minds as to put away doubt and fear; putting away hate and malice, jealousy and those things that cause man to err. Replace these with the desire to help, with hope, with the willingness to divide self and self's surroundings with those who are less fortunate; putting on the whole armor of God—in righteousness.

5749-13

No matter how valid, how well, how good a condition may be, there must be on the part of self the desire and the *will* to fill, to find, to do that which *will* enable self to be aroused to that ability of being a channel of blessing to someone.

That is the purpose for which the Creator has brought each individual into being, that they—through their ability to serve—may be a fit companion in those realms, those glories He would have them share. Hence, the decision is in self.

The field is truly ripe, the harvest is nigh. Will ye be a laborer in that vineyard, and fill, and give, and aid self *and* others? for in our approach to the Throne of grace it will be leaning upon the arm of someone we have attempted, sincerely, to serve and aid.   **2733-2**

If you would have love, you must show yourself lovely. If you would have others [be] kind to thee, be kind to others. Be patient, be long-suffering, show forth brotherly love. Thy choice in the present may not appear important, but ye can use thy experiences as a means for endearing thyself to everyone ye meet.   **5005-1**

Then, in thy daily dealings with others, forget not to interpret the lesson, the problem of the day, from a *spiritual* angle. Not that as of a goody-

goody manner; not that as of rote for rote's sake, but—as is expressed in nature—step by step, line by line, precept upon precept, *because* it gives such security in life and its expressions in the earth as to make same more worth while . . .

Know that it is an unchangeable law—they that would be the greatest among any group will be able to serve that group the more. This requires policy, tact, as well as psychological analyses of material and mental surroundings. Yet . . . there are the abilities and urges toward the beautiful, the ability to see the best in everyone, and that approach as for the universal consciousness—or as to things and peoples and groups and masses.   **1204–3**

(Q) How can I make the most of my remaining years in service to my fellow man?
(A) As has been indicated, help here and there to make the paths straight; to light the light to those who sit in darkness; to raise the hopes of those who have been discouraged, in that those who love Him—their seed shall not beg bread.

This may be done in writing, in speaking, in *doing!* For the experience, or this or that influence ye have seen or may see, is not the important thing—but what have ye done, and what are ye doing, and what *will* ye do *about same!*   **1598–1**

Remember . . . no one gives a cup of cold water in His name without receiving a reward. This is not as the buying of position or of conditions, but those who give ungrudgingly, those who give willingly of themselves that others may attain, that others may have the opportunity to learn of and to know that good, that purity, that love, that unselfishness exists in a material world, are complying with the law of love—which is manifested by and in the mercy, love and grace which the loving heavenly Father gives to individuals. Thus such individuals through the law of love receive joy and happiness in return.   **5018–1**

 . . . it is not all just to have faith, nor to be good; but have faith *in* something sufficient to put it into *practical* application in the daily experience; to be good not only as for the ease, the satisfaction it may bring, but being good *for* something; expending self, as it were, *abasing* self in the service of others—*this* is worth while, and brings joy, contentment, and an experience that is worth while.   **657–2**

Spiritual advice

Begin in the beginning. Learn thy relationships with God. Stand oft and look thyself in the mirror and see if you see an image of the God you worship. If you don't, change it. Change your disposition, smile more. Don't hate anyone. Don't begrudge anyone. And you will find life different.   **3544–1**

(Q) Give the body any spiritual advice . . .
(A) To thine own self be true, in the affairs of the mental, spiritual and physical forces of the body. Keep thine eye single in its aspirations towards those of the spiritual things in life, remembering that in an attitude of hopefulness and helpfulness may the greater blessings in every manner come to the body.   **5431–2**

A.R.E. PRESS

The A.R.E. Press publishes books, videos, and audiotapes meant to improve the quality of our readers' lives—personally, professionally, and spiritually. We hope our products support your endeavors to realize your career potential, to enhance your relationships, to improve your health, and to encourage you to make the changes necessary to live a loving, joyful, and fulfilling life.

For more information or to receive a free catalog, call:

1–800–723–1112

Or write:

A.R.E. Press
215 67th Street
Virginia Beach, VA 23451–2061

BAAR PRODUCTS

A.R.E.'s Official Worldwide Exclusive Supplier of Edgar Cayce Health Care Products

Baar Products, Inc., is the official worldwide exclusive supplier of Edgar Cayce health care products. Baar offers a collection of natural products and remedies drawn from the work of Edgar Cayce, considered by many to be the father of modern holistic medicine.

For a complete listing of Cayce-related products, call:

1–800–269–2502

Or write:

Baar Products, Inc.
P.O. Box 60
Downingtown, PA 19335 U.S.A.

Customer Service and International: 610–873–4591
Fax: 610–873–7945
Web Site: www.baar.com   E-mail: cayce@baar.com

THE OLD FARMER'S ALMANAC

CALCULATED ON A NEW AND IMPROVED PLAN FOR THE YEAR OF OUR LORD

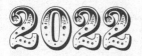

Being 2nd after Leap Year and (until July 1) 154th year of Canadian Confederation

FITTED FOR OTTAWA, WITH SPECIAL CORRECTIONS
AND CALCULATIONS TO ANSWER FOR ALL THE CANADIAN PROVINCES.

Containing, besides the large number of Astronomical Calculations and
the Farmer's Calendar for every month in the year, a variety of
NEW, USEFUL, & ENTERTAINING MATTER.

ESTABLISHED IN 1792
BY ROBERT B. THOMAS (1766–1846)

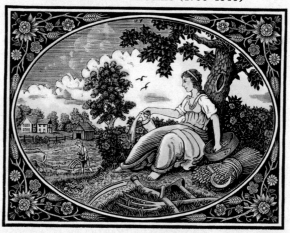

*There are only two days in the year when nothing can be done. One is called Yesterday and
the other is called Tomorrow. Today is the right day to Love, Believe, Do, and mostly Live.*
–His Holiness the 14th Dalai Lama, Tenzin Gyatso, Tibetan Buddhist monk (b. 1935)

Cover design registered
U.S. Trademark Office

Copyright © 2021 by Yankee Publishing Incorporated,
An Employee-Owned Company
ISSN 0078-4516

Library of Congress
Card No. 56-29681

Cover illustration by Steven Noble • Original wood engraving (above) by Randy Miller

The Old Farmer's Almanac • Almanac.ca
P.O. Box 520, Dublin, NH 03444 • 603-563-8111

CONTENTS

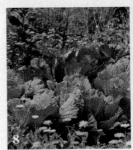

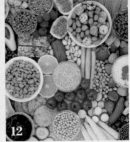

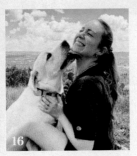

2022 TRENDS
Facts to Ponder and Forecasts to Watch For   6

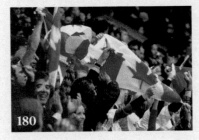

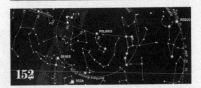

74

42

58

PREVAILING CUSTOMS

Had it not been the prevailing custom to usher these periodical pieces into the world by a preface, I would have excused myself the trouble of writing, and you of reading one to this: for if it be well executed, a preface will add nothing to its merit; if otherwise, it will be far from supplying its defects.

So wrote the founder of this Almanac, 26-year-old farmer and teacher Robert Bailey Thomas (the gentleman pictured at right on our cover) on this page of his first edition on the eve of its publication in Sterling, Massachusetts, on September 15, 1792.

He believed that his Almanac—"calculated on a new and improved plan for the year of our Lord, 1793"—needed no introduction.

He offered it as a comprehensive and trustworthy package of "new, useful, and entertaining matter" to an agrarian New England populace eager for exactly that: reliable Moon phase and sunrise/-set times (so important to planting traditions and farm chores), no-nonsense reminders and advisories (e.g., February: "If you neglected cutting timber last month, be sure to cut it now"), timesaving recipes ("a new method of making butter"), home remedies (for ailments afflicting people and animals), court dates, distances between places, math challenges, ac-counts of remarkable events (e.g., in 1571, England's Marcley Hill continuously moved for 2 days, carrying with it trees, hedges, and cattle), and more—all in a mere 46-page booklet.

Thomas's first edition was indeed well executed and without defect. Fulfilling his lifelong goal, it sold out, thus launching him on a career that would last another 53 years (edition years for which he wrote prefaces, later dubbed "To Patrons" in appreciation of readers' patronage) and setting the title—*The [Old] Farmer's Almanac*—on a course that would eventually establish the book as the oldest continuously published periodical in North America.

This is how the Almanac that you hold in your hands began and the reason why its execution—accuracy, relevance, usefulness, and entertainment—continues, we hope, to meet (or exceed!) the expectations of readers—*patrons*—like you. Thank you for your patronage!

–J. S., JUNE 2021

However, it is by our works and not our words that we would be judged. These, we hope, will sustain us in the humble though proud station we have so long held in the name of
Your obedient servant,

Rob. B. Thomas.

2022 TRENDS

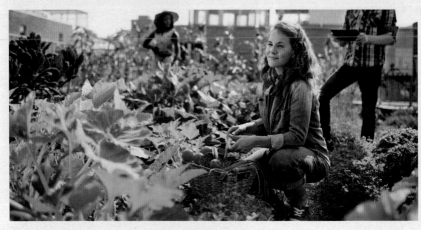

ON THE FARM

> "Municipal and national policies are advancing urban agriculture."
> *–Michael Levenston, executive director, City Farmer, Vancouver, B.C.*

FORWARD-THINKING FARMERS AND RANCHERS ARE:

- renting out livestock to families to teach children responsibility or to other farmers to try before buying
- using Web sites to accept nutritional assistance programs and arrange food pickup or delivery
- inviting volunteers to do farm chores for increased fitness

BUZZWORD
Farmfluencer: a farmer who promotes the farming lifestyle

CONSUMER-CONSCIOUS FARMERS ARE:

- getting the word out on their environmentally friendly practices:

"More farmers are using programs that offer traceability through the supply chain."
–Gary Joiner, Texas Farm Bureau

- getting food to people who order directly from the farm:

"Farmers are trying to obtain an economically feasible solution to selling online, with delivery or safe central pickup."
–Phil Blalock, executive director, National Association of Farmers' Market Nutrition Programs

 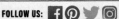

FACTS TO PONDER AND FORECASTS TO WATCH FOR

Compiled by Stacey Kusterbeck

ECO-CONSCIOUS FARMERS ARE:

- leaving grasslands undisturbed to leave carbon in the soil, in exchange for carbon credits (which companies buy to offset their own emissions)
- joining neighbors to convert a portion of their land to bee habitat

TECH TOOLS

In-demand software features for U.S. and Canadian farmers . . .

- yield mapping
- crop-input record-keeping
- imagery (satellite, plane, or drone)
- weather data

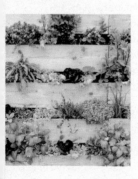

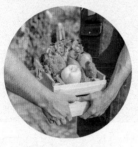

PATIENCE, PLEASE!

"Order-to-grow will emerge as a new way to reduce food waste."

–Cecelia Girr, director of cultural strategy, TBWA Worldwide

THE FUTURE OF FARMING

- Vertical farms, hydroponics, aquaponics, and greenhouses are surging.

"More controlled-environment agriculture projects will be launched."

–Sylvain Charlebois, director, Dalhousie University's Agri-Food Analytics Lab, Halifax, N.S.

COMING SOON

Apps that track who is growing our food and its maturity stage

(continued)

BY THE NUMBERS

$580: 6 months' rent for two egg-laying hens and a chicken coop

$4,100: average cost of U.S. cropland per acre

2.76 million: square footage of the world's largest greenhouse (in Morehead, Ky.)

More bees, please:

82.9 million: pounds of honey produced annually by Canada's honeybees

$1.5 billion: value that wild bee pollination contributes to seven U.S. crops (apples, highbush blueberries, sweet and tart cherries, almonds, watermelons, pumpkins)

20%: increase in yield if almond trees are bee-pollinated

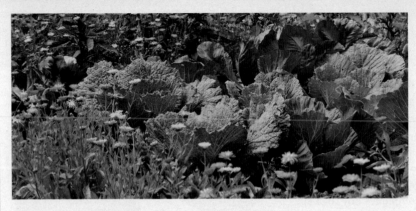

IN THE GARDEN

> "Gardeners are planting in stripes—
> one row vegetables, one row flowers."
>
> *–C. L. Fornari, author,* The Cocktail Hour Garden *(St. Lynn's Press, 2016)*

GARDENER GARB

- pants with wraparound hip pockets and/or reinforced knees
- kimono-style jackets
- field shirts with extra pockets

NEW VEGGIE VARIETIES

- 'Hampton' one-cut lettuce
- 'Prospera' Italian large leaf (4-inch) DMR basil
- disease-resistant 'Marciano' red butterhead lettuce
  –Johnny's Selected Seeds
- sweet 'Bitesize' hybrid brussels sprouts
- 'Blue Prince' hybrid pumpkin
- 'Depurple' hybrid cauliflower
  –Jung Seed
- compact 'Hasta La Pasta' winter squash
- 'Veranda Red' cherry tomato (a windowsill houseplant)

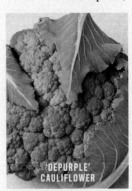

'DEPURPLE' CAULIFLOWER

- early-ripening 'Midnight Moon' hybrid eggplant
  –W. Atlee Burpee & Company

HARVEST HACKS

- Backyard growers are saving seeds to grow and/or swap— thus saving money and getting rare varieties.

- Companies are installing gardens in yards of people who pay for weeding, tending, and harvesting.

MADE FOR THE SHADE

"Shade-loving plants are in demand in

(continued)

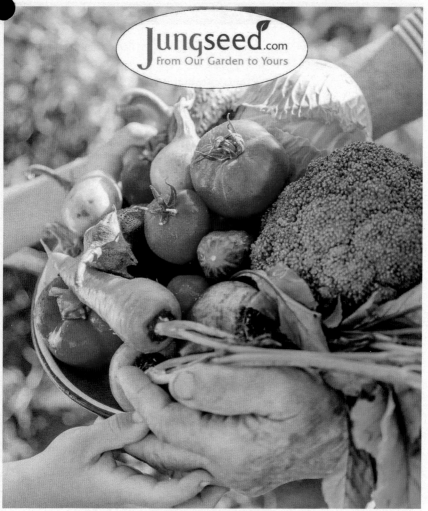

urban areas without sunny growing space."
–*Katie Rotella, Ball Horticultural*

- Carnival series 'Cinnamon Stick' and 'Burgundy Blast' compact coral bells (*Heuchera*)

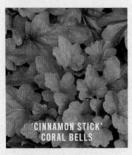

'CINNAMON STICK' CORAL BELLS

NATURAL IS NICE
"Rewilding" gardeners are . . .
- returning a portion or all of their yard to its natural state
- leaving gaps in fences to allow passage by rabbits and other small wildlife

IN-DEMAND HOUSEPLANTS
- Australian tree fern
- *Calathea orbifolia*
- council tree
- 'Fabian' aralia
- ruffled fan palm
–*Hilton Carter, plant stylist and author of* Wild Creations (CICO Books, 2021)

TINY IS TOPS
"As new gardeners learn the ropes, tiny plants that grow faster are all the rage."
–*Katie Dubow, president, Garden Media Group*

Multiseason smaller solutions:
- 'Autumn Starburst' and 'Autumn Majesty' dwarf azaleas that

BY THE NUMBERS

1.7% of Canadians grow all of the fruit and vegetables that they eat.

23.1 million U.S. adults have converted some lawn to a natural or wildflower landscape.

36.8 million U.S. adults have bought at least one plant because it was native to their area.

flower across three seasons
–*Encore Azalea*

- 'Little Miss Figgy', which bears figs in spring and fall
–*Southern Living Plant Collection*

SMALL-SPACE GARDENERS ARE . . .
Hanging in baskets:
- 'Midnight Cascade' blueberries with white, bell-shape flowers
–*Bushel and Berry*

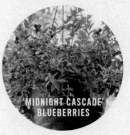

'MIDNIGHT CASCADE' BLUEBERRIES

Planting in small pots:
- 'Red Velvet' and 'Cocoa' tomatoes
–*PanAmerican Seed*

NO FLOWERS? NO WORRIES!
"The no-flower 'boom without the bloom' foliage look is trending."
–*Katie Rotella*

- Indoor/outdoor varieties include 'Shangri La' philodendron and 'Gryphon' begonia
(continued)

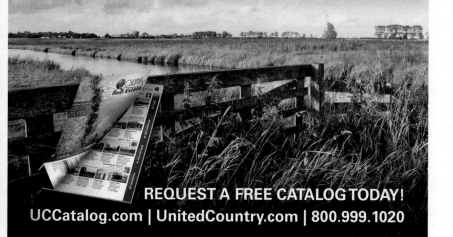

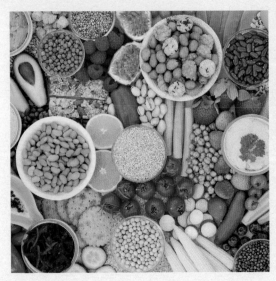

GOOD EATS

"Consumers will balance their desire for plant-based alternatives with actual plants to maximize nutritional benefits and watch their wallets."
–Melanie Bartelme, global food analyst, Mintel Food & Drink

GOOD FOR THE GLOBE

"There's more prominence and appreciation of regional ingredients from parts of the world that are often overlooked."
–Denise Purcell, Specialty Food Association

- from Cambodia: chile pastes
- from Senegal: fonio (an ancient grain)
- from Nigeria: cassava grits

HERE NOW

- grocery stores that sell only plant-based products
- peel-and-stick patches that keep takeout food from getting soggy
- "upcycled" food products using *(continued)*

BY THE NUMBERS

Food stats, for Canada:

80% of consumers will pay extra for produce that's locally grown.

$12,667: amount that households spend on food, annually

600,000: the vegan population

$1,766: value of food waste, per household

20% of consumers never eat food past its expiration date.

Snack stats, for the U.S.:

7% of consumers snack all day rather than consume meals.

2.7: number of food and beverage items consumed each time people snack

530: number of between-meal snacks, per capita, annually, in 2020

FOLLOW US:

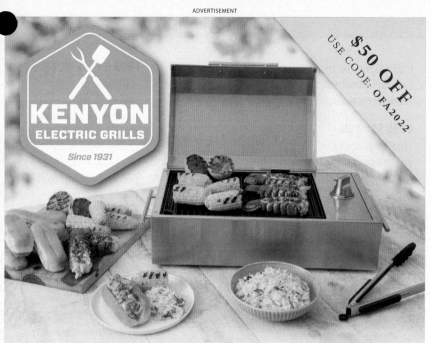
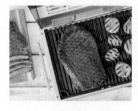
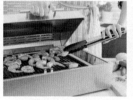
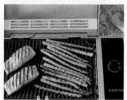
13

ingredients or by-products that would have been wasted

GOOD FOR YOU

Health-conscious shoppers are buying more legumes and other veggies, plus other whole foods—for example:

- chickpea flour
- meat-free "jerky"
- nut butters made with powdered mushrooms

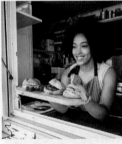

"Carts and food trucks will collaborate with grocery and hardware stores to create shopping events."
–Dana McCauley, director of new venture creation, Research Innovation Office, University of Guelph, Ont.

SERVING UP SUCCESS

Restaurant chefs are meeting customers' needs . . .

BUZZWORD
Restaurmart: eatery selling its own packaged food onsite for takeout
–Phil Lempert, Supermarket Guru.com

- *offsite:* by setting up curbside pop-ups in high-traffic locations
- *virtually:* by teaching how to make favorite dishes online
- *at home:* by providing music playlists and plating instructions for takeout meals to replicate the ambiance of the restaurant where they were made
–Dana McCauley

FLAVORS WE'RE CRAVING

- maple syrup with edible glitter
- flash-frozen cups of coffee (as is or to be reconstituted with hot water)
- oat milk powder (after oats are pressed for milk)
- vacuum-fried salmon skins (left over after the fish are filleted)
–Denise Purcell

FOOD ON THE MOVE

- Mobile grocery stores in trucks visit neighborhoods, and shoppers stroll through trailer "aisles." Trucks are then restocked before heading to the next location.
- Groceries in temperature-controlled boxes are delivered to homes at any time, without worry about food spoilage.
- Restaurant kitchens built for takeout orders are occupying former retail spaces and parking lots.

VAUNTED VENDING

The most tempting vending machines . . .

- offer fresh, healthy food, restocked daily
- cook pizza, quiche, and croissants on demand
- grind coffee beans to order *(continued)*

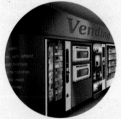

FOLLOW US:

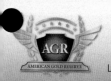

AMERICAN GOLD RESERVE
WEALTH PRESERVATION
LEGAL TENDER MINTED BY THE U.S. MINT • AUTHORIZED BY CONGRESS

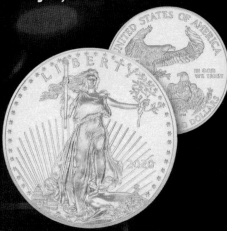

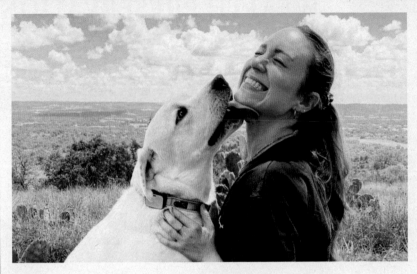

OUR ANIMAL FRIENDS

"The ability to interface directly with veterinarians will become a new standard for pet wearables."

–Daniel Granderson, Packaged Facts

CATS AND DOGS ARE DINING ON . . .
- pet food with insect-based protein (fly larvae that are fed food waste; crickets)
- ancient grains (quinoa, millet, buckwheat)
- plant-based ingredients (kale, blueberries, spinach)

FLYING OFF SHELVES
- breed-specific subscription pet food services

BY THE NUMBERS

84.9 million U.S. households have at least one pet.

14% of current pet owners got a dog in 2020.

12% of current pet owners got a cat in 2020.

47% of pet owners are buying lower-cost store brands of pet food more frequently.

- pet bowls that automatically reorder food
- toys, leashes, and collars made from recycled materials

HEALTHY PETS ARE HAPPY PETS
"There is increasing demand for products touting mental health benefits for pets."
–Daniel Granderson

- supplements to calm pets during noisy times or travel

(continued)

FOLLOW US:

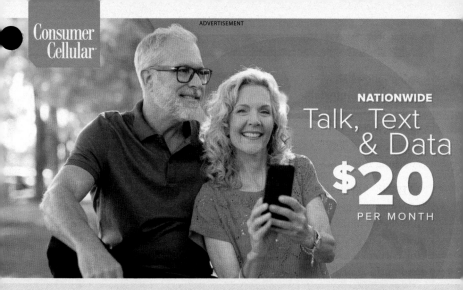

Consumer Cellular

NATIONWIDE

Talk, Text & Data

$20

PER MONTH

PREMIUM COVERAGE
We operate on two of the largest wireless networks—offering the same great service.

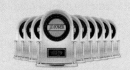

AWARDED BY J.D. POWER 10 TIMES IN A ROW
"#1 in Customer Service among Wireless Value MVNOs."

TOP PHONES & DEVICES
Choose from the latest technology from Apple, Samsung, Motorola— or, bring your own device!

FLEXIBLE, NO-CONTRACT MONTHLY PLANS DELIVER SUPERB VALUE
Popular Options for *Two Lines* include:

$**20**.00 MONTH/LINE	UNLIMITED TALK + TEXT / 500MB SHARED DATA	
$**22**.50 MONTH/LINE	UNLIMITED TALK + TEXT / 3GB SHARED DATA	
$**37**.50 MONTH/LINE	UNLIMITED TALK + TEXT / UNLIMITED SHARED DATA	

Activation on our service is *FREE!* Sign up 100% risk-free: try us 30 days with zero obligation.

AARP MEMBERS RECEIVE A 5% DISCOUNT ON MONTHLY SERVICE.

CALL CONSUMER CELLULAR
(888) 270-8608

VISIT US ONLINE
StartCC.com

AVAILABLE AT **TARGET**

- dog pillows shaped for a more comfortable head position and calmer sleep

- crates that play soothing music

NATURAL, NATURALLY

"Consumers are interested in pet food labels. They're looking for natural ingredients and nothing artificial."
–Glenn A. Polyn, editor in chief, Pet Age

PET TECH

In-demand devices monitor a pet's activities, vital signs, body functions, and location.
–Daniel Granderson

FELINE FRENZY

"Cats are an underserved demographic in the pet food and pet durables market. We'll see more and better products and services

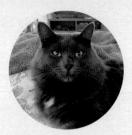

and more marketing attention for cats."
–David Lummis, lead pet analyst, Packaged Facts

HEY, SPORT!

More than ever, we're working out alongside our pets . . .

- *kayaking* with canine life vests featuring top-mounted handles for owners to grab in case of emergency

- *running* with leashes that cinch around waists for hands-free exercise

- *hiking* with boots on dogs that protect paws and provide traction

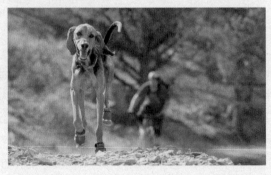

- *camping* with sleeping bags made to fit dogs

PET PERKS

"Pet products are focusing more on environmental friendliness and the use of quality, human-grade items and ingredients."
–Jamie Baxter, American Pet Products Association

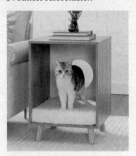

Pet-centric homes feature . . .
- end tables that double as pet beds

- litter-box planters

- pet-size Murphy beds

- in-ground dog waste composting units

TALK TO ME!

- Collars can identify a dog's mood based on the sound of its bark.

- Owners are training pets to use push-button audio devices to "speak." *(continued)*

ADVERTISEMENT

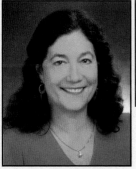
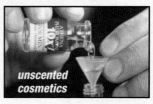
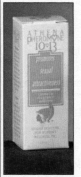
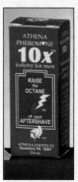

YOUR HEALTH OUTLOOK

"The 'food as medicine' approach will topple our reliance
on pharmaceuticals. Doctor and farmer
collaborations will have us trading pills for produce."

–Skyler Hubler, cultural strategist, TBWA Worldwide

FOR SAVVIER SHUT-EYE

- Practice "Circadian eating": Eat in daylight, stop after dark.
- Wear blue light–blocking glasses at night.
- Don sleepwear that adjusts its temperature.
- Use kill switches to shut off all lights and Wi-fi in a room.
- Use lights that automatically go from bright blue-light in daytime to warmer hues at night to boost melatonin levels.

BY THE NUMBERS

51% of consumers are very or extremely likely to tell their doctors when they disagree with them.

50% of people who use fitness- and health-tracking devices share the data with their doctors.

MANDATORY MENTAL HEALTH DAYS

Companies are offering extra "holidays" and requiring that stressed-out employees take them.

IN DEVELOPMENT

- technology to reprogram cells to speed up healing

FOOD TO HELP YOU FEEL BETTER

- Community health programs are connecting low-income residents with local produce.
- Doctors are writing prescriptions for produce redeemable at farmers' markets.

(continued)

 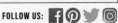

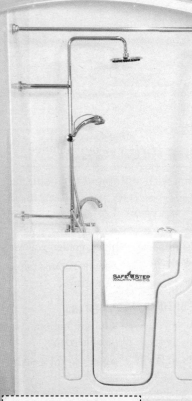
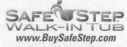

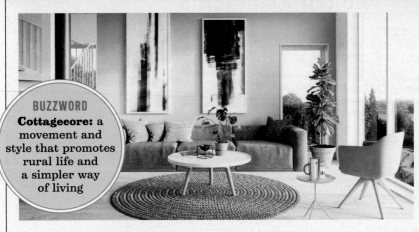

BUZZWORD
Cottagecore: a movement and style that promotes rural life and a simpler way of living

AROUND THE HOUSE

> "We're seeing sleek, minimal rooms with statement furnishings."
> *–Ana Cummings, president, Alberta chapter, Decorators and Designers Association of Canada*

SPACING OUT

"We are utilizing all of our available spaces in our home. Rooms that are adaptable, ergonomic, and private are important as we connect our health with our physical spaces."
–Kelly DeVore, chair, interior architecture & design, Columbus College of Art & Design

DOUBLE DUTY

- Underutilized walk-in closets are being converted to workout spaces, offices, or guest rooms.
- Greenhouses are becoming dining rooms.

- Tables with adjustable heights are used as desks or dining tables.

HOME OFFICE OPTIONS

- refitted garden sheds
- leased pods on lawns
- free-standing buildings, with French doors and covered porches

COLORS FOR HOMES

- kitchens: green marble countertops and bright blue cabinets
- bedrooms: cobalt blues; beige with black accents

- bathrooms: pale blues; golden yellows
- living rooms: teals; light grays

IN DEMAND

- multifunction, flexible rooms
- electric car docking stations
–American Institute of Architects Home Design Trends Survey

IN DEVELOPMENT

- windows of transparent wood, which is safer during extreme winds—being nonshattering—and more efficient than glass
(continued)

FOLLOW US:

FIREWOOD ALERT!

You have the power to protect forests and trees!

BUY IT WHERE YOU BURN IT.

Pests like the invasive emerald ash borer can hitchhike in your firewood. You can prevent the spread of these damaging insects and diseases by following these firewood tips:

▶ Buy locally harvested firewood at or near your destination.

▶ Buy certified heat-treated firewood ahead of time, if available.

▶ Gather firewood on site when permitted.

What might be in your firewood?

GYPSY MOTH is a devastating pest of oaks and other trees. Female moths lay tan patches of eggs on firewood, campers, vehicles, patio furniture — anything outside! When these items are moved to new areas, this pest gets a free ride.

SPOTTED LANTERNFLY sucks sap from dozens of tree and plant species. This pest loves tree-of-heaven but will feed on black walnut, white oak, sycamore, and grape. Like the gypsy moth, this pest lays clusters of eggs on just about any dry surface, from landscaping stone to firewood!

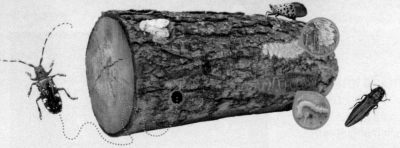

ASIAN LONGHORNED BEETLE will tunnel through, and destroy, over 20 species of trees — especially maple trees. The larvae of this beetle bore into tree branches and trunks, making it an easy pest to accidentally transport in firewood.

EMERALD ASH BORER — the infamous killer of ash trees — is found in forests and city trees across much of the eastern and central United States. This insect is notoriously good at hitching rides in infested firewood. Don't give this tree-killing bug a ride to a new forest, or a new state!

DONT MOVE FIREWOOD.org

This graphic is for illustrative purposes only. Many of these pests will only infest certain types of trees, making it very unlikely for a single log to contain all species as shown.

Visit dontmovefirewood.org for more information.

NODS TO NATURE

"Biophilic design is the future. Ideas that help to merge indoor and outdoor are extremely vital."

We'll see . . .

- terrarium lamps
- plants in hammocks over beds
- plants replacing chandeliers

–Hilton Carter

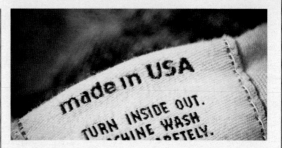

MONEY MATTERS

"U.S. consumers are specifically shopping for products that are made in the USA, even if this means paying a little more."

–Gabrielle Pastorek, retail analyst, Finder.com

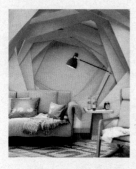

INTERIOR WISH LISTS

- *On walls:* 3D artwork in trapezoidal and rhombus shapes
- *In bedrooms:* dressers with carved scalloped or fluted edges; walls covered in upholstered fabric
- *In bathrooms:* full marble, from walls to molding to counter and sink—all in the same color

–Ana Cummings

PEOPLE ARE TALKING ABOUT . . .

- realtors selling houses with pets included
- financial therapists helping with both money problems and emotions

(continued)

BY THE NUMBERS

10% of people have a credit card that they keep secret from their partner.

70% of employees say that they got a raise after asking for one.

35% of parents admit to trying to "keep up with the Joneses."

$8.75: average amount of pocket money parents give kids each week

21: number of U.S. states that require a personal finance course for high school graduation

$120,230: the maximum amount of debt that women will accept while still continuing a romantic relationship

$109,127: the amount of similar debt that a man will accept

FOLLOW US:

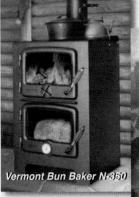
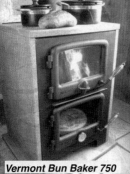
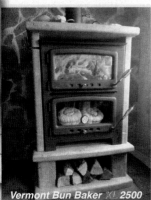
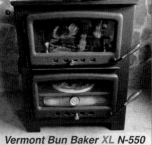
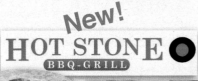
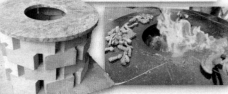

25

Choose Life
Grow Young with HGH

From the landmark book Grow Young with HGH comes the most powerful, over-the-counter health supplement in the history of man. Human growth hormone was first discovered in 1920 and has long been thought by the medical community to be necessary only to stimulate the body to full adult size and therefore unnecessary past the age of 20. Recent studies, however, have overturned this notion completely, discovering instead that the natural decline of Human Growth Hormone (HGH), from ages 21 to 61 (the average age at which there is only a trace left in the body) and is the main reason why the body ages and fails to regenerate itself to its 25 year-old biological age.

Like a picked flower cut from the source, we gradually wilt physically and mentally and become vulnerable to a host of degenerative diseases, that we simply weren't susceptible to in our early adult years.

Modern medical science now regards aging as a disease that is treatable and preventable and that "aging", the disease, is actually a compilation of various diseases and pathologies, from everything, like a rise in blood glucose and pressure to diabetes, skin wrinkling and so on. All of these aging symptoms can be stopped and rolled back by maintaining Growth Hormone levels in the blood at the same levels HGH existed in the blood when we were 25 years old.

There is a receptor site in almost every

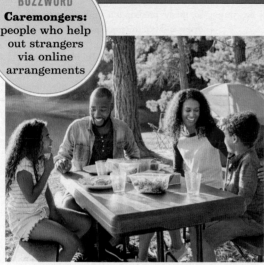

CULTURE

"The fastest-growing industries are artificial intelligence, healthcare, robotics, and travel."
–Daniel Levine, Avant-Guide Institute

COMING SOON
- artificial intelligence to sort nonrecyclable plastics for reuse as fuels
- roads that alert cars of hazards—e.g., black ice, potholes
- biodegradable "plastics" made from trees

GROUP EFFORTS
- firms setting up compost hubs where residents can drop off food waste

- companies exchanging collected compost scraps for produce from local farms for a fee

PEOPLE ARE TALKING ABOUT . . .
- mobile work vans with a desk, chair, and built-in coffee machine
- "random" camping (for free, on public land)
- hotels providing waterproof books for guests to read in pools

- laundromats playing soothing music
- "dark sky" locations (with no light pollution) for stargazing

MORE REUSE NEWS
"We will see more grocery subscription services with items delivered in reusable containers that are picked up at the next delivery."
–*Michael G. Luchs, professor, Raymond A. Mason School of Business, College of William & Mary*

(continued)

BY THE NUMBERS
1,000 miles: maximum distance achieved in 1 day by a hybrid solar/electric car

45 miles: maximum distance achieved from one full solar-only charge of such a car

17% of U.S. consumers think that self-driving cars will be safer than those with human drivers.

FOLLOW US:

Train at home to

Work at Home

Be a Medical Coding & Billing Specialist

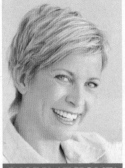

WORK AT HOME!

✓ Be home for your family
✓ Be your own boss
✓ Choose your own hours

SAVE MONEY!

✓ No day care, commute, or office wardrobe/lunches
✓ Possible tax breaks
✓ Tuition discount for eligible military and their spouses
✓ Military education benefits & MyCAA approved

Train at home in as little as 5 months to earn up to $42,630 a year!*

Now you can train in the comfort of your own home to work in a medical office, or from home as your experience and skills increase.

Make great money…up to $42,630 a year with experience! It's no secret, healthcare providers need Medical Coding & Billing Specialists. **In fact, the U.S. Department of Labor projects 8% growth, 2019 to 2029, for specialists doing coding and billing.

10 Years	**8%**
5 Years	**Increase In Demand!**

No previous medical experience required. Compare the money you can make!

Coders earn great money because they make a lot of money for the people they work for. Entering the correct codes on medical claims can mean the difference in thousands of dollars in profits for doctors, hospitals and clinics. Since each and every medical procedure must be coded and billed, there's plenty of work available for well-trained Medical Coding & Billing Specialists.

Get FREE Facts. Contact Us Today!

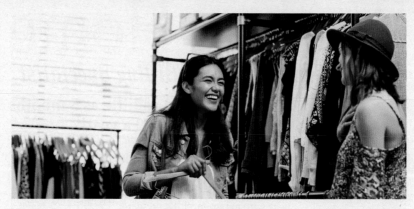

FASHION

"Retailers will offer the best of human and automated services—the beginning of a truly 'bionic' customer experience."

–Achim Berg, global leader, Apparel, Fashion, & Luxury Group, McKinsey

SUSTAINABLE NOTIONS

"Cradle-to-cradle concepts will really start to take off."
–Kelly DeVore

Products will get a second life:
- Jeans will be transformed into housing insulation.
- Shoes will be made out of soda bottles.

We'll also see . . .
- "leather" clothing and shoes made from mushroom roots
- naturally dyed sneakers
- technology that identifies fabric so that it can be recycled before ending up in a landfill

LET'S FACE IT

"Consumers will see stories and photos of farmers and clothing sewers on hangtags, Web sites, and QR codes, to put a face behind the fashion products that we buy."
–Andrea Kennedy, faculty, LIM College Fashion Merchandising Dept.

"USED" IS MAKING NEWS

"Secondhand apparel retailing will become the fastest growing segment of the Canadian retail apparel market."
–Randy Harris, president, Trendex North America

Clothing brands are offering "take back" programs: Customers return items to be cleaned, repaired, and resold, instore or online.
–Andrea Kennedy ∎

> **BY THE NUMBERS**
>
> **69%** of consumers want to know how their clothing was manufactured.
>
> **53%** of consumers give unwanted clothes to others for reuse.

Photo: Goodboy Picture Company/Getty Images

FOLLOW US: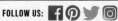

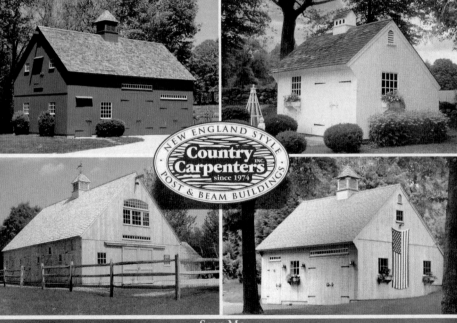

When it's built by *hand,*

It's connected to the *Heart.*

For three generations, the builders, blacksmiths, and craftsmen at Country Carpenters have put their hands and their hearts into designing and building the finest New England Style buildings available. Hand-selected materials, hand-forged hardware, all hand-built and hand-finished by real people. You can feel the difference in your heart.

NEW ENGLAND STYLE
Country Carpenters INC.
since 1974
POST & BEAM BUILDINGS

Scan to Receive $500 Off Your
Purchase of a Country Barn,
Carriage House or Outbuilding*

Scan Me

Use PROMO Code AYOFA22
*Offer Valid with Deposit Paid
before Oct. 1, 2022

COUNTRY BARNS, CARRIAGE HOUSES, POOL & GARDEN SHEDS, CABINS
Visit our models on display! We ship nationwide!
326 Gilead Street, Hebron, CT 06248 • **860.228.2276** • **countrycarpenters.com**

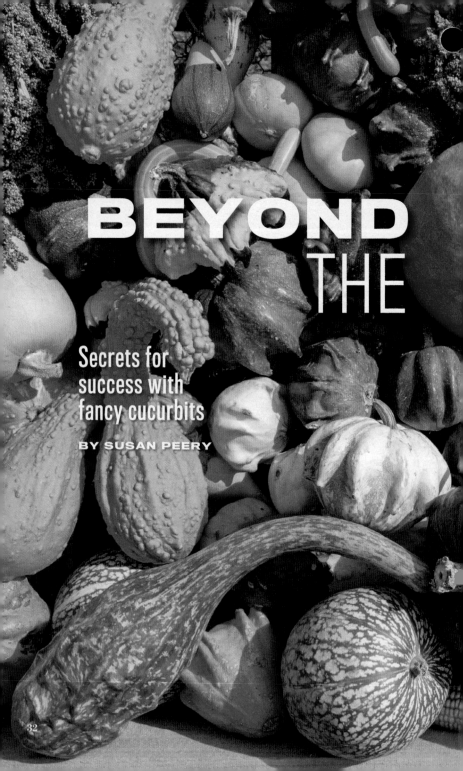

BEYOND
THE

Secrets for success with fancy cucurbits

BY SUSAN PEERY

PUMPKIN
PATCH

**SHOW OFF
YOUR SQUASHES!**
Post pics of your
pumpkins and squashes at
📷 @theoldfarmersalmanac

Photo: Evgeniya Vlasova/GAP Photos

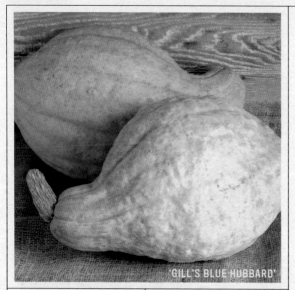

'GILL'S BLUE HUBBARD'

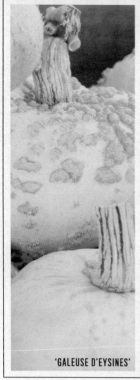

'GALEUSE D'EYSINES'

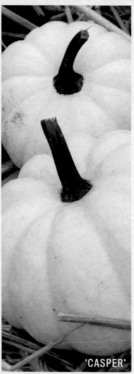

'CASPER'

Autumn brings out the cucurbit beauties. A field of orange pumpkins in October, a pyramid of butternut and acorn squashes at the farmers' market: To a gardener, what could be more inspiring? Only these: a warty 'Galeuse d'Eysines' squash (the bumps are the measure of sweetness) or a smooth white 'Casper' pumpkin (developed in Canada as a container plant, both edible and ornamental); a jade-color 'Gill's Blue Hubbard' (cousin of the Boston Marrow, the quintessential New England pie pumpkin); or a turbaned 'Kindred' (born and raised in Kindred, North Dakota, and as sweet as it is handsome). With care, you can grow these and other fancy fruit.

Pumpkin- and squash-growing is a pleasure and an accomplishment that will make you proud, but it can also be fraught with setbacks. Plant

Photos, clockwise from top: Johnny's Selected Seeds; emer1940/Getty Images; AlpamayoPhoto/Getty Images

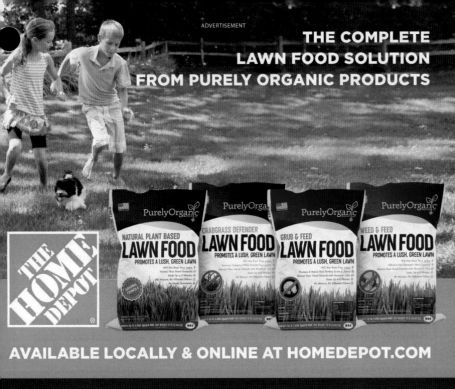
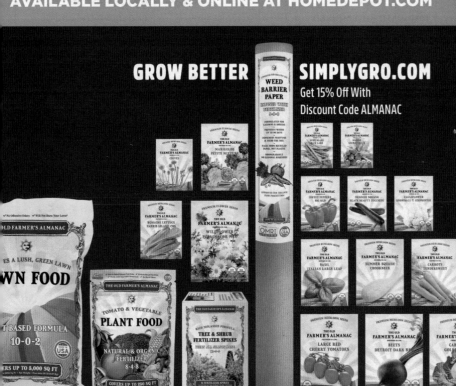

scientists at Purdue University say that they get more questions about pumpkin diseases than on any other crop. Blights and rots and spots and wilts are out there, lurking. Striped and spotted cucumber beetles, squash bugs, and squash vine borers can attack without warning. The weather is beyond any gardener's control. But don't despair! Here are a few strategies for pumpkin and squash success. We encourage you to try planting some of the more unusual heirloom varieties listed; this gardening advice applies to all types.

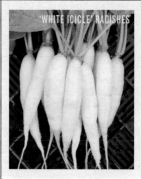

'WHITE ICICLE' RADISHES

1. EDGE WITH ICICLE RADISHES

Early in the season, plant a large circle of 'White Icicle' radishes around the perimeter of your pumpkin patch. By the time the radishes go to seed, it will be warm enough to plant the cucurbits. As an additional benefit, the adult clearwing moth, which emerges from last year's squash borer cocoon, dislikes radishes and will not try to lay eggs or overwinter in this spot.

2. PLANT PROPITIOUSLY

It can be tempting to be the first in your neighborhood to get the garden planted. But look at a soil thermometer, not the calendar, and do not plant pumpkin or squash seeds until the soil registers 70°F at a depth of 1 to 2 inches. In northern gardening zones, and depending on the weather, this can mean the end of June. This helps the harvest in four ways.

FIRST, male blossoms (the ones with a straight stem) must open first so that their pollen will be

MEET THE FAMILY

All pumpkins and squashes originated in Central and South America, cultivated first as livestock food. Seeds from the sweetest, least watery specimens were saved and replanted over generations. In eastern North America, Native Americans shared their life-sustaining crop with the early settlers.

Pumpkins, squashes, and some gourds belong to the genus *Cucurbita* and are now grown worldwide for their edible fruit. The three main species of pumpkins and winter squashes are *C. pepo*, which includes acorn squashes and jack-o'-lantern—type pumpkins (notably the classic 'Connecticut Field' pumpkin, an heirloom); *C. moschata* (the butternut squash family); and *C. maxima*, which is soft-stemmed and less fibrous and includes varieties ranging from the celebrated Cinderella pumpkin 'Rouge Vif d'Étampes' (translation from the French: "vivid red from Étampes") and the whole Hubbard squash family to the giant (if inedible) pumpkins grown for competitions.

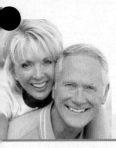

Breakthrough
Joint Pain Discovery

Doctor's Formula Eases Joint Issues

If you're over 40 or 50, odds are you suffer pain or stiffness in at least one of your body's 230 joints.

In fact, over 21 million Americans suffer from "wear and tear" concerns such as:

- **Joint pain or stiffness**
- **Restricted motion in joints**
- **Grinding, crackling**
- Mild joint swelling or warmth
- **Enlargement of joints**

These issues can make it difficult to climb stairs, clean house, do yardwork, enjoy hobbies, or even just keep up with the grandkids.

Many doctors tell you pain is just part of growing older. They say you should learn to "live with it."

Don't Ignore Joint Pain

Renowned holistic doctor David Brownstein, M.D., decided to search for new natural strategies to help soothe and comfort aching joints.

After seeing so many patients take handfuls of expensive but low-quality joint supplements, Dr. Brownstein formulated **LIMBEX®**.

This advanced joint support formula contains 11 premium ingredients to improve and maintain healthy joints, cartilage, and connective tissue.

ApresFlex® Starts Helping Joints in as Little as 5 Days!

LIMBEX contains ApresFlex, a new next-generation boswellia extract that quickly helps balance the body's inflammatory response. There are 10 more hard-working ingredients in **LIMBEX** that support healthy joints, including bromelain, turmeric, glucosamine, chondroitin, holy basil, green tea, pomegranate, piperine, and vitamins C & E.

These ingredients work to reduce inflammation, block damaging enzymes, and lubricate joints. They improve blood flow to damaged joints while reducing swelling, pain, and stiffness.

The Simple Solution for Joint Health Support

LIMBEX now makes it easy to help support and soothe your joints.

Get back to living your life again with less pain and stiffness. Try **LIMBEX** today, at no cost!

RISK-FREE Trial of LIMBEX

DR. BROWNSTEIN

We're offering a risk-free trial supply at NO COST. That's a $39.95 value!

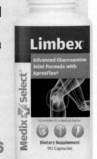

Limbex
Advanced Glucosamine
Joint Formula with
ApresFlex®

Medix Select

Formulated by a Medical Doctor

Dietary Supplement
90 Capsules

Toll-Free:
800-347-5116

Online:
TryLimbex.com/Almanac

Joint Pain Sufferers Love LIMBEX

"The pain in my hip is all but gone. I can get up from a chair and walk without limping." *Carol T. from Texas*

"Wonderful! When I don't take it, my knees kill me. I absolutely love **LIMBEX**!" *Caridad W. from Maryland*

*Trial offer requires enrollment in SmartShip program. See Website for details. These statements have not been evaluated by the Food and Drug Administration. This product is not intended to diagnose, treat, cure, or prevent any disease. Testimonials are from actual customers who have used our products. Testimonials reflect their experience but may not be representative of all those who will use our product.

accessible when the female flowers (which have a bulge at the base) appear. Male blossoms are especially sensitive to nighttime temperatures below 65° and are more prolific once it warms up.

SECOND, bacterial wilt and squash mosaic virus are carried by the cucumber beetle, a

spotted in the West.)

THIRD, downy mildew, a fungus-like organism, germinates from spores in the cool and moist conditions of spring. Waiting until the soil warms up and dries out before planting seeds makes the pathogen less likely to thrive.

FOURTH, the squash

waiting until July to plant can shorten your growing season enough that a frost can come before the pumpkins are ready to harvest, if you regularly get frosts in September. Pumpkins and winter squashes usually need a minimum of 100 days from planting to harvest.

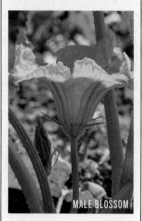

MALE BLOSSOM

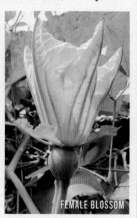

FEMALE BLOSSOM

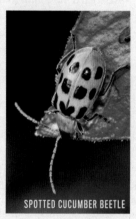

SPOTTED CUCUMBER BEETLE

ubiquitous insect that is the bane of all vining plants. Although these beetles chew tender leaves, their role as a disease vector, or transmitter, is the most damaging. This beetle is most active in May and early June and usually dies out by late June. (Cucumber beetles are striped east of the Rocky Mountains and

vine borer, which is the larval stage of a clearwing moth, tunnels into tender vines to eat in late spring and then buries itself in the soil to form a cocoon until the next year. Waiting to plant until later in its life cycle can save your pumpkin vines.

A caveat: In garden Zones 4 and colder,

3. SEEDS OR SEEDLINGS?

Most growers agree that planting pumpkin and squash seeds directly into warm soil, either into hills for better drainage (thin to two or three plants once seeds have sprouted) or rows (allow 6 feet in every direction between seeds), will yield the most robust plants.

(continued)

Photos, from left: Liudmyla/Getty Images; Subas chandra Mahato/Getty Images; johnandersonphoto/Getty Images

HEIRLOOM HALL OF FAME

In addition to the varieties already mentioned, consider growing these unusual pumpkins and squashes, all open-pollinated (they will produce true to type).

'Pennsylvania Dutch Crookneck' *(C. moschata):* Excellent keeper and best for pies and soups. After harvest, hook the squash over a pole to cure in a warm place. Close relative of the 'Canada Crookneck' and favorite of homesteaders in the 19th century.

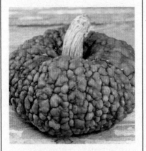

The bumps are also called "sugar warts" because of the concentration of sugars below the skin. Born to be stuffed into ravioli. Also known as Chioggia sea pumpkin.

'Blue Banana' and 'Pink Banana' *(C. maxima):* These oblong pumpkins, introduced in the United States in the 1890s, may have originated in Peru more than 800 years ago. The flesh is intensely sweet. Some say that 'Sibley' (aka 'Pike's Peak'), introduced by Hiram Sibley & Co., of Rochester, New York, in 1887, is the best of this Banana group.

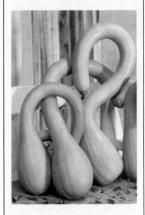

'Marina di Chioggia' *(C. maxima):* This gorgeous green pumpkin, warts and all, started in South America and was developed in Chioggia, on the Adriatic coast of what is now Italy, in the 1600s.

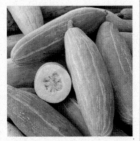

'Cutchogue Flat Cheese' *(C. moschata):* Cousin to 'Long Island Cheese' (which is larger) and 'Musquee de Provence' (also larger, with a darker rind, and good flavor). The cheese pumpkin is known strictly for its looks (it resembles a wheel of cheese), not its

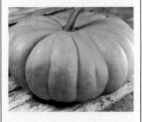

taste, and for its longevity. Beautiful on your doorstep long after other pumpkins have turned to glop.

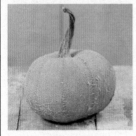

'Winter Luxury Pie' *(C. pepo):* Lauded by pumpkin expert and *The Compleat Squash* (Artisan, 2004) author Amy Goldman for making "the smoothest and most velvety pumpkin pie" ever. Introduced in 1893.

Photos: EdenBrothers.com (Blue Banana); Nova Photo Graphik/GAP Photos (Crookneck); Baker Creek Heirloom Seeds (all others)

4. USE MULCH AND/OR ROW COVERS

These will conserve soil moisture, warm the soil, and protect young plants from insects and windborne spores. Once vining and flowering begin, be sure to remove row covers during the day

You can even gently vacuum the leaves to remove the eggs. A hand vacuum is perfect for this. Vigilance early in the growing season will really pay off. Wrap aluminum foil around the base of stems as an additional deterrent to squash

stem. They are fragile at this stage and will bruise or nick easily. Bring the plump beauties into a heated space and let them cure for 2 to 3 weeks at temperatures of 60° to 70°. This toughens the skins, lowers the water content, and helps the

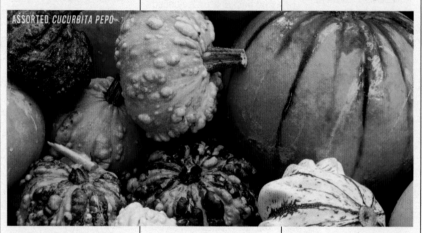

ASSORTED, *CUCURBITA PEPO*

so that pollinators can do their work. Once pumpkins and squashes form, slip an old shingle or piece of cardboard under them if the soil is soggy.

5. BE PICKY

That is, if you spot eggs of squash bugs or cucumber beetles on the top or underside of leaves, pick them off by hand and destroy them.

borers. Plant nasturtiums nearby, as these repel squash bugs.

6. DON'T WAIT FOR FROST ON THE PUMPKIN

Cold temperatures (under 50°F) reduce the quality and keeping power of your pumpkins and squashes, and freezing is fatal. Harvest by cutting the fruit from the vine, leaving a few inches of

crop to keep longer. As squashes and pumpkins age, enzymes convert starches to sugars, making them much tastier than when first harvested. Once cured, store them at 50° to 60°. The traditional advice is to put them under a bed in an unheated bedroom. ∎

Susan Peery is a regular contributor to Almanac publications.

THE OLD FARMER'S GUIDE TO
SEEDS, PLANTS, AND BULBS

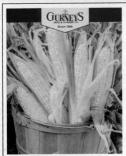
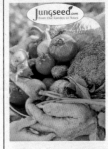
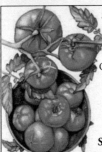
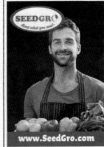
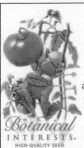
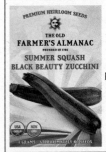
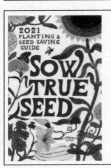
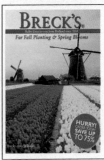
41

Dazzling Dahlias,
DARLINGS OF SUMMER

**DAZZLE US WITH
YOUR DAHLIAS!**
Post pics at
@ @theoldfarmersalmanac

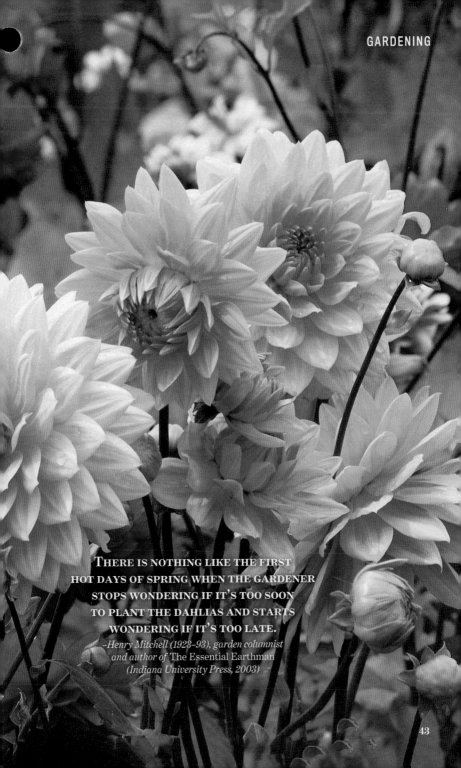

THERE IS NOTHING LIKE THE FIRST
HOT DAYS OF SPRING WHEN THE GARDENER
STOPS WONDERING IF IT'S TOO SOON
TO PLANT THE DAHLIAS AND STARTS
WONDERING IF IT'S TOO LATE.

–Henry Mitchell (1923–93), garden columnist
and author of The Essential Earthman
(Indiana University Press, 2003)

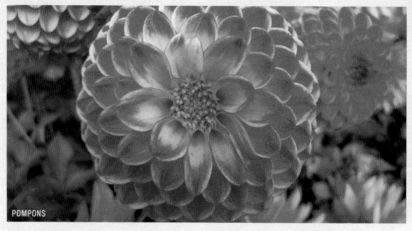

POMPONS

Dahlias have a place in any sunny garden with a growing season that's at least 120 days long.

Want to grow something spectacular? Plant dahlias. Unlike perennials and flowering shrubs, dahlias go from nothing to big in one season and make a sensational finish. As Scott Kunst, former proprietor of Old House Gardens in Ann Arbor, Michigan, once observed: "Dahlias get more and more charged up. They're like fireworks—they can animate and transform the garden."

Although not well suited to ex-

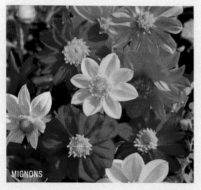

MIGNONS

tremely hot and humid climates (as in much of Texas and Florida), dahlias have a place in any sunny garden with a growing season that's at least 120 days long. Resolve to make your garden pop by planting dahlias now, because it may take you a while to choose a few from the amazing array of options—20,000 by one count!

These relatives of daisies and sunflowers brighten up the garden after so many ornamentals begin to wane. More important, there is a size—both in plant height and bloom dimension—to suit almost any situation or imagination.

COLOR YOUR WORLD

Picking a favorite dahlia is next to impossible for many people, so wildly varied are the blooms in color and form. The American Dahlia Society (ADS) recognizes 15 color categories, but the spectrum of flower colors includes all shades of white,

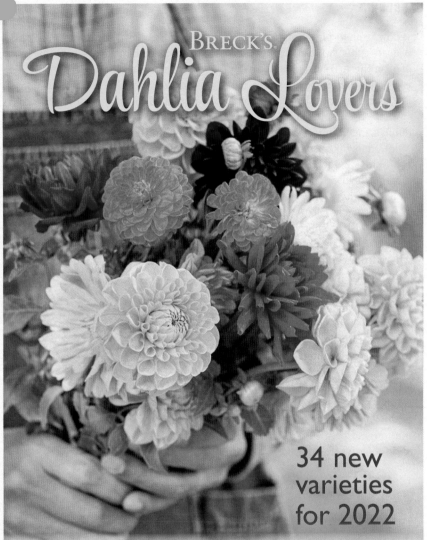

BRECK'S. Dahlia Lovers

34 new varieties for 2022

We offer an extensive selection of outstanding dahlia varieties—all grown in Holland and shipped directly to you. They produce lush, gorgeous, mid- to late-season blooms in a countless combination of colours, forms and sizes.

For a limited time, you can **save up to 75%** on your dahlia order from Breck's and **enjoy free shipping**. To claim this special offer, enter the code **DAHLIA22** at checkout!

Brecks.com/dahlialovers

yellow, orange, pink, red, purple, and bronze—plus two-tones and blends of all of these. (Blue dahlias don't exist.) A few dahlias bear a sweet, mellow scent, but most lack fragrance.

There are many classifications of dahlias, including . . .

- flat, daisylike, *single* and smaller (under 2 inches wide) *mignon* blooms, beloved by pollinators as well as planters
- *collarettes,* small to medium-size flowers with a short ruff of inner ("collar") petals, bred for everywhere from bedding to balcony
- *anemones,* prolific multipurpose plants with a wreath of petals evoking a pincushion
- lollipop-style, nearly round, 2-inch *pompons* and slightly larger but flatter *balls* that brighten beds, borders, and bouquets
- fantastically frilly *decoratives* in two bloom styles: *informal,* with generally flat petals in an irregular formation and best suited for borders and containers, and *formal,* with

regularly placed or perfectly packed petals, which make eye-catching arrangements as cut flowers
- *cactuses,* with dense cushions of quilled petals in profusions of blooms from 2 to 12 inches wide on stems up to 6 feet in height, which can play many roles
- the exotically delicate-looking and slightly fragrant *orchid* style, both single- and double-flower, which displays well in the ground, in containers, or in a vase
- *peony* dahlias, which yield multipetaled blossoms around prominent

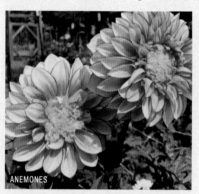

ANEMONES

Collarettes are bred for everywhere from bedding to balcony.

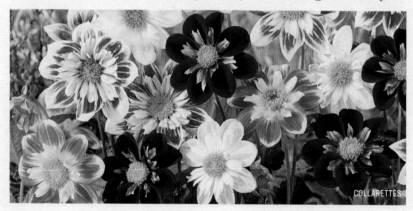

COLLARETTES

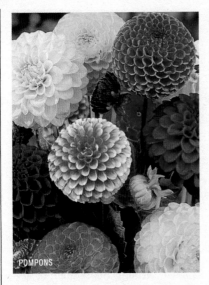

POMPONS

centers that are all the more striking above often blackish stems and foliage

PREP FOR PERFECTION

Dahlias prefer at least half a day of sun, fertile soil with good drainage, and a bit of protection from wind.

Don't be in a hurry to plant; dahlias will struggle in cold soil. Plant them shortly after tomato plants go in; in Zone 6, this is in early June. (Some gardeners start tubers indoors a month ahead to get a jump on the season.)

Avoid dahlia tubers that appear wrinkled or rotten. A little bit of green growth is a good sign.

Don't break or cut individual dahlia tubers as you would potatoes. Plant them whole, with the growing points, or "eyes," facing up, about 6 to 8 inches deep.

There's no need to water the soil

until the dahlia plants appear; in fact, overwatering can cause tubers to rot.

Dahlias tend to be tall plants that need anchoring. It's a good idea to plant a tuber with a sturdy stake right in the planting hole. Like many large-flower hybrids, the big dahlias may need extra attention before or after rain, when open blooms tend to fill up with water or take a beating from the wind.

FINDING A FEEDING PATTERN

Dahlias are heavy feeders and, arguably, finicky; it's difficult to generalize about fertilizing requirements from one region to another. Some professional growers advise feeding dahlias a month after they sprout with a low-nitrogen fertilizer, such as bonemeal or any 5-10-10 or 10-20-20 balanced product. Too much nitrogen (represented by the first number in the NPK formula) results in big leaves and stalks but not optimum flowering. A grower on Cape Cod (Mass.) for years noted that his

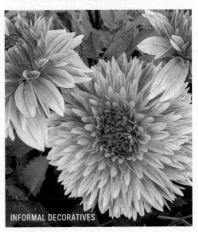

INFORMAL DECORATIVES

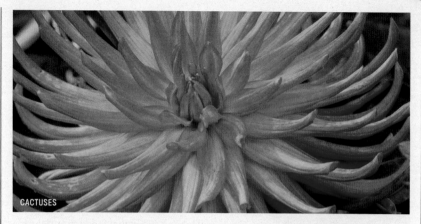

CACTUSES

In cold climates of North America, dahlias are known as tender perennials: They do not handle frost well.

dahlias needed more manure than he could conveniently supply, while an avid Maryland dahlia devotee claimed that gardeners who have sandy soil and frequent rain or irrigation need to be sure that they supply enough water-soluble nutrients (primarily potassium and sulfur) during the growing season. Be sure to withhold fertilizer about a month before frost; this will help the tubers to keep better over the winter.

BED BUG BITES

Dahlias sometimes fall prey to disease, frequently spread by mites and aphids. Pesky mites may appear on plants toward the end of summer; they start on the bottom of the plant, where they cause the leaves to yellow, and work their way up to the top. Leaves chewed by mites have a gritty feel. Remedies include spraying plants with conventional insecticides from mid-

August through September or using alternative soap sprays against mites and neem oil on aphids. Unfortunately, deer, slugs, and groundhogs may also discover the joy of a dahlia.

COLD STORAGE

In cold climates of North America, dahlias are known as tender perennials: They do not handle frost well. In cold regions (generally Zone 7 and northward), if you wish to save your plants, you have to dig up the tubers in early fall and store them over the winter.

To avoid the risk of injury to the tubers from the cold, cut back the foliage and dig up the plants before the first killing frost. Use a spading fork and gently shake the soil off the tubers. Cut rotten or mummified tubers off the clump and discard them. Don't let the tubers dry out too much before packing

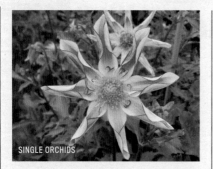

SINGLE ORCHIDS

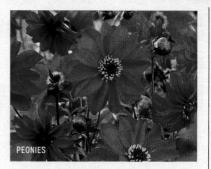

PEONIES

them up in some sort of loose, fluffy material. The possibilities for packing materials are many, including pet-shop animal bedding, coarse vermiculite, wood shavings, and newspaper. (For years, coarse peat moss was recommended, but the impact of its harvest on the environment has caused it to fall out of favor.) The ADS suggests common kitchen plastic wrap (see Dahlia.org for details). Bear in mind that what works in one case may not work in another, so experiment.

For storage over the winter, temperatures in the 40° to 45°F range are ideal, with 35° to 50° acceptable. Warmer conditions tend to cause rot, although shriveling seems to be a more common complaint.

Take out the tubers in the spring, separate them from the parent clump, swap favorites with friends, and begin again. Too much bother? You can skip digging and storing and just start over by buying new tubers in the spring. ■

–with assistance from Rosalie Davis

DAHLIA DIEHARDS GO THE DISTANCE(S)

The many-colored varieties of garden dahlias are hybrids, descendants of wild species with red to yellow single-flower heads that were first cultivated by the Aztecs. Botanical literature from the 16th century shows that they used the stems medicinally. Dahlia seeds were introduced to Europeans in the late 18th century through the Madrid (Spain) Royal Botanical Garden; although such efforts came to naught, it was hoped that the bitter but starchy tubers would serve as a food crop. By the mid-19th century, the acclaim generated by dahlias' ornamental qualities had led to the development of many garden varieties in England as well as continental Europe. This popularity spread back to America, where they remained a staple of flower gardens at least through the 1950s. Amazingly enough, in the early 1980s, horticultural trendsetters began to scoff at bold tropicals like dahlias in favor of more refined perennials and hardy bulbs. Nonetheless, true fans of these exuberant summer flowers have never forsaken them.

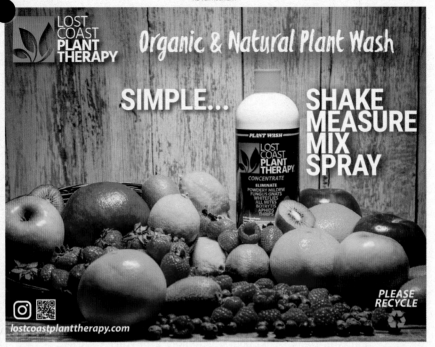
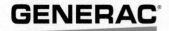
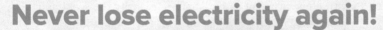
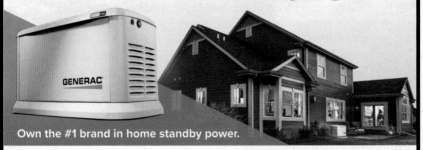

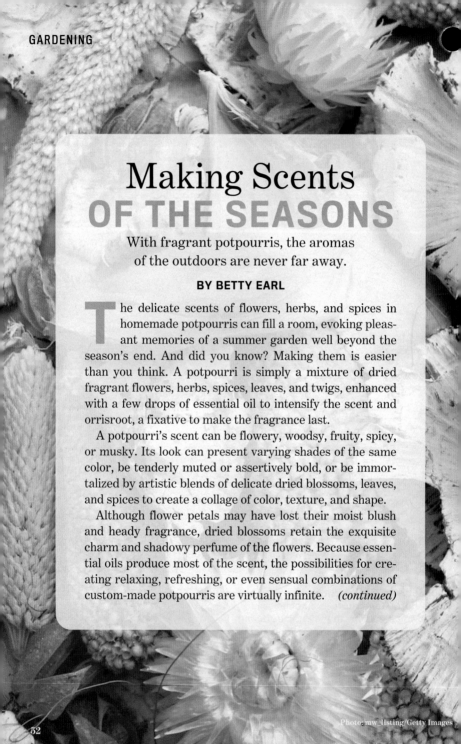

Making Scents
OF THE SEASONS

With fragrant potpourris, the aromas
of the outdoors are never far away.

BY BETTY EARL

The delicate scents of flowers, herbs, and spices in homemade potpourris can fill a room, evoking pleasant memories of a summer garden well beyond the season's end. And did you know? Making them is easier than you think. A potpourri is simply a mixture of dried fragrant flowers, herbs, spices, leaves, and twigs, enhanced with a few drops of essential oil to intensify the scent and orrisroot, a fixative to make the fragrance last.

A potpourri's scent can be flowery, woodsy, fruity, spicy, or musky. Its look can present varying shades of the same color, be tenderly muted or assertively bold, or be immortalized by artistic blends of delicate dried blossoms, leaves, and spices to create a collage of color, texture, and shape.

Although flower petals may have lost their moist blush and heady fragrance, dried blossoms retain the exquisite charm and shadowy perfume of the flowers. Because essential oils produce most of the scent, the possibilities for creating relaxing, refreshing, or even sensual combinations of custom-made potpourris are virtually infinite.   *(continued)*

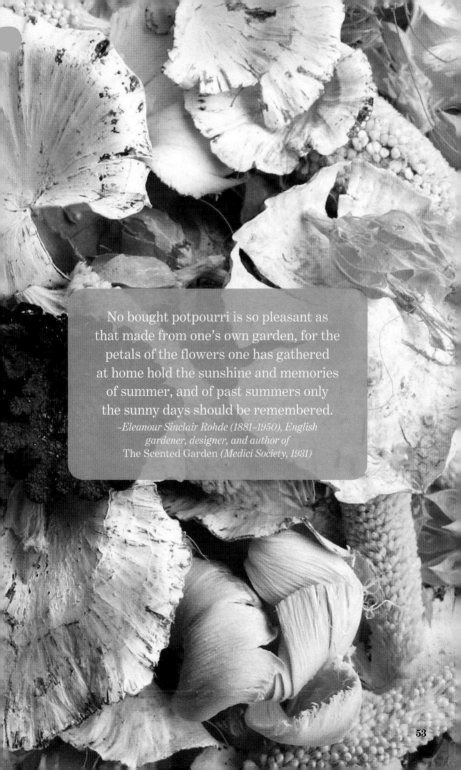

No bought potpourri is so pleasant as
that made from one's own garden, for the
petals of the flowers one has gathered
at home hold the sunshine and memories
of summer, and of past summers only
the sunny days should be remembered.

–Eleanour Sinclair Rohde (1881–1950), English
gardener, designer, and author of
The Scented Garden *(Medici Society, 1931)*

POPULAR POTPOURRIS

FLORAL

Rose, jasmine, and orange blossom are the primary scents of floral potpourris. They retain their scents when dried and are used for color and texture. Other fragrant favorites include heliotrope, honeysuckle, jonquil, lilac, lily-of-the-valley, mock orange, nicotiana, peony, pinks, dame's rocket, stock, violet, and sweet William. The best flowers for color are black-eyed Susan, borage, cornflower, delphinium, geranium, hydrangea, larkspur, marigold, nasturtium, periwinkle, poppy, and zinnia.

Pick flowers on a sunny day after the dew has evaporated. Use petal colors of yellow, pink, rose, and purple, which retain their colors best when dried. White petals can turn an unsightly brown, and some red flowers become very dark.

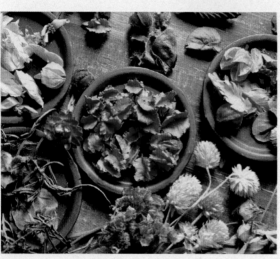

HERBAL

Pungently aromatic and heady, herbs add color, bulk, and texture. Lavender, the most popular herb, is almost a standard addition to most potpourri mixtures. Other good choices include sweet herbs such as the pink flower heads of chives; the leaves of artemisia, bay, lemon verbena, sage, and scented geranium; and the flowers and leaves of chamomile, hyssop, marjoram, monarda, oregano, sweet woodruff, and thyme. Consider also mentholated herbs, including eucalyptus, evergreen, and peppermint (but use these with discretion).

CITRUS

Peels of lemon, lime, orange, and tangerine are prized for their fresh, clean scents. If you don't have these growing at home, find what you need at the grocery store.

WOODLAND

Outdoorsy aromas come from ingredients that you can purchase or find in your neighborhood. Allspice berries, cardamom seeds, cinnamon sticks, cloves, coriander, cumin seeds, mace, nutmeg, star anise, and vanilla beans are all effective. Include bits of wood and cones, such as acorns, cedar wood shavings, gingerroot, sandalwood chips, and small cones from alder, larch, and pine. Don't forget colorful elderberries, hawthorn berries, juniper berries, and rose hips.

(continued)

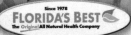

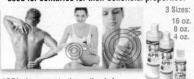
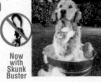
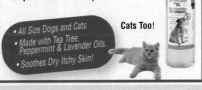
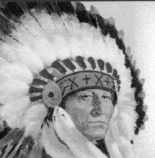

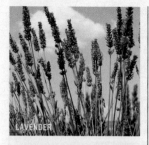
LAVENDER

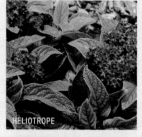
HELIOTROPE

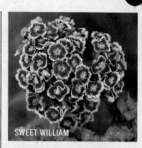
SWEET WILLIAM

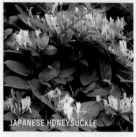
JAPANESE HONEYSUCKLE

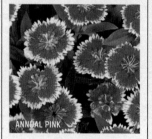
ANNUAL PINK

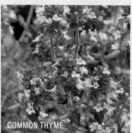
COMMON THYME

PLANT A POTPOURRI GARDEN

Make space in a bed or container to grow some of your own ingredients.

LAVENDER (*Lavandula angustifolia* 'Hidcote'): This perennial produces gray-green foliage and thick spikes of deep violet-blue blossoms in early summer. Grow it in full sun and average, well-drained, preferably alkaline soil. Give plants a light to medium trimming each spring just as new growth starts.

HELIOTROPE (*Heliotropium arborescens* 'Marine'): Producing flowers in a bewitching shade of dark violet-blue, this annual likes full sun and rich, well-drained soil.

SWEET WILLIAM (*Dianthus barbatus*): A biennial in the North, sweet William often behaves as a perennial in warmer areas. It's prized for its sweet-scented small flowers and densely packed heads. Plant in full sun and average to rich soil.

JAPANESE HONEYSUCKLE (*Lonicera japonica* 'Halliana'): Although this climbing perennial vine can become a rampant pest, its hauntingly fragrant pure white flowers turn soft yellow with age. Provide it with a fence or pergola and plant in sun or shade and rich, well-drained soil.

ANNUAL PINK (*Dianthus chinensis* 'Telstar Picotee'): A fast grower, this easy annual produces white-edged red flowers in great profusion. Plant it in full sun and well-drained, alkaline soil and pick the flowers diligently to encourage a long season of bloom.

COMMON THYME (*Thymus vulgaris*): Use both the aromatic foliage and rose-purple flowers of this perennial herb. It prefers full sun and well-drained soil.

(continued on page 196)

Photos, clockwise from top left: Pixabay; Gratysanna/Getty Images; Pixabay; Pixabay; All-America Selections; Aftabbanoori/Wikimedia

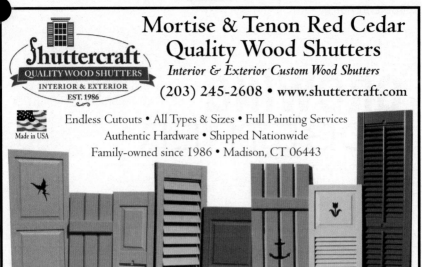
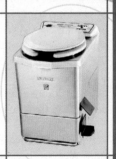

GROWING
TOGETHER

FARMERS SHARE THEIR STORIES, INSPIRATION, DREAMS, AND ADVICE.

By Stacey Kusterbeck
and Karen Davidson

SU'S FARMING
SIMCOE, ONTARIO

"If I'm awake, I'm working," says Henry Su, a Canadian-born Chinese farmer. He grew up on his immigrant parents' farm in Simcoe and while a teenager enjoyed a career as a competitive figure skater.

Figure eights behind him, he's continuing the family brand started 30 years ago; today, he nurtures 7 to 10 acres of eggplants (aka aubergines) and several more of zucchini.

Producing eggplants with perfectly glossy purple skin is a summerlong challenge. As Su explains, wind-whipped leaves can easily scratch the fruit's complexion, so about midseason, the lower leaves are removed by hand to ensure the produce's appeal to the diverse population of the Toronto area.

While Italians seem to favor thick-skin Sicilian varieties of eggplant, Asians prefer the thin, violet-color Chinese long varieties or round, midnight-purple Indian eggplants for their softer flesh. These are also in demand by the green grocers and restaurateurs who buy wholesale at the Ontario Food Terminal—or at least did until the COVID-19 virus struck.

Restaurants closed. Neighborhood stores had little foot traffic. Zucchini and aubergines had no takers. Su was skating on thin ice.

"In 2019, the buyers said, 'We can take all of the zucchini that you can grow.' In 2020, we couldn't give it away," says Su wistfully.

While pandemic economics saw eggplants and zucchini fall out of favor for food businesses, Su continues to hope that consumers will try more adventuresome ingredients in home cooking. Asian eggplant is an appealing option.

"Eggplant is the perfect vessel for flavor,' says Su, who remains determined to carry on.

After all, one bad year is a blip in the history of the eggplant, which has been grown in China since at least the T'ang dynasty—A.D. 618. Undaunted, Su plans to perpetuate its legacy.

(continued)

Photo: Su's Farming

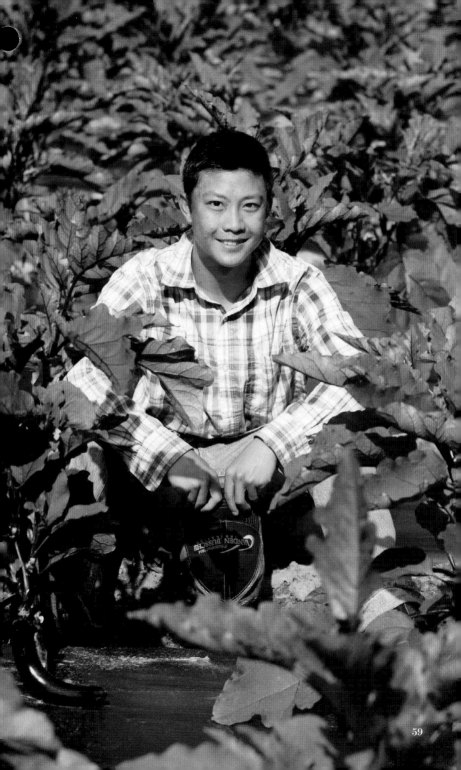

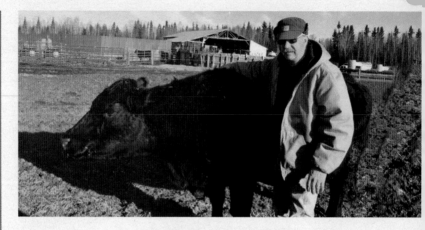

MUGRAGE HAY & CATTLE
DELTA JUNCTION, ALASKA

With experience in the South and Midwest behind him, veteran cattleman Scott Mugrage at first had little interest when in 2013 his son pointed out an ad for a 550-acre farm in Alaska—but he couldn't get the idea out of his mind. Both the challenge and the slower-paced lifestyle sounded appealing. Mugrage traveled to see the place in an uncharacteristically warm late July and was struck by the extraordinary beauty of the site, with mountains on both sides of a valley. "In every direction you look, it's like a photograph on the wall," observes Mugrage.

His operation now boasts the largest private herd of cattle (650 Black Angus and Scottish Highland) in the state and is its only large-scale finisher of beef as well as biggest beef supplier. Most is sold wholesale. The farm produces most of the grain needed to keep the herd fed through 7-month winters, but they buy from local producers, too.

While Mugrage found ways to cope with Alaska's short growing seasons and abundant wildlife, the lack of infrastructure to support agriculture turned out to be more daunting. "All of our input costs are higher, from fuel to fertilizer to parts," he notes. "Most of our equipment is from an era that allows us to still work on it, and we just keep repairing it."

Still, Mugrage sees potential everywhere: He continually tries new crops in order to improve soil quality and eliminate weeds. "There is so much good-quality land and such a diverse variety of crops," he says. "I can see Alaska becoming the breadbasket of the nation."

Experiential agritourism is promising. In the works is a cattle drive across the wilderness. "Riders will travel hundreds of miles and likely never cross privately owned land," he says. "That's something you can't do in the Lower 48." *(continued)*

Photo: Mugrage Hay & Cattle

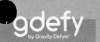

KALALA ORGANIC ESTATE WINERY
WEST KELOWNA, BRITISH COLUMBIA

Karnail Sidhu is that rarest of grape growers: He is intolerant of alcohol. "I do taste, but I don't drink," he says, savoring a 2019 award from the British Columbia Grapegrowers' Association as viticulturalist of the year.

Fortunately, Sidhu's aversion to alcohol has not detoured a 30-year career path that started with a post as an electrical engineer in India's Punjab state and has now evolved to include the role of Canadian vineyard/winery owner.

Today, his combined 70-acre organic vineyards, Oliver and Osoyoos, are known for their viticulture practices. One intervention is to hand-pull the lower leaves of the grapevines in mid-June. By this time of year, leafhoppers have laid eggs on the undersides of the leaves. If they are allowed to hatch, the leaves will be sucked dry of nutrients.

While his workers remove the hosts of these voracious pests, Sidhu allows other beneficial insects to thrive in the unmowed grass lanes that burst with spring dandelions. While the vineyards may appear unruly, they are thriving with plant and insect diversity.

"We work with the ecosystem in the vineyards," notes Sidhu. "We deal with whatever comes from nature."

Besides his capable hand at canopy management, Sidhu has a nose for wine—and specifically for the aromas that might signal a fermentation process gone awry. A whiff of wet dog, for example, or rotten eggs will tell him that there may not be enough oxygen for yeast to survive. Early detection of such defects can be fixed by his winemaker.

Since 2008, Kalala Organic Estate Winery has produced a number of acclaimed vintages, including a Chardonnay ice wine. However, it turns out that Sidhu's favorite is Zweigelt, a disease-resistant, medium-body red first cultivated in Austria. "It's our signature sip," he reports. *(continued)*

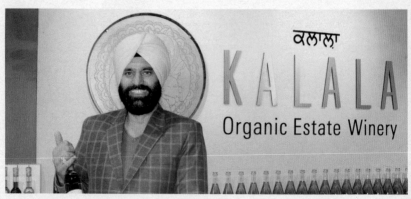

कलाला

KALALA
Organic Estate Winery

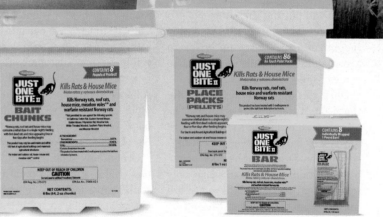

The taste rats and house mice just die for!®

JUST ONE BITE II

Rodents in your barn aren't up to anything good. Put an end to feed contamination and waste, damage to equipment and electrical wiring, and risk of serious disease.

It's time to take action with **Just One Bite®* II** rodent bait made especially for agricultural use to effectively control rodents and help prevent reinfestation.

Reclaim your barn! Visit justonebitebrand.com to find a retail location near you.

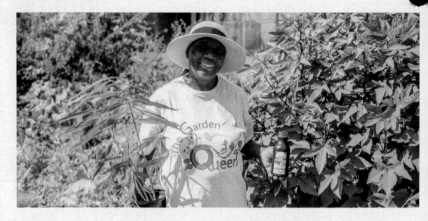

WEST END COMMUNITY GARDEN
ATLANTA, GEORGIA

After moving to New York City from Jamaica at age 14, Haylene Green ("The Garden Queen") found her favorite pastime to be breaking off small pieces of plants and putting them into pots to see if they would grow. "I was never taught to farm. I grew up loving to grow things," recalls Green, who comes from a long line of farmers.

During a family reunion in Atlanta, the region's plentiful trees caught her attention. "I assumed that they were for fruit or bark or leaves for eating," says Green. Drawn to the good growing conditions, she moved south, only to find that the trees that she had admired weren't for edibles after all.

Green searched at markets for the tropical produce of her childhood—not just to eat, but also for its seeds. Soon, turmeric, tropical pumpkins, pomegranates, persimmons, ackee, breadfruit, and peach, plum, and pear trees were springing up on her half-acre plot of land.

"I was just growing for fun—people were the ones who turned it into a business," recalls Green. Passersby took note of the fruit; some offered money for them. Green soon set up a small stand to sell her hibiscus sorrel tea—after a free sample and conversation, one customer offered her a grant from the Southern Foodways Alliance. The money allowed her to build a greenhouse and hire some help. With the first harvest, neighbors became customers.

Green now sells fruit and vegetables, the tea, and tropical pumpkin soup at five farmers' markets. Over 300 schoolchildren have visited the farm, where a "garden therapy" program also connects seniors with young people. Green never tires of teaching the joys of growing healthy food. "As long as I am alive," she vows, "I am going to be teaching the young ones how to grow." *(continued)*

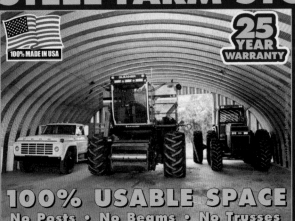
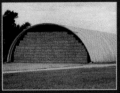

65

TEES BEES
TEES, ALBERTA

Home to about 300,000 beehives in 2019, the province of Alberta is the largest honey producer in Canada. The COVID-19 crisis threatened this distinction when borders closed, delaying international shipments of queen bees as well as the travel of temporary foreign workers and completely halting imported replacement stock.

The year 2020 was the second bad one in a row for overwintering survival and honey production, says Jeremy Olthof, president of the Alberta

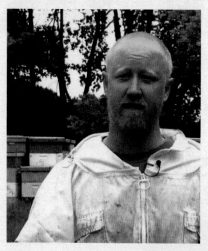

Beekeepers Commission. In 2019, a wet, cool spring delayed the foraging of bees. In 2020, the delay of trained seasonal workers compounded the stress. Of eight Mexican workers booked, only six arrived at Olthof's Tees, Alberta, farm.

Many of these workers have a

decade of experience in the care of bee "livestock" (bees are considered food producers). Explains Olthof: "It requires an early, 1:00 A.M. rise to move the hives in the cool of night and drive 3 to 4 hours before even working the bees."

Starting in late June, the men round up nearly a quarter of Olthof's beehives and move them to pollinate hybrid canola fields. Honeybee hives are placed in the dryland corners of irrigated fields at a stocking density of one per acre, depending on whether leafcutting bees (an important native pollinator) are placed throughout the field as well. Then the honeybees fan out to forage among the yellow-petal blooms. From mid-July through September, the workers are busy extracting honey from the hives' frames.

Olthof's goal is 150 pounds of honey per hive. In 2020, he did not expect to meet it: "We'll be lucky to get 120 pounds of honey per hive," he observed that October. This low forecast stung, but there was a balm: higher prices of $1.80 to $2.00 per pound, up from $1.40. Olthof's bottom line was also cushioned by another source of revenue: His bees pollinate commercial hybrid seed canola.

While ups and downs are part of the profession, the beekeeper takes comfort in knowing that canola country will continue to be an annual opportunity for his apiary.

RESENDIZ BROTHERS PROTEA GROWERS
FALLBROOK, CALIFORNIA

In his two decades of working on a protea ("sugarbush") farm (eventually becoming manager) after immigrating from Mexico with his three brothers, Ismael "Mel" Resendiz learned to grow—and love—the huge and bright but little-known blooms. In 1999, he started his own operation on a 10-acre parcel. "I never considered doing anything else," says Resendiz. "I love what I am doing."

Sales were slow at first, with just a few local wholesalers as customers. Then Resendiz devised a new marketing strategy: Over a few years, he showed off his own protea varieties (created by cross-pollinating flowers and grafting ones he especially liked onto more vigorous root stock) at trade shows and also began serving as president of both the California and International Protea Associations.

Soon the farm was shipping flowers throughout the state and nationally, as well as to Canada, China, Korea, and Japan. Today, it consists of some 250 acres across 15 parcels; some of the land is very steep, but it has the good drainage that the flowers require. Finding good labor and growing in extreme weather (up to 120°F in summer) are constant challenges. On the hottest days, Resendiz works day and night to irrigate the plants.

During the pandemic, special events slowed to a trickle. Fortunately, online sales boomed, fueled by social media posts of gorgeous protea arrangements. "More people are buying direct, which is better, because they get fresher flowers," Resendiz reports. A typical order was once hundreds of boxes of flowers shipped to a wholesaler—now, it's more often a single bouquet sent to someone's home.

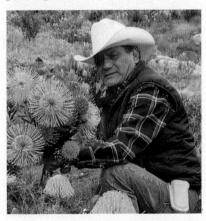

Answering dozens of phone calls from customers each day requires friendliness, patience, and plenty of time. "But you have to go where the business is," says business manager Diana Roy. Their proteas are sold at only one farmers' market currently, but others are knocking at their door. "Our goal is to teach people about proteas," says Roy. "Food feeds the body, but flowers feed the soul." ■

U.S. profiles are by **Stacey Kusterbeck**, a regular contributor to the Almanac. Canadian profiles are by **Karen Davidson**, editor of *The Grower*, a leading Canadian horticultural magazine, and frequent contributor to the Almanac.

FOUR SEASONS OF GREAT TASTE

BY SARAH PERREAULT, ALMANAC FOOD EDITOR

Whether fall, winter, spring, or summer, each season brings its own bounty of flavors and benefits. Not only do fresh fruit and vegetables taste better in season, but also they are often more nutritious than produce that has been stored for weeks or even months. Choose and use each season's best with a little help from these recipes. As the year rolls along, be sure to check out additional seasonal recipes by searching for key ingredients at Almanac.com/Cooking.

FALL
PUMPKIN PICKLES

Use a "cooking" type of pumpkin—usually called "sugar pumpkins" or "pie pumpkins." They're round and small.

4 cups pumpkin, peeled and cut into bite-size cubes
1½ cups sugar
1½ cups apple cider vinegar
10 whole cloves
2 sticks cinnamon

Steam pumpkin until barely tender, about 10 minutes (don't let pumpkin touch the boiling water or it will get mushy). Drain thoroughly and set aside.

In a saucepan, combine sugar, vinegar, cloves, and cinnamon and simmer, covered, for 20 minutes. Add pumpkin, return to a simmer, cover, and cook for 3 minutes more. Remove from heat and leave pumpkin in the syrup; refrigerate for 24 hours.

Heat mixture to simmering and cook for 5 minutes. Remove spices and pack pumpkin into sterilized pint jars, then fill with the syrup. Seal and process for 10 minutes in a boiling water bath.

Makes about 3 pints.

(continued)

WHAT'S IN SEASON?

This depends on where you live. Your local farmers' markets and co-ops will always have the best tastes of the season. Also, many grocery stores now have an "in season" area in the produce section.

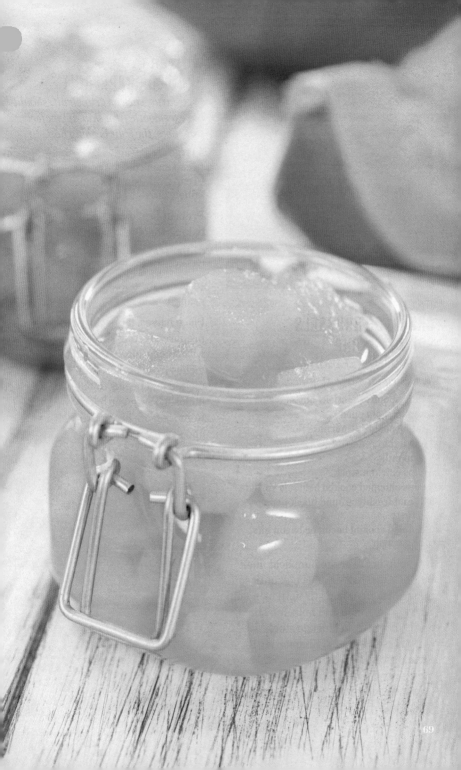

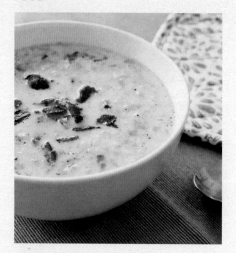

FALL
CREAM OF BRUSSELS SPROUTS SOUP

Brussels sprouts have more flavor if harvested after a frost or two.

4 tablespoons (½ stick) butter
2 shallots, chopped
3 tablespoons all-purpose flour
1 cup light cream
½ cup milk
5 cups chicken stock
4 cups chopped cooked brussels sprouts
salt and freshly ground black pepper, to taste
crumbled cooked bacon or bacon bits, for garnish

In a soup pot over medium heat, melt butter. Add shallots and cook until soft. Sprinkle in flour and stir until blended. Slowly add cream and milk and stir until smooth. Add chicken stock and brussels sprouts. Simmer for 10 minutes, uncovered. Do not boil. Taste, then season with salt and pepper. Garnish each serving with bacon.

Makes 4 to 6 servings.

WINTER
BROILED GRAPEFRUIT

Ripe citrus, such as grapefruit, should have a smooth, firm skin. If you feel soft spots, the fruit is going bad.

4 large grapefruit
¼ cup maple or white sugar
¼ cup fresh mint, whole leaves or finely diced

Preheat broiler to high. Line a baking sheet with aluminum foil.

Cut a thin slice of rind (don't cut into fruit) off each end of grapefruit so that halves will lie flat. Cut grapefruit in half.

Place halves, large cut sides up, on prepared baking sheet. Sprinkle with maple sugar. Cook 3 to 4 inches from broiler, until sugar has melted and begins to bubble. Watch it closely, as sugar burns easily. Remove from broiler, top with mint, and serve.

Makes 8 servings.

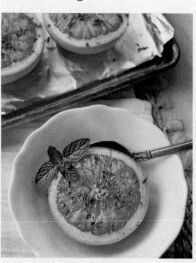

Photos: Samantha Jones/Quinn Brein Communications

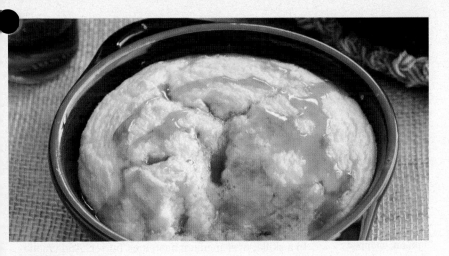

WINTER
TURNIP SOUFFLÉ

Turnips can be eaten raw, baked, boiled, roasted, or mashed.
Try them as an alternative to potatoes.

1 pound turnips, peeled and cut into chunks
½ cup heavy cream
2 whole cloves
1 bay leaf
pinch of freshly grated nutmeg
4 tablespoons (½ stick) unsalted butter
3 tablespoons all-purpose flour
pinch of kosher salt
pinch of white pepper (optional)
4 eggs, separated
maple syrup, for serving

Preheat oven to 375°F. Butter six 6-ounce ramekin dishes.

In a pot of boiling salted water, cook turnips for 20 minutes, or until tender. Drain and pat dry. Press through a food mill or ricer. Set aside.

In a saucepan over medium heat, combine cream, cloves, bay leaf, and nutmeg. When cream is scalded, strain it and discard the solids.

In a separate saucepan over medium heat, melt butter. Whisk in flour and cook for 1 minute. Whisk in strained cream, half at a time. Whisk in turnips. Cook, stirring constantly, until mixture thickens. Season with salt and white pepper (if using). Cool to room temperature.

In a bowl, beat egg yolks. Fold in one-third of the turnip mixture. Fold in remaining turnip mixture.

In a chilled bowl, beat egg whites until stiff. Fold egg whites into turnip mixture.

Spoon mixture into prepared dishes and place on a baking sheet. Bake for 18 to 20 minutes, or until soufflés are browned and rise 1 inch or more.

Serve with maple syrup.

Makes 6 servings.   *(continued)*

SPRING
RISOTTO WITH ASPARAGUS AND SCALLOPS

Asparagus does not keep for very long after it's picked,
so be sure to eat it within 2 to 3 days of harvest.

1 bunch asparagus, trimmed and cut into 2-inch pieces

½ pound bay or sea scallops

6 to 8 cups chicken broth

3 tablespoons butter

1 onion, chopped

1½ cups arborio rice

2 tablespoons heavy cream

½ cup grated Parmesan cheese

salt and freshly ground black pepper, to taste

Steam asparagus briefly and set aside. For thin asparagus, this will take only 3 to 5 minutes. The pieces should be bright green in color and just slightly tender (not hard).

In a saucepan, bring 3 cups of lightly salted water to a boil. Add scallops and cook (poach) until white and firm. Drain, set aside, and keep warm.

In a separate saucepan, heat chicken broth.

In a skillet over medium heat, melt butter. Add onions and sauté until soft. Add rice to the skillet, reduce heat, and stir for 3 minutes. Add hot broth, half a cup at a time, stirring until liquid is absorbed before adding more. Continue cooking and stirring for about 20 minutes, or until rice is tender. Remove from heat. Add cream, Parmesan, scallops, and asparagus. Season with salt and pepper.

Makes 8 servings. *(continued on page 198)*

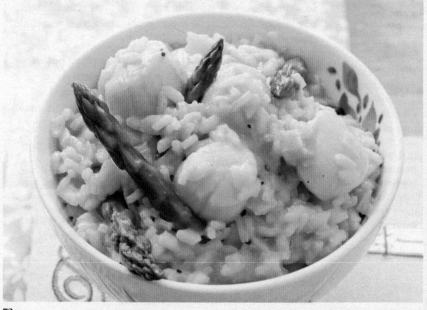

Photo: Becky Luigart-Stayner

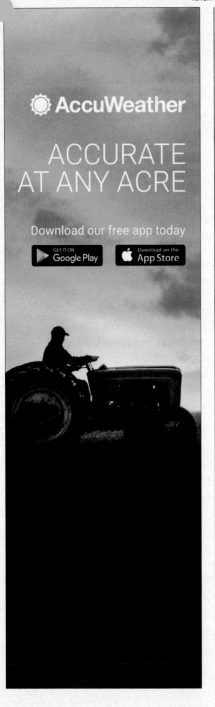
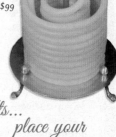
73

RECIPE CONTEST WINNERS

Last year, we asked you for your best recipes using five or fewer ingredients (salt and pepper excluded), and we received a record amount of entries! Our most sincere thanks go out to all of you who took the time to enter.

**STYLING AND PHOTOGRAPHY:
SAMANTHA JONES/QUINN BREIN COMMUNICATIONS**

FIRST PRIZE: $300

APRICOT SRIRACHA-GLAZED BABY BACK RIBS

4 to 5 pounds baby back pork ribs
2 tablespoons Cajun spice blend
¾ cup apricot preserves
1 tablespoon sriracha sauce
1 tablespoon soy sauce

Remove ribs from packaging and rinse with cold water. Pat dry with paper towels. Rub Cajun spice all over the ribs. Place in a large baking pan and cover tightly with foil. Keep in the refrigerator for 4 hours, or overnight. Bring to room temperature 30 minutes before cooking.

Preheat oven to 325°F.

Leave baking pan covered and bake for 1½ hours.

While ribs are cooking, combine apricot preserves, sriracha, and soy sauce in a saucepan over medium heat. Cook for 3 minutes, stirring frequently, until melted and syrupy.

Remove ribs from the oven and brush with the glaze, reserving about ½ cup. Increase oven temp to 375°F and cook ribs, uncovered, for an additional 30 to 40 minutes, or until meat falls off the bone easily. Brush with the remaining sauce and serve immediately.

Makes 6 servings.

–Pamela Gelsomini, Wrentham, Massachusetts

(continued)

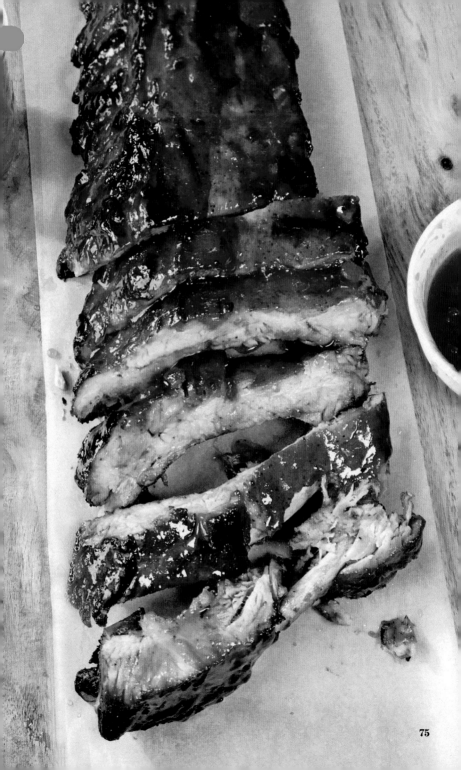

SECOND PRIZE: $200

EASY LATTE TRUFFLES

¾ cup white chocolate chips

¾ cup heavy whipping cream

2 teaspoons instant coffee granules

1 cup milk chocolate melting wafers, divided

Line a standard loaf pan with parchment paper.

Place white chocolate chips in a heatproof bowl.

In a saucepan over medium heat, warm the cream. Add instant coffee and mix well until combined. Once cream starts to bubble, turn off heat and pour over white chocolate chips. Let sit for a few minutes, then stir until the white chocolate chips are melted. Continue stirring until mixture thickens and resembles a very sticky dough.

Transfer truffle mixture to the prepared pan and press with a spatula to even out. Let sit at room temperature for 1 to 2 hours, or until set.

Lift parchment paper out of baking pan and cut truffles into desired shapes.

In the top of a double boiler, melt ½ cup of chocolate wafers. Once they are fully melted, remove from heat and add in remaining ½ cup of chocolate wafers. Stir until melted.

Using a fork or spoon, dip truffles in melted chocolate, then place on parchment paper. If desired, melt more white chocolate chips and decorate the truffles. Let sit at room temperature for 2 to 4 hours, or until set. Store in an airtight container for up to 3 days.

Makes 16 pieces.

–Kiran Upadhyayula, Folsom, California
(continued)

ENTER THE 2022 RECIPE CONTEST: BANANAS

Got a great recipe using bananas (that's not banana bread!)?
Send it in and it could win! See contest rules on page 251.

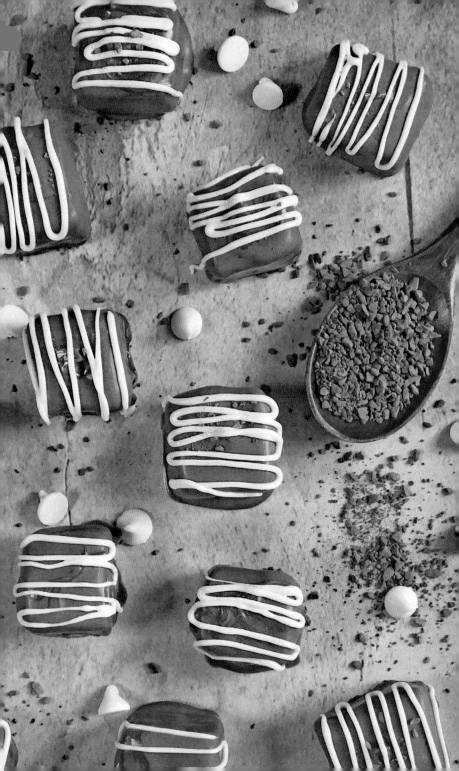

THIRD PRIZE: $100

PESTO RICOTTA WITH ASPARAGUS ON TOAST

1 cup ricotta
cheese

¼ cup plus
2 teaspoons
basil pesto

salt and freshly
ground black
pepper, to
taste

16 asparagus
spears

4 slices hearty
white, whole
wheat, or
Panella bread

4 eggs

In a bowl, combine ricotta, ¼ cup of pesto, and salt and pepper.

Break ends off asparagus. Place spears in a shallow, nonstick pan with a lid. Add enough water to just cover asparagus. Cover and cook over medium-high heat for 6 to 8 minutes, or until crisp tender. Remove asparagus from water and blot with paper towels to dry. Sprinkle with salt and pepper. Drain water from pan and set aside for cooking the eggs.

While asparagus is cooking, toast bread slices in a toaster or under the broiler until golden brown.

Put remaining 2 teaspoons of pesto into the pan and spread out evenly. Over medium-high heat, cook eggs for about 1 to 2 minutes on one side and 30 seconds to 1 minute on the other. (You want the yolk to be runny.)

Spread one-quarter of the ricotta mixture on top of a piece of toast, then add four asparagus spears and top with an egg. Repeat for the rest of the pieces of toast. **Makes 4 servings.**

–Renee Seaman, Andover, New Jersey

(continued on page 200)

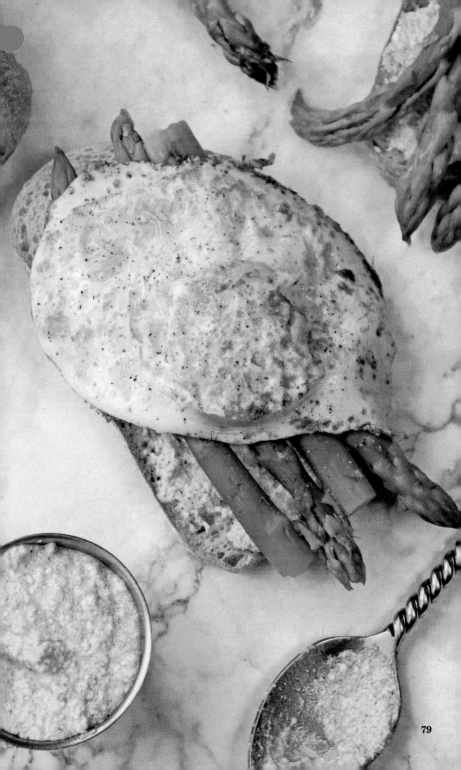

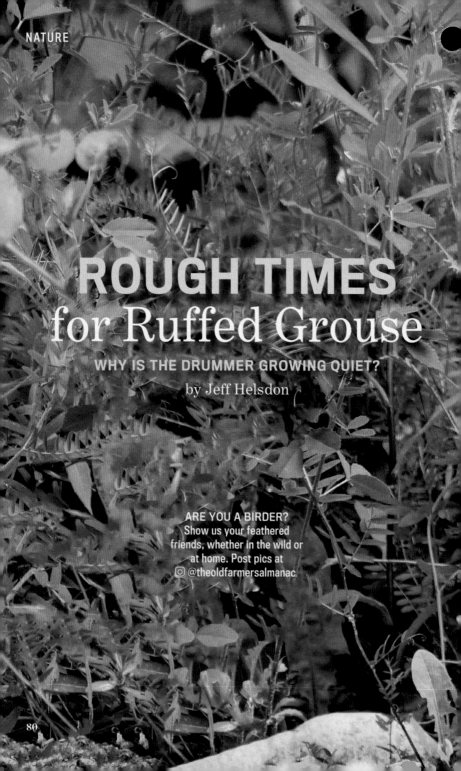

ROUGH TIMES
for Ruffed Grouse

WHY IS THE DRUMMER GROWING QUIET?

by Jeff Helsdon

ARE YOU A BIRDER?
Show us your feathered
friends, whether in the wild or
at home. Post pics at
@theoldfarmersalmanac

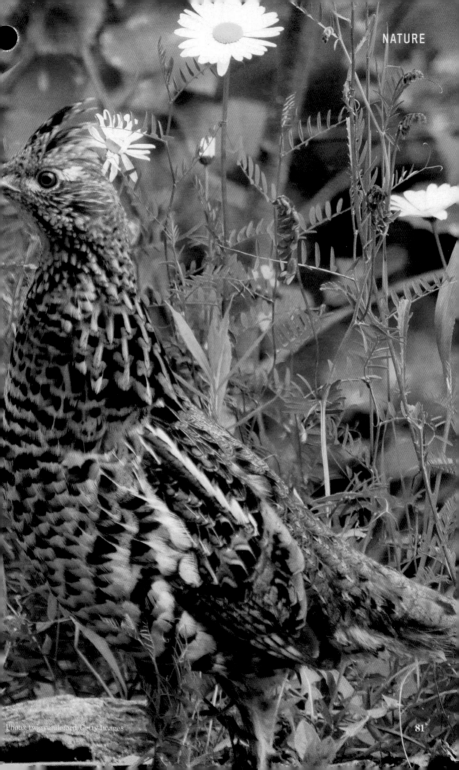

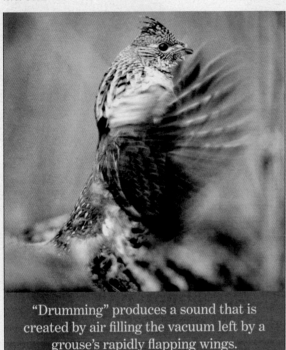

"Drumming" produces a sound that is created by air filling the vacuum left by a grouse's rapidly flapping wings.

Like the call of the loon, the sound of a ruffed grouse's drumming echoing through woodlots has an almost mystical quality that speaks of wild places. Starting slowly at first, the pace picks up before stopping, beating a rhythm that is eons old.

Drumming is the mating call of the ruffed grouse, intended to attract females and ward off other males. Called (in translation) the "carpenter bird" by some Native Americans because they thought that the bird was beating its wing against the log where drumming takes place, the bird produces a sound that is actually more like a sonic boom created by air filling the vacuum left by its rapidly flapping wings.

While this sound was once a commonplace sign of spring, it is being heard less and less across the ruffed grouse's range. Knowing more about the ruffed grouse is the key to understanding its plight.

A "RUFF" LIFE

The most common upland game bird in North America, the ruffed grouse has a range that stretches from Alaska and the Yukon Territory in the north down across the American Midwest to the Appalachians.

Average ruffed grouse are about 16 to 19 inches in length and weigh 17 to 25 ounces, or about 1 to 1½ pounds. Their main background color can be either gray or reddish brown. "Ruff" refers to the male's darker-color neck feathers, which are puffed out when the bird is displaying to a hen or defending its territory. A darker band is also found on the tail of both sexes, in both color phases.

One unique adaptation that grouse have to survive the winter is small lateral extensions of the scales on their feet that act like snowshoes.

(continued)

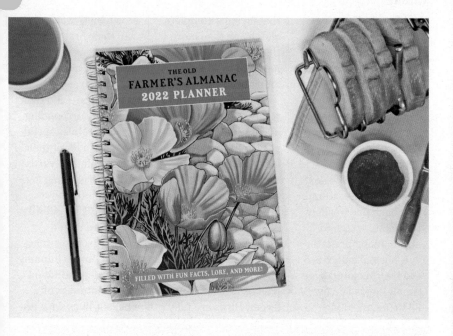
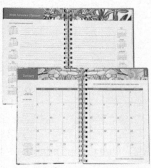
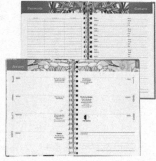

After finding a drumming male and participating in a brief courtship, the hen searches for a nest site. Ruffed grouse are ground-nesting birds, usually making their nests in a hollowed depression in leaves. Nests are usually next to a tree trunk, stump, or a bush pile to allow the hen to watch for approaching predators.

A normal clutch is 8 to 14 buff-colored eggs. A new egg is laid every 36 hours, meaning that laying a complete clutch can take more than 2 weeks. Chicks hatch 24 to 26 days after the last egg is laid.

At hatching, ruffed grouse chicks are about the size of a person's thumb. Chicks leave the nest after they dry off and begin feeding themselves immediately. The young birds eat insects in the first few weeks, before gradually switching to plants and fruit as they become larger. Birds are fully grown by 17 weeks.

In their first fall, young males start looking for a drumming log—ideally, a fallen mature tree—and then claim the surrounding territory. Males spend the remainder of their lives within 300 yards of their drumming log.

CHALLENGES ABOUND

The ruffed grouse's reaction to humans varies, depending on the remoteness of where it lives with its

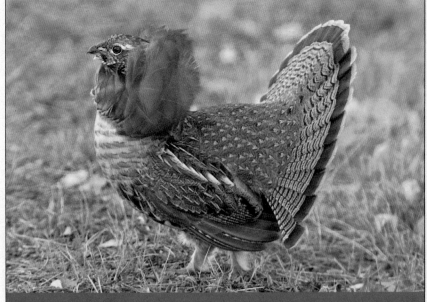

"Ruff" refers to the male's darker-color neck feathers, which puff out when it's displaying to a hen or defending its territory.

GROW BETTER WITH A HAND FROM US!

Created for aspiring growers, novices, green thumbs, and old hands alike, The Old Farmer's Almanac *gardening publications and programs always root for your success!*

Vegetable Gardener's Handbook

"Down-to-earth" guidance on cultivating, harvesting, and storing 30+ veggies, plus advice on soil, water, fertilizer, seed-saving, pests, and more

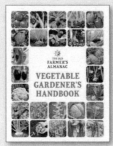

Gardening Webinars

Exclusive: Experts share techniques and tips for beginning gardens, container plants, attracting pollinators, thwarting pests, hydroponics, and more, both live and recorded for later reference

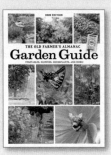

Garden Guide

120+ inspiring pages on edibles and ornamentals, landscaping and decorating, and new products and DIY projects, plus recipes and essential reference tables

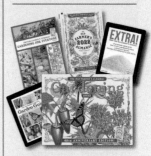

EARLY SPRING 2022—Flower Gardener's Handbook

Essential information about growing 30+ blooming plants and shrubs, plus advice on native plants, pollinators, plot-planning, cutting and drying flowers, easy maintenance, and more

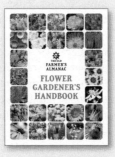

The Gardening Club

Exclusive (U.S. only): Members get the annual *Old Farmer's Almanac,* best-selling Gardening Calendar, *Gardening for Everyone* magazine, and *EXTRA!* monthly e-magazine

PRINT PRODUCTS AVAILABLE WHEREVER BOOKS AND MAGAZINES ARE SOLD. ONLINE, GO TO ALMANAC.COM OR AMAZON. FOR WEBINARS AND CLUB, VISIT ALMANAC.COM.

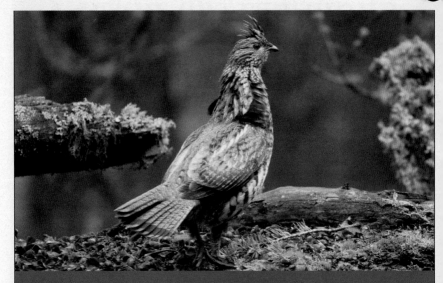

Grouse thrive in areas with a comparatively greater number of tree stems per acre of forest. An important component of grouse habitat is a fallen mature tree for drumming.

surroundings. In more populated areas, it will hold perfectly still, hoping that its camouflage will conceal it, before bursting into the air in a heart-stopping flush. The same bird is unafraid of humans in remote areas and can be approached to within feet.

The grouse was an important food source for early settlers and still is in northern areas. Its natural predators include the bobcat, fisher, fox, goshawk, and great horned owl.

Ruffed grouse are a bird of secondary growth or early transitional forest, although they use all forest stages. They thrive in areas with a comparatively greater number of tree stems per acre of forest. An important component of grouse habitat is a fallen mature tree for drumming.

A serious problem is that young forest is disappearing from the United States and southern parts of Canada. This type of forest is caused by clear-cutting, a practice that is often frowned upon, and fire, which is suppressed. As the forest matures, young forest growth diminishes. To have good habitat for grouse as well as other species dependent on early successional (age-diverse) forest, repeated disturbances are needed. However, there is a societal swing toward managing for mature forestland.

(continued)

START EACH DAY WITH A SMILE!

Just like this Almanac, our free **DAILY ALMANAC** newsletter is "useful, with a pleasant degree of humor"!

Written by the editors of this Almanac, this daily email arrival is full of ideas and inspirations that are specific to each day, including verse and timely articles on the topics you love—weather, gardening, nature, astronomy, recipes, natural remedies, humor, and more. The **DAILY ALMANAC**, sent straight to your Inbox first thing in the morning, will get you thinking about, talking, sharing, and doing things that brighten your day.

PLUS . . .

With the **DAILY ALMANAC**, you'll be the first to know when new Almanac publications and products are available and get details on exclusive special offers—like this one: Sign up now for the **DAILY ALMANAC**, and you will receive our free *Beginner Gardening Guide!*

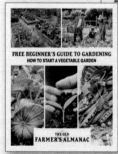

Make every "Good morning!" even better with Almanac wit and wisdom!

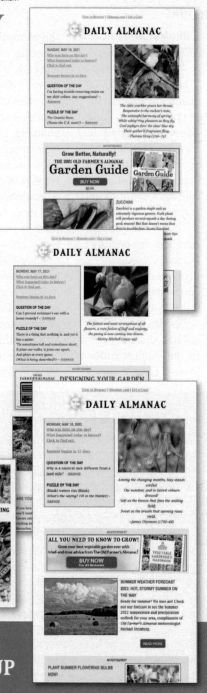

Sign up today! Go to
ALMANAC.COM/SIGNUP

87

A DRUMBEAT OF ALARM

The situation is dire. Grouse are listed as a species of concern in 18 states, and Indiana has recently listed the bird as an endangered species. (Grouse were once found in all of Indiana's counties but can now be found in only a few.) While grouse numbers are healthy in most Canadian provinces, there is concern in southern Ontario and Quebec.

Besides diminishing habitat, there are other factors against ruffed grouse. Grouse survive the winter by snow roosting, a technique whereby the birds literally dive into a snowbank for warmth. One concern is that a changing climate—for example, less snow in mountainous regions of the lower Appalachian states and more freeze-and-thaw cycles in the Great Lakes states, resulting in a crust on the snow—is making survival more challenging for grouse. Research is also pointing to West Nile virus negatively affecting grouse populations, especially in areas of marginal habitat.

What can you do? To learn more about ruffed grouse and/or their habitat, visit Ruffedgrousesociety .org (in the U.S.), Rgs .ca (in Canada), or Audubon.org.

To hear and see a ruffed grouse drumming, visit Allaboutbirds.org. ■

Jeff Helsdon is a freelance writer and photographer based in Ontario. He writes for several publications in the United States and Canada, including *Ontario OUT of DOORS.*

GROUSE FACTS

• The ruffed grouse's Latin name, *Bonasa umbellus,* literally means "good when roasted" and "sunshade." The latter refers to the ruff on its neck.
• The ruffed grouse is the state bird of Pennsylvania.
• A group of grouse is referred to as a chorus, covey, drumming, grumbling, or leash.
• Ruffed grouse don't mate for life, and males can mate with several females in a season.
• Although ruffed grouse can survive up to 10 years, they rarely live more than a year or two due to predation and disease.
• Ruffed grouse populations in Newfoundland and Nevada were established through introduction by wildlife authorities.
• Ruffed grouse are one of 10 grouse species native to North America.
• A male grouse can be discerned from a female by looking at the feathers on its upper side, in front of the tail. Two or three whitish spots indicate a male. If there are no spots or only one, it is a female.
• The ruffed grouse is known to many Americans and Canadians as a partridge. Many attribute the origin of the term "partridge" to early European settlers, who were familiar with the partridge of their homelands. The two birds are not the same.

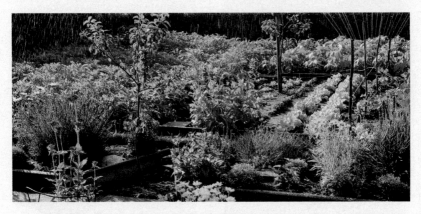
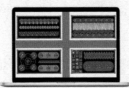
89

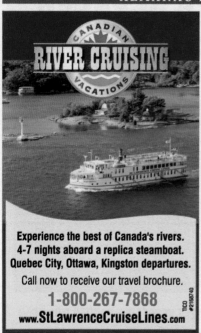
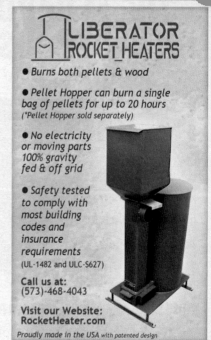
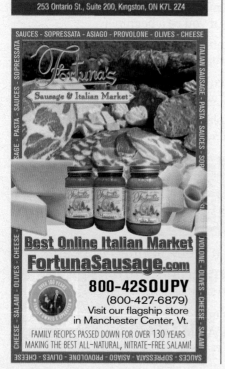
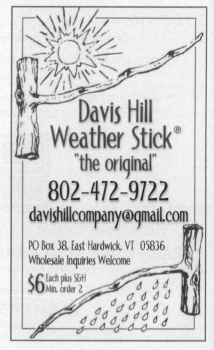

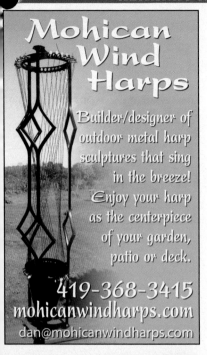
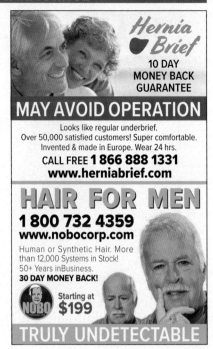
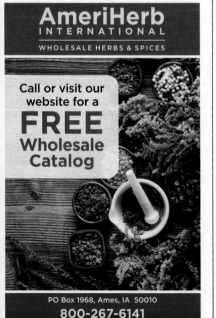
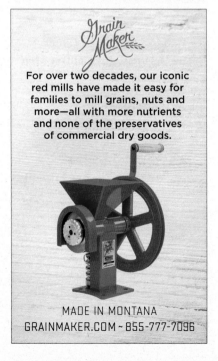

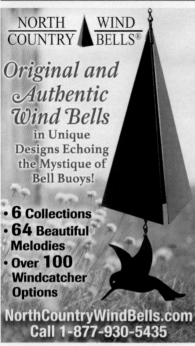
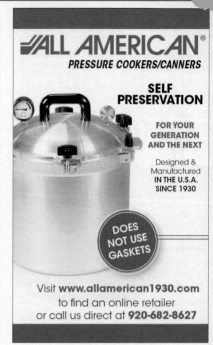
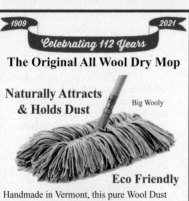
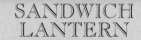
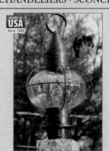

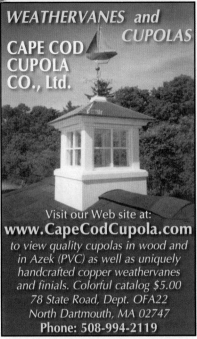
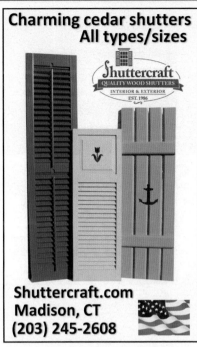
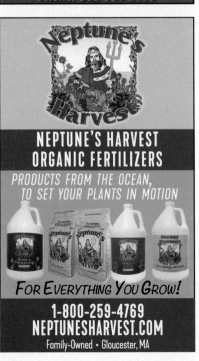
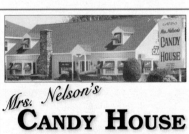

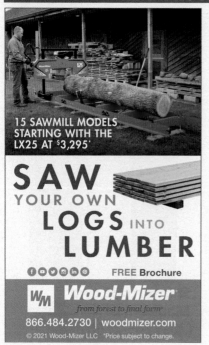
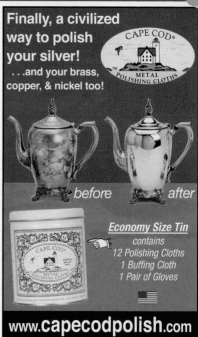
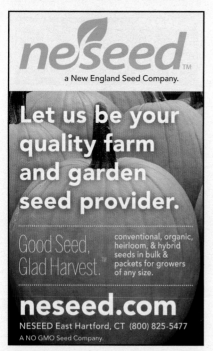
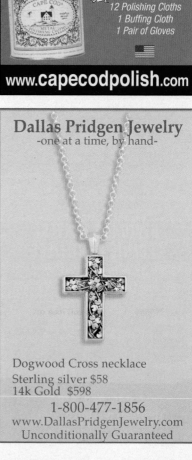

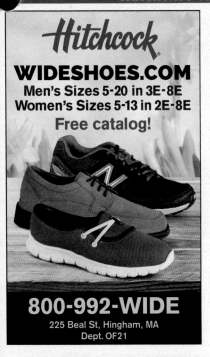
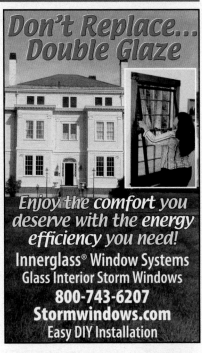
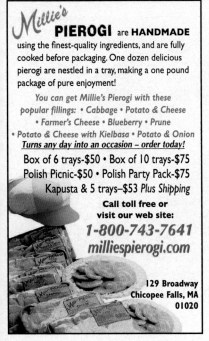
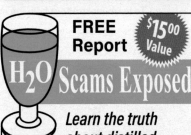

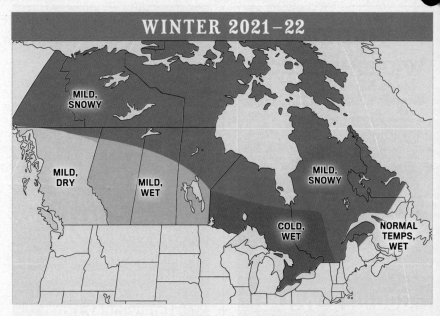

WINTER 2021–22

MILD, SNOWY

MILD, DRY

MILD, WET

MILD, SNOWY

COLD, WET

NORMAL TEMPS, WET

These weather maps correspond to the winter and summer predictions in the General Weather Forecast (opposite) and on the regional forecast pages, 211–216. To learn more about how we make our forecasts, turn to page 209.

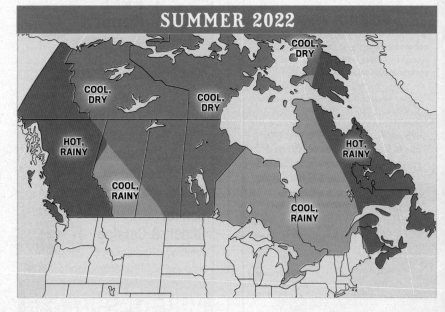

SUMMER 2022

COOL, DRY

COOL, DRY

COOL, DRY

HOT, RAINY

COOL, RAINY

HOT, RAINY

COOL, RAINY

Maps: AccuWeather, Inc.

THE GENERAL WEATHER REPORT AND FORECAST

FOR REGIONAL FORECASTS, SEE PAGES 211–216.

W hat's shaping the weather? We are currently in the early stages of Solar Cycle 25, which is expected to reach its maximum peak at around July 2025. Cycle 24 was the smallest in more than 100 years, while Cycle 25 is expected to also bring very low solar activity. Although low levels of solar activity have historically been associated with cooler temperatures across Earth, recent rising temperature trends mean that winter temperatures, on average, will be above normal in most of Canada.

Important factors in coming weather patterns include a weak La Niña, a continued warm phase in the Atlantic Multidecadal Oscillation (AMO), a neutral to positive phase in the North Atlantic Oscillation (NAO), and the Pacific Decadal Oscillation (PDO) in the early stages of its warm cycle.

WINTER temperatures will average below normal from central Quebec westward through Ontario and near or above normal elsewhere. Precipitation will be below normal in northern Atlantic Canada and British Columbia and above normal elsewhere. Snowfall will be greater than normal from western Atlantic Canada into eastern Quebec and in the Yukon, Northwest Territories, and Nunavut and below normal in most other areas.

SPRING temperatures will be near or above normal throughout the nation. Precipitation will be below normal from Atlantic Canada westward through Quebec and above normal elsewhere.

SUMMER temperatures will be cooler than normal from Quebec westward to Alberta and northward to the Arctic Ocean and hotter than normal elsewhere. Precipitation will be below normal in Manitoba, most of Saskatchewan, northern Alberta, the Northwest Territories, and western and central Nunavut and above normal elsewhere.

AUTUMN temperatures will be below normal in Quebec and near or above normal elsewhere. Precipitation will be below normal in the Yukon and above normal elsewhere.

WEATHER

How Accurate Was Our Forecast Last Winter?

O ur temperature forecasts for the November through March winter season were accurate to within 1.3 degrees C in forecasting the direction of change in temperature departure from normal in six of the seven regions, which computes to an 85.7% accuracy rate. Our forecasts for the change in precipitation were correct in five of the seven regions, which computes to a 71.4% accuracy rate. Our overall combined accuracy rate of 78.5% was slightly below our traditional accuracy rate of 80%. Snowfall was generally less than we had forecast.

As shown on the table below using one representative city from each region, the average difference between our winter season temperature forecasts and the actual temperatures was 1.19 degrees C.

REGION/ CITY	Nov.–Mar. Temp Departure From Normal (degrees)		REGION/ CITY	Nov.–Mar. Temp Departure From Normal (degrees)	
	PREDICTED	ACTUAL		PREDICTED	ACTUAL
1. Halifax, NS	0.6	0.9	5. Vancouver, BC	–0.3	0.9
2. Quebec, QC	–0.4	0.8	6. Mayo, YK	–0.2	0.7
3. Toronto, ON	–0.3	2.4	7. Yellowknife, NWT	–1.0	0.3
4. Edmonton, AB	0.2	0.9			

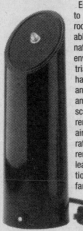
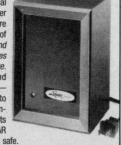

THE OLD FARMER'S ALMANAC

FOUNDED IN 1792

Established in 1792 and published every year thereafter
ROBERT B. THOMAS, *founder* (1766–1846)

YANKEE PUBLISHING INC.
EDITORIAL AND PUBLISHING OFFICES
P.O. Box 520, 1121 Main Street, Dublin, NH 03444
Phone: 603-563-8111 • Fax: 603-563-8252

EDITOR *(13th since 1792):* Janice Stillman
ART DIRECTOR: Colleen Quinnell
MANAGING EDITOR: Jack Burnett
SENIOR EDITORS: Sarah Perreault, Heidi Stonehill
ASSISTANT EDITOR: Benjamin Kilbride
WEATHER GRAPHICS AND CONSULTATION:
AccuWeather, Inc.

V.P., NEW MEDIA AND PRODUCTION:
Paul Belliveau
PRODUCTION DIRECTOR: David Ziarnowski
PRODUCTION MANAGER: Brian Johnson
SENIOR PRODUCTION ARTISTS:
Jennifer Freeman, Rachel Kipka, Janet Selle

WEB SITE: ALMANAC.CA
SENIOR DIGITAL EDITOR: Catherine Boeckmann
ASSOCIATE DIGITAL EDITOR: Christopher Burnett
NEW MEDIA DESIGNER: Amy O'Brien
DIGITAL MARKETING SPECIALIST: Holly Sanderson
E-MAIL MARKETING SPECIALIST: Samantha Caveny
E-COMMERCE DIRECTOR: Alan Henning
PROGRAMMING: Peter Rukavina

CONTACT US

We welcome your questions and comments about articles in and topics for this Almanac. Mail all editorial correspondence to Editor, The Old Farmer's Almanac, P.O. Box 520, Dublin, NH 03444-0520; fax us at 603-563-8252; or contact us through Almanac.ca/Feedback. *The Old Farmer's Almanac* can not accept responsibility for unsolicited manuscripts and will not acknowledge any hard-copy queries or manuscripts that do not include a stamped and addressed return envelope.

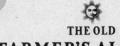

THE OLD
FARMER'S ALMANAC
FOUNDED IN 1792

OUR CONTRIBUTORS

Bob Berman, our astronomy editor, leads annual tours to Chilean observatories as well as to view solar eclipses and the northern lights. He is the author of *Earth-Shattering: Violent Supernovas, Galactic Explosions, Biological Mayhem, Nuclear Meltdowns, and Other Hazards to Life in Our Universe* (Little Brown, 2019).

Julia Shipley, a journalist and poet, wrote the Farmer's Calendar essays that appear in this edition. She raises animals and vegetables on a small farm in northern Vermont.

Tim Clark, a retired English teacher from New Hampshire, has composed the weather doggerel on the Calendar Pages since 1980.

Bethany E. Cobb, our astronomer, is an Associate Professor of Honors and Physics at George Washington University. She conducts research on gamma-ray bursts and specializes in teaching astronomy and physics to non–science majoring students. When she is not scanning the sky, she enjoys rock climbing, figure skating, and reading science fiction.

Celeste Longacre, our astrologer, often refers to astrology as "a study of timing, and timing is everything." A New Hampshire native, she has been a practicing astrologer for more than 25 years. Her book, *Celeste's Garden Delights* (2015), is available for sale on her Web site, www.celestelongacre.com.

Michael Steinberg, our meteorologist, has been forecasting weather for the Almanac since 1996. In addition to college degrees in atmospheric science and meteorology, he brings a lifetime of experience to the task: He began predicting weather when he attended the only high school in the world with weather Teletypes and radar.

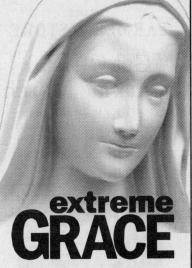

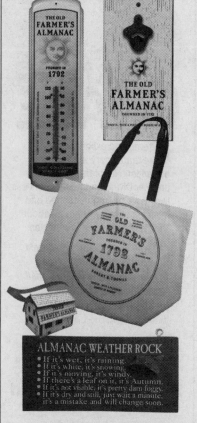
THE OLD
FARMER'S ALMANAC

Established in 1792 and published every year thereafter

ROBERT B. THOMAS, *founder* (1766–1846)

YANKEE PUBLISHING INC.
P.O. Box 520, 1121 Main Street, Dublin, NH 03444
Phone: 603-563-8111 • Fax: 603-563-8252

PUBLISHER *(23rd since 1792):* Sherin Pierce
EDITOR IN CHIEF: Judson D. Hale Sr.

FOR DISPLAY ADVERTISING RATES
Go to Almanac.ca/AdvertisingInfo or
call 800-895-9265, ext. 109

Stephanie Bernbach-Crowe • 914-827-0015
Steve Hall • 800-736-1100, ext. 320

FOR CLASSIFIED ADVERTISING
Cindy Levine, RJ Media • 212-986-0016

AD PRODUCTION COORDINATOR:
Janet Selle • 800-895-9265, ext. 168

PUBLIC RELATIONS
Quinn Brein • 206-842-8922
Ginger Vaughan • ginger@quinnbrein.com

FOR ONLINE ORDERS,
go to Amazon.ca

RETAIL SALES
Stacey Korpi • 800-895-9265, ext. 160
Janice Edson, ext. 126

DISTRIBUTORS
NATIONAL: Comag Marketing Group
Smyrna, GA
BOOKSTORE: Thomas Allen & Son Ltd.
Markham, ON
NEWSSTAND CONSULTANT: PSCS Consulting
Linda Ruth • 603-924-4407

Old Farmer's Almanac publications are available
for sales promotions or premiums. Contact Beacon
Promotions, info@beaconpromotions.com.

YANKEE PUBLISHING INCORPORATED
AN EMPLOYEE-OWNED COMPANY

Jamie Trowbridge, *President;* Paul Belliveau,
Ernesto Burden, Judson D. Hale Jr.,
Brook Holmberg, Jennie Meister, Sherin Pierce,
Vice Presidents.

Natural Pill Shocker Beats Out Other Powerful Joint Treatments

2022's first major breakthrough is a new pill that uses the science behind an immune modulating botanical that "drastically reduces joint discomfort"

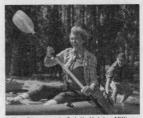

A New Discovery is Quietly Helping Millions Maintain Vital Joint Health

From comfort to mobility, the relief users report continues to amaze the millions who seek non-pharma therapies for joint comfort.

The pill, sold as VeraFlex®, contains a concentrated dose of a patented natural flavonoid. Scientific studies show it promotes immune modulation, which supports healthy inflammation response, a key function to prevent further joint deterioration, and improve comfort.

"Our customers say the first thing they notice is within days of using there's greater mobility and comfort around joints. Users may also feel less bloated and experience far less digestive discomfort," explains Dr. Liza Leal, a board-certified pain-management specialist and spokesperson for VeraFlex.

"It's why they love the product. It helps relieve excess discomfort, especially around stiff and degrading joints. It's remarkable."

An Amazing Breakthrough

Until now, many doctors have overlooked the idea of combining ingredients from different health categories, specifically linking joint health to gut health.

But researchers at the University of Rochester Medical Center provided the first evidence that bacteria in your gut could be the key driving force behind joint discomfort.

And VeraFlex is proving it may be the only way going forward.

"Most of today's top treatments are financially out of reach. That's why millions of adults are still in excruciating discomfort most days or willing to accept potentially devastating side effects," explains Dr. Leal.

"VeraFlex is a cost-effective way for virtually anyone looking to improve joint mobility and comfort."

Support Immune Health and Fight Joint Discomfort

Sufferers across the country are eager to get their hands on the new pill and according to the research, they should be.

This is because the other patented ingredient in VeraFlex is called Maxcell®, a bioenhancer made from a blend of aloe vera (acid buffer), jujube (immune support), black pepper (helps absorption), and licorice root (supports digestive health).

Studies have found that this special blend has the remarkable ability to protect the active ingredient through the digestive system and simultaneously support healthy immune function!

The Science Behind VeraFlex

Research shows that the joint soreness and discomfort are likely caused by certain enzymes released by the body's immune system.

The featured ingredient in VeraFlex supports a healthy immune response that can inhibit the production of these enzymes. The results can be a dramatic improvment in comfort and mobility.

This immune supporting characteristic is why researchers believe people experience relief so quickly.

VeraFlex users can generally expect to start to see more flexibility in just a few days...and with continued use, a tremendous improvement to overall joint function that may help them move more like they did years prior," explains Dr. Leal. "I recommend this product because it works."

Rapid Results & Lasting Comfort

The secret behind VeraFlex is its active ingredient UP446 which is protected by 8 patents and is backed by over $2 Million in safety studies. It's also undergone two double blind placebo controlled clinical trials, with 8 different research publications confirming the incredible results.

In the first, 60 participants were randomly placed into four groups.

The data collected by researchers was stunning.

The groups taking the VeraFlex ingredient reported staggering improvements over a 30-, 60-, and 90-day period including flexibility, improved comfort, and joint mobility.

A second study was conducted to ensure the data was accurate. But this time, the study was done to see how quickly it worked and again the results participants experienced while taking the VeraFlex compound blew away researchers.

Shockingly, both men and women experienced an improvement in flexibility in as little as 3 days, which was 2 days faster than the group using powerful traditional treatments.

The ingredients create a triple play for supporting joint health. First is accelerated action that's clinically shown to improve comfort and mobility...second is lasting comfort... and third is long-term safety without known side effects.

This would explain why so many users are experiencing impressive results so quickly. Because each dose of VeraFlex delivers the same amount of UP446 as the clinical studies, readers can now experience the same affordable comfort with daily use.

"The science and clinical studies are remarkable," explains Dr. Leal. "This product starts working incredibly fast. Users should expect to be highly satisfied with the results."

How to Claim Three Free Months of VeraFlex

This is the official nationwide release of the new VeraFlex pill. And so, the company is offering our readers up to 3 FREE bottles with their order.

This special give-away is available for only a limited time so don't wait. All you have to do is call toll free **1-800-997-5967** and provide the operator with the Approval Code: VF2104. The company will do the rest.

The company is so confident it will work that each order is backed by our 100% satisfaction guarantee; if you don't love the results, we'll refund the purchase price, no questions asked.

With such an incredible offer this is expected to sell out. Don't wait to call, US operators are standing by.

THESE STATEMENTS HAVE NOT BEEN EVALUATED BY THE FDA. THESE PRODUCTS ARE NOT INTENDED TO DIAGNOSE, TREAT, CURE OR PREVENT ANY DISEASE. RESULTS MAY VARY. OFFER NOT AVAILABLE TO RESIDENTS OF IOWA

ECLIPSES

There will be four eclipses in 2022, two of the Sun and two of the Moon. Solar eclipses are visible only in certain areas and require eye protection to be viewed safely. Lunar eclipses are technically visible from the entire night side of Earth, but during a penumbral eclipse, the dimming of the Moon's illumination is slight. See the **Astronomical Glossary, page 110,** for explanations of the different types of eclipses.

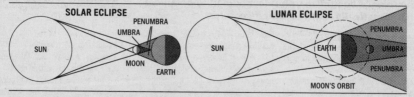

APRIL 30: PARTIAL ECLIPSE OF THE SUN. This eclipse is not visible from North America. (The partial solar eclipse is visible from the southeastern Pacific Ocean, the Antarctic Peninsula, and southern South America.)

MAY 15–16: TOTAL ECLIPSE OF THE MOON. This eclipse is visible from North America, except in northwestern regions. The Moon will enter the penumbra at 9:31 P.M. EDT on May 15 (6:31 P.M. PDT) and leave it at 2:52 A.M. EDT on May 16 (11:52 P.M. PDT on May 15).

OCTOBER 25: PARTIAL ECLIPSE OF THE SUN. This eclipse is not visible from North America. (The partial solar eclipse is visible from Greenland, Iceland, Europe, northeastern Africa, the Middle East, western Asia, India, and western China.)

NOVEMBER 8: TOTAL ECLIPSE OF THE MOON. This eclipse is visible from North America, although the Moon will be setting during the eclipse for observers in eastern regions. The Moon will enter the penumbra at 3:01 A.M. EST on November 8 (12:01 A.M. PST) and leave it at 8:58 A.M. EST (5:58 A.M. PST).

TRANSIT OF MERCURY. Mercury's proximity to the Sun makes it difficult to observe. The planet can be seen for only a few weeks before and after times of greatest elongation. Near its greatest eastern and western elongations, Mercury is observable during evening twilight and morning twilight, respectively. In 2022, Mercury is best viewed from the Northern Hemisphere just after sunset from mid-April to early May and shortly before sunrise during the first 3 weeks of October. Look for a conjunction between Mercury and Saturn on the morning of March 2 and between Mercury and Jupiter on the morning of March 20.

THE MOON'S PATH

The Moon's path across the sky changes with the seasons. Full Moons are very high in the sky (at midnight) between November and February and very low in the sky between May and July.

FULL-MOON DATES (ET)

	2022	2023	2024	2025	2026
JAN.	17	6	25	13	3
FEB.	16	5	24	12	1
MAR.	18	7	25	14	3
APR.	16	6	23	12	1
MAY	16	5	23	12	1 & 31
JUNE	14	3	21	11	29
JULY	13	3	21	10	29
AUG.	11	1 & 30	19	9	28
SEPT.	10	29	17	7	26
OCT.	9	28	17	6	26
NOV.	8	27	15	5	24
DEC.	7	26	15	4	23

ake your home more comfortable than ever

"To you, it's the **perfect lift chair.** To me, it's the **best sleep chair** I've ever had."

— J. Fitzgerald, VA

NOW also available in **Genuine Italian Leather** *(and new Chestnut color)*

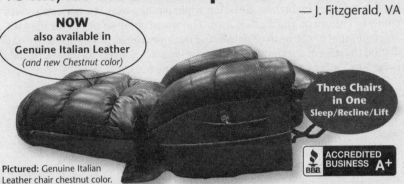

Three Chairs in One Sleep/Recline/Lift

ACCREDITED BUSINESS A+

Pictured: Genuine Italian Leather chair chestnut color.

You can't always lie down in bed and sleep. Heartburn, cardiac problems, hip or back aches – and dozens of other ailments and worries. Those are the nights you'd give anything for a comfortable chair to sleep in: one that reclines to exactly the right degree, raises your feet and legs just where you want them, supports your head and shoulders properly, and <u>operates at the touch of a button</u>.

Our **Perfect Sleep Chair®** does all that and more. More than a chair or recliner, it's designed to provide total comfort. **Choose your preferred heat and massage settings, for hours of soothing relaxation.** Reading or watching TV? Our chair's recline technology allows you to pause the chair in an infinite number of settings. You'll love the other benefits, too. It helps with correct spinal alignment and promotes back pressure relief, to prevent back and muscle pain. The overstuffed, oversized biscuit style back and unique seat design will cradle you in comfort. Generously filled, wide armrests provide enhanced arm support when sitting or reclining. **It even has a battery backup in case of a power outage.**

White glove delivery included in shipping charge. Professionals will deliver the chair to the exact spot in your home where you want it, unpack it, inspect it, test it, position it, and even carry the packaging away! You get your choice of Genuine Italian leather, stain and water repellent custom-manufactured DuraLux™ with the classic leather look or plush MicroLux™ microfiber in a variety of colors to fit any decor. **New Chestnut color only available in Genuine Italian Leather. Call now!**

The Perfect Sleep Chair®
1-888-849-1623

Mention code 115047 when ordering.

BRIGHT STARS

TRANSIT TIMES

This table shows the time (ET) and altitude of a star as it transits the meridian (i.e., reaches its highest elevation while passing over the horizon's south point) at Ottawa on the dates shown. The transit time on any other date differs from that of the nearest date listed by approximately 4 minutes per day. To find the time of a star's transit for your location, convert its time at Ottawa using Key Letter C **(see Time Corrections, page 240)**.

STAR	CONSTELLATION	MAGNITUDE	JAN. 1	MAR. 1	MAY 1	JULY 1	SEPT. 1	NOV. 1	ALTITUDE (DEGREES)
Altair	Aquila	0.8	**1:09**	9:17	6:17	2:18	**10:10**	**6:10**	56.3
Deneb	Cygnus	1.3	**1:59**	10:07	7:08	3:08	**11:00**	**7:00**	92.8
Fomalhaut	Psc. Aus.	1.2	**4:16**	**12:24**	9:24	5:24	1:20	**9:16**	17.8
Algol	Perseus	2.2	**8:26**	**4:34**	**1:34**	9:34	5:30	1:31	88.5
Aldebaran	Taurus	0.9	**9:53**	**6:01**	**3:01**	11:01	6:58	2:58	64.1
Rigel	Orion	0.1	**10:31**	**6:39**	**3:40**	11:40	7:36	3:36	39.4
Capella	Auriga	0.1	**10:34**	**6:42**	**3:42**	11:42	7:39	3:39	93.6
Bellatrix	Orion	1.6	**10:42**	**6:50**	**3:50**	11:50	7:47	3:47	54.0
Betelgeuse	Orion	var. 0.4	**11:12**	**7:20**	**4:20**	**12:20**	8:17	4:17	55.0
Sirius	Can. Maj.	-1.4	12:06	**8:10**	**5:10**	**1:10**	9:06	5:06	31.0
Procyon	Can. Min.	0.4	1:00	**9:04**	**6:04**	**2:04**	10:00	6:01	52.9
Pollux	Gemini	1.2	1:06	**9:10**	**6:10**	**2:10**	10:07	6:07	75.7
Regulus	Leo	1.4	3:28	**11:33**	**8:33**	**4:33**	**12:29**	8:29	59.7
Spica	Virgo	var. 1.0	6:45	2:53	**11:49**	**7:49**	**3:45**	11:46	36.6
Arcturus	Boötes	-0.1	7:35	3:43	12:43	**8:39**	**4:36**	**12:36**	66.9
Antares	Scorpius	var. 0.9	9:49	5:57	2:57	**10:53**	**6:49**	**2:49**	21.3
Vega	Lyra	0	11:55	8:03	5:03	1:04	**8:56**	**4:56**	86.4

TIME OF TRANSIT (ET) — BOLD = P.M. LIGHT = A.M.

RISE AND SET TIMES

To find the time of a star's rising at Ottawa on any date, subtract the interval shown at right from the star's transit time on that date; add the interval to find the star's setting time. To find the rising and setting times for your city, convert the Ottawa transit times above using the Key Letter shown at right before applying the interval **(see Time Corrections, page 240)**. Deneb, Algol, Capella, and Vega are circumpolar stars—they never set but appear to circle the celestial north pole.

STAR	INTERVAL (H.M.)	RISING KEY	DIR.*	SETTING KEY	DIR.*
Altair	6 36	B	EbN	E	WbN
Fomalhaut	3 59	E	SE	D	SW
Aldebaran	7 06	B	ENE	D	WNW
Rigel	5 33	D	EbS	B	WbS
Bellatrix	6 27	B	EbN	D	WbN
Betelgeuse	6 31	B	EbN	D	WbN
Sirius	5 00	D	ESE	B	WSW
Procyon	6 23	B	EbN	D	WbN
Pollux	8 01	A	NE	E	NW
Regulus	6 49	B	EbN	D	WbN
Spica	5 23	D	EbS	B	WbS
Arcturus	7 19	A	ENE	E	WNW
Antares	4 17	E	SEbE	A	SWbW

*b = "by"

SCIATICA BACK PAIN?

Are radiating pains down the back of your leg, or pain in your lower back or buttocks making it uncomfortable to sit, walk or sleep? Millions of people are suffering unnecessarily because they are not aware of this effective, topical treatment.

MagniLife® Leg & Back Pain Relief Cream combines seven active ingredients including Colocynthis to relieve burning pains and tingling sensations. This product is not intended to *treat or cure* sciatica, but can relieve painful symptoms. *"It provided me with the only relief for my sciatica."* - Mary.

MagniLife® Leg & Back Pain Relief Cream is **sold at Walgreens, CVS, Rite Aid and Amazon**. Order risk free for $19.99 +$5.95 S&H for a 4 oz jar. Get a **FREE** jar when you order two for $39.98 +$5.95 S&H. Send payment to: MagniLife SC-FA2, PO Box 6789, McKinney, TX 75071 or call **1-800-993-7691**. Money back guarantee. Order now at **www.LegBackCream.com**

BURNING FOOT PAIN?

Do you suffer from burning, tingling or stabbing pain in your feet? You should know help is available. Many are suffering from these symptoms and live in pain because they are not aware of this proven treatment.

MagniLife® Pain Relieving Foot Cream contains eucalyptus oil and yellow jasmine, known to relieve tingling, burning, and stabbing pain while also restoring cracked, damaged, and itchy skin. *"It's the ONLY product that helps relieve the burning, and tingling feeling in my feet!"* - Mabel, NY

MagniLife® Pain Relieving Foot Cream is **sold at Walgreens, CVS, Rite Aid and Walmart** in footcare and diabetes care. Order risk free for $19.99 +$5.95 S&H for a 4 oz jar. **Get a FREE jar** when you order two for $39.98 +$5.95 S&H. Send payment to: MagniLife NC-FA2, PO Box 6789, McKinney, TX 75071, or call **1-800-993-7691**. Satisfaction guaranteed. Order at **www.MDFootCream.com**

PSORIASIS ITCH OR PAIN?

Is itchy, painful, red or scaly skin causing you discomfort or embarrassment? Millions of Americans now suffer from psoriasis, which is becoming more prevalent among older adults. New treatments are now available without steroids or prescriptions.

MagniLife® Psoriasis Care+ can be used on the scalp, knees, elbows and body and contains Oat-derived Beta Glucan to relieve itching, pain and redness. Moisturizing gel deeply hydrates for visibly healthier skin. *"...for me this will take away the pain and burning overnight."* - Jessica.

MagniLife® Psoriasis Care+ is sold at **Walgreens** stores and **Amazon**. Order risk free for $17.99 +$5.95 S&H for a 2 oz jar. Get a FREE jar when you order two for $35.98 +$5.95 S&H. Send payment to: MagniLife OC-FA2, PO Box 6789, McKinney, TX 75071 or call **1-800-993-7691**. Satisfaction guaranteed. Order now at **www.PsoriasisCareGel.com**

THE TWILIGHT ZONE/METEOR SHOWERS

Twilight is the time when the sky is partially illuminated preceding sunrise and again following sunset. The ranges of twilight are defined according to the Sun's position below the horizon. **Civil twilight** occurs when the Sun's center is between the horizon and 6 degrees below the horizon (visually, the horizon is clearly defined). **Nautical twilight** occurs when the center is between 6 and 12 degrees below the horizon (the horizon is distinct). **Astronomical twilight** occurs when the center is between 12 and 18 degrees below the horizon (sky illumination is imperceptible). When the center is at 18 degrees (**dawn** or **dark**) or below, there is no illumination.

LENGTH OF ASTRONOMICAL TWILIGHT (HOURS AND MINUTES)

LATITUDE	JAN. 1–APR. 10	APR. 11–MAY 2	MAY 3–MAY 14	MAY 15–MAY 25	MAY 26–JULY 22	JULY 23–AUG. 3	AUG. 4–AUG. 14	AUG. 15–SEPT. 5	SEPT. 6–DEC. 31
37°N to 42°N	1 33	1 39	1 47	1 52	1 59	1 52	1 47	1 39	1 33
43°N to 47°N	1 42	1 51	2 02	2 13	2 27	2 13	2 02	1 51	1 42
48°N to 49°N	1 50	2 04	2 22	2 42	–	2 42	2 22	2 04	1 33
50°N to 55°N	1 54	2 15	2 52	3 25	–	3 11	2 37	2 10	1 53
56°N to 60°N	2 12	3 04	–	–	–	–	–	2 46	2 11

TO DETERMINE THE LENGTH OF TWILIGHT: The length of twilight changes with latitude and the time of year. See the **Time Corrections, page 240,** to find the latitude of your city or the city nearest you. Use that figure in the chart above with the appropriate date to calculate the length of twilight in your area.

TO DETERMINE ARRIVAL OF DAWN OR DARK: Calculate the sunrise/sunset times for your locality using the instructions in **How to Use This Almanac, page 116.**

Subtract the length of twilight from the time of sunrise to determine when dawn breaks. Add the length of twilight to the time of sunset to determine when dark descends.

EXAMPLE:
OTTAWA, ONT. (LATITUDE 45°25')

Sunrise, August 1	5:47 A.M. ET
Length of twilight	– 2 13
Dawn breaks	3:34 A.M.
Sunset, August 1	8:31 P.M. ET
Length of twilight	+2 13
Dark descends	10:44 P.M.

PRINCIPAL METEOR SHOWERS

SHOWER	BEST VIEWING	POINT OF ORIGIN	DATE OF MAXIMUM*	NO. PER HOUR**	ASSOCIATED COMET
Quadrantid	Predawn	N	Jan. 4	25	–
Lyrid	Predawn	S	Apr. 22	10	Thatcher
Eta Aquarid	Predawn	SE	May 4	10	Halley
Delta Aquarid	Predawn	S	July 30	10	–
Perseid	Predawn	NE	Aug. 11–13	50	Swift-Tuttle
Draconid	Late evening	NW	Oct. 9	6	Giacobini-Zinner
Orionid	Predawn	S	Oct. 21–22	15	Halley
Northern Taurid	Late evening	S	Nov. 9	3	Encke
Leonid	Predawn	S	Nov. 17–18	10	Tempel-Tuttle
Andromedid	Late evening	S	Nov. 25–27	5	Biela
Geminid	All night	NE	Dec. 13–14	75	–
Ursid	Predawn	N	Dec. 22	5	Tuttle

*May vary by 1 or 2 days   **In a moonless, rural sky   **Bold** = most prominent

NEW PROSTATE PILL HELPS RELIEVE SYMPTOMS WITHOUT DRUGS OR SURGERY

Combats all-night bathroom urges and embarrassment... *Yet most doctors don't even know about it!*

By Health Writer, Peter Metler

Thanks to a brand new discovery made from a rare prostate relief plant; thousands of men across America are taking their lives back from "prostate hell". This remarkable new natural supplement helps you:

- **MINIMIZE** constant urges to urinate
- **END** embarrassing sexual "let-downs"
- **SUPPORT** a strong, healthy urine flow
- **GET** a restful night of uninterrupted sleep
- **STOP** false alarms, dribbles
- **ENJOY** a truly empty bladder

More men than ever before are dealing with prostate problems that range from annoying to downright EMBARRASSING! But now, research has discovered a new solution so remarkable that helps alleviate symptoms associated with an enlarged prostate (sexual failure, lost sleep, bladder discomfort and urgent runs to the bathroom). Like nothing before!

Yet 9 out of 10 doctors don't know about it! Here's why: Due to strict managed health care constrictions, many MD's are struggling to keep their practices afloat. "Unfortunately, there's no money in prescribing natural products. They aren't nearly as profitable," says a confidential source. Instead, doctors rely on toxic drugs that help, but could leave you sexually "powerless" (or a lot worse)!

On a CNN Special, Medical Correspondent Dr. Steve Salvatore shocked America by quoting a statistic from the prestigious Journal of American Medical Association that stated, "... about 60% of men who go under the knife for a prostatectomy are left UNABLE to perform sexually!"

PROSTATE PROBLEM SOLVED!

But now you can now beat the odds. And enjoy better sleep, a powerful urine stream and a long and healthy love life. The secret? You need to load your diet with essential Phyto-Nutrients, (traditionally found in certain fruits, vegetables and grains).

The problem is, most Phyto-Nutrients never get into your bloodstream. They're destroyed

HERE ARE 6 WARNING SIGNS YOU BETTER NOT IGNORE

✓ Waking up 2 to 6 times a night to urinate
✓ A constant feeling that you have to "go"... but can't
✓ A burning sensation when you do go
✓ A weak urine stream
✓ A feeling that your bladder is never completely empty
✓ Embarrassing sputtering, dripping & staining

by today's food preparation methods (cooking, long storage times and food additives).

YEARS OF RESEARCH

Thankfully, a small company (Wellness Logix™) out of Maine, is on a mission to change that. They've created a product that arms men who suffer with prostate inflammation with new hope. And it's fast becoming the #1 Prostate formula in America.

Prostate IQ™ gives men the super-concentrated dose of Phyto-Nutrients they need to beat prostate symptoms. "You just can't get them from your regular diet" say Daniel. It's taken a long time to understand how to capture the prostate relieving power of this amazing botanical. But their hard work paid off. *Prostate IQ*™ is different than any other prostate supplement on the market...

DON'T BE FOOLED BY CHEAP FORMULATIONS!

Many hope you won't notice, but a lot of prostate supplements fall embarrassingly short with their dosages. The formulas may be okay, but they won't do a darn thing for you unless you take 10 or more tablets a day. *Prostate IQ*™ contains a whopping 300mg of this special "Smart Prostate Plant". So it's loaded with Phyto-Nutrients. Plus, it gets inside your bloodstream faster and stays inside for maximum results!

TRY IT RISK-FREE

SPECIAL OPPORTUNITY

Get a risk-free trial supply of *Prostate IQ*™ today - just for asking. But you must act now, supplies are limited!

Call Now, Toll-Free at:

1-800-380-0925

THE VISIBLE PLANETS

Listed here for Ottawa are viewing suggestions for and the rise and set times (ET) of Venus, Mars, Jupiter, and Saturn on specific days each month, as well as when it is best to view Mercury. Approximate rise and set times for other days can be found by interpolation. Use the Key Letters at the right of each listing to convert the times for other localities (see pages 116 and 240).

FOR ALL PLANET RISE AND SET TIMES BY POSTAL CODE, VISIT ALMANAC.CA/2022.

VENUS

Venus will appear as a dazzling morning star, especially in February and March. The year opens with Venus low in the west in evening twilight, only to sink and vanish a few days later. Venus then emerges as a morning star in mid-January and remains striking through the summer, while gradually fading from its mid-February brilliance at magnitude –4.9. It plummets even lower until it sinks too low in September and finally vanishes behind the Sun in its superior conjunction on October 22. It slowly emerges again as an evening star to be glimpsed low in the western twilight in December. After forming a triangle with Jupiter and the Moon on April 27, it has a predawn conjunction with Jupiter on the 30th.

Jan. 1	set	**5:38**	B	Apr. 1	rise	5:01	D	July 1	rise	3:26	A	Oct. 1	rise	6:30	C
Jan. 11	rise	7:00	D	Apr. 11	rise	4:51	D	July 11	rise	3:29	A	Oct. 11	rise	6:57	C
Jan. 21	rise	5:56	D	Apr. 21	rise	4:40	C	July 21	rise	3:38	A	Oct. 21	set	6:11	B
Feb. 1	rise	5:08	D	May 1	rise	4:27	C	Aug. 1	rise	3:56	A	Nov. 1	set	**5:59**	B
Feb. 11	rise	4:43	D	May 11	rise	4:13	C	Aug. 11	rise	4:17	A	Nov. 11	set	**4:52**	B
Feb. 21	rise	4:29	D	May 21	rise	3:59	B	Aug. 21	rise	4:41	A	Nov. 21	set	**4:50**	A
Mar. 1	rise	4:23	D	June 1	rise	3:46	B	Sept. 1	rise	5:10	B	Dec. 1	set	**4:54**	A
Mar. 11	rise	4:16	D	June 11	rise	3:35	B	Sept. 11	rise	5:37	B	Dec. 11	set	**5:05**	A
Mar. 21	rise	5:10	D	June 21	rise	3:28	A	Sept. 21	rise	6:03	C	Dec. 21	set	**5:24**	A
												Dec. 31	set	**5:47**	A

MARS

Mars achieves its brightest appearance on December 8, when it is higher in the sky for Northern Hemisphere observers than anytime in the past 15 years. The Red Planet starts the year as a predawn object subdued by dawn's twilight glare, shining at nearly its dimmest at magnitude 1.6. It slowly inches farther from the Sun and by April reaches the first magnitude. Steadily brightening as it glides eastward, it breaks the zero-magnitude threshold in August in Aries. Brightening through the summer as it crosses into Taurus, it starts rising before midnight and comes up soon after nightfall in November. Mars is closest on November 30 and reaches opposition on December 8 at a magnitude of –1.9, when it rises at sunset, is out all night long, and displays a disk 17 arc seconds in width.

Jan. 1	rise	5:42	E	Apr. 1	rise	4:58	D	July 1	rise	1:30	B	Oct. 1	**rise**	**9:55**	A
Jan. 11	rise	5:38	E	Apr. 11	rise	4:38	D	July 11	rise	1:07	B	Oct. 11	**rise**	**9:26**	A
Jan. 21	rise	5:32	E	Apr. 21	rise	4:16	D	July 21	rise	12:44	B	Oct. 21	**rise**	**8:51**	A
Feb. 1	rise	5:24	E	May 1	rise	3:54	D	Aug. 1	rise	12:19	B	Nov. 1	**rise**	**8:07**	A
Feb. 11	rise	5:14	E	May 11	rise	3:31	C	Aug. 11	**rise**	**11:55**	B	Nov. 11	**rise**	**6:21**	A
Feb. 21	rise	5:03	E	May 21	rise	3:07	C	Aug. 21	**rise**	**11:33**	A	Nov. 21	**rise**	**5:28**	A
Mar. 1	rise	4:52	E	June 1	rise	2:41	C	Sept. 1	**rise**	**11:09**	A	Dec. 1	**rise**	**4:32**	A
Mar. 11	rise	4:36	E	June 11	rise	2:17	C	Sept. 11	**rise**	**10:46**	A	Dec. 11	set	7:32	E
Mar. 21	rise	5:19	E	June 21	rise	1:54	C	Sept. 21	**rise**	**10:22**	A	Dec. 21	set	6:37	E
												Dec. 31	set	5:46	E

BOLD = P.M. LIGHT = A.M.

JUPITER

Jupiter opens the year as an evening star in Aquarius, low in the southwest evening. By month's end, it has sunk too low to be easily seen, but it reappears as a morning star in mid-April. Jupiter has a conjunction with Venus on April 30 in the predawn east and rises 2 hours earlier each month thereafter, until rising before midnight in August. Jupiter's opposition occurs on September 26, when it has a magnitude of –2.9. In autumn, it is increasingly an evening sky object. Jupiter remains visible in the west after sunset through the end of the year.

Jan. 1	set	8:42	B	Apr. 1	rise	6:08	C	July 1	rise	12:45	C	Oct. 1	set	6:38	C
Jan. 11	set	8:13	B	Apr. 11	rise	5:34	C	July 11	rise	12:07	C	Oct. 11	set	5:52	C
Jan. 21	set	7:46	B	Apr. 21	rise	4:59	C	July 21	rise	11:25	C	Oct. 21	set	5:07	C
Feb. 1	set	7:16	B	May 1	rise	4:24	C	Aug. 1	rise	10:42	C	Nov. 1	set	4:19	C
Feb. 11	set	6:49	B	May 11	rise	3:49	C	Aug. 11	rise	10:03	C	Nov. 11	set	2:36	C
Feb. 21	set	6:22	B	May 21	rise	3:14	C	Aug. 21	rise	9:22	C	Nov. 21	set	1:56	C
Mar. 1	set	6:01	B	June 1	rise	2:35	C	Sept. 1	rise	8:37	C	Dec. 1	set	1:17	C
Mar. 11	rise	6:20	D	June 11	rise	1:59	C	Sept. 11	rise	7:56	C	Dec. 11	set	12:40	C
Mar. 21	rise	6:46	C	June 21	rise	1:22	C	Sept. 21	rise	7:14	C	Dec. 21	set	12:04	C
												Dec. 31	set	11:27	C

SATURN

Saturn starts the year low in the west at dusk, in Capricornus. Its rings are angled in open configuration easily observable through any telescope using more than 30× magnification. Saturn vanishes into solar glare by late January, reappears in the predawn east in March, and then rises 2 hours earlier each month. The Ringed Planet comes up before midnight in late June and slightly brightens until it reaches its opposition on August 14, when it is out all night. The Moon is near Saturn on May 22, June 18, and July 15 and closely meets Mars in the predawn hours of April 4 and 5 while standing 15 degrees high.

Jan. 1	set	7:02	B	Apr. 1	rise	5:03	D	July 1	rise	11:09	D	Oct. 1	set	2:44	B
Jan. 11	set	6:29	B	Apr. 11	rise	4:26	D	July 11	rise	10:29	D	Oct. 11	set	2:04	B
Jan. 21	set	5:55	B	Apr. 21	rise	3:48	D	July 21	rise	9:48	D	Oct. 21	set	1:24	B
Feb. 1	set	5:19	B	May 1	rise	3:11	D	Aug. 1	rise	9:03	D	Nov. 1	set	12:41	B
Feb. 11	rise	7:02	D	May 11	rise	2:33	D	Aug. 11	rise	8:22	D	Nov. 11	set	10:59	B
Feb. 21	rise	6:25	D	May 21	rise	1:54	D	Aug. 21	set	5:39	B	Nov. 21	set	10:22	B
Mar. 1	rise	5:56	D	June 1	rise	1:12	D	Sept. 1	set	4:51	B	Dec. 1	set	9:46	B
Mar. 11	rise	5:20	D	June 11	rise	12:32	D	Sept. 11	set	4:08	B	Dec. 11	set	9:10	B
Mar. 21	rise	5:43	D	June 21	rise	11:49	D	Sept. 21	set	3:26	B	Dec. 21	set	8:36	B
												Dec. 31	set	8:01	B

MERCURY

Mercury dashes from the morning to the evening sky every few months. To observe Mercury, it must be at least 5 degrees above the horizon 40 minutes after sunset or before sunrise, at a time when its brightness exceeds magnitude 0.5. This year, its most favorable evening star conditions occur in twilight during the last half of April. It may be glimpsed less favorably as an evening star in the first half of January and from July 25 to September 1. In the eastern sky, Mercury is best seen as a morning star during the first 3 weeks of October, in the first 3 weeks of March, the last half of June, and from October 10 to 25.

DO NOT CONFUSE: *Mars with Saturn during their conjunction on April 4 and 5. Mars is orange, Saturn is brighter. • Jupiter with Venus on April 30 and during February through May, when both are visible before dawn. Venus is brighter. • Saturn with Mercury on February 2, low in the east before dawn. Mercury is slightly orange. • Venus, Mars, and Saturn when they form a triangle before dawn from March 24 to 26. Venus is brighter than the others, while Saturn is brighter than Mars.*

APHELION (APH.): The point in a planet's orbit that is farthest from the Sun.

APOGEE (APO.): The point in the Moon's orbit that is farthest from Earth.

CELESTIAL EQUATOR (EQ.): The imaginary circle around the celestial sphere that can be thought of as the plane of Earth's equator projected out onto the sphere.

CELESTIAL SPHERE: An imaginary sphere projected into space that represents the entire sky, with an observer on Earth at its center. All celestial bodies other than Earth are imagined as being on its inside surface.

CIRCUMPOLAR: Always visible above the horizon, such as a circumpolar star.

CONJUNCTION: The time at which two or more celestial bodies appear closest in the sky. **Inferior (Inf.):** Mercury or Venus is between the Sun and Earth. **Superior (Sup.):** The Sun is between a planet and Earth. Actual dates for conjunctions are given on the **Right-Hand Calendar Pages, 121–147**; the best times for viewing the closely aligned bodies are given in **Sky Watch** on the **Left-Hand Calendar Pages, 120–146.**

DECLINATION: The celestial latitude of an object in the sky, measured in degrees north or south of the celestial equator; comparable to latitude on Earth. This Almanac gives the Sun's declination at noon.

ECLIPSE, LUNAR: The full Moon enters the shadow of Earth, which cuts off all or part of the sunlight reflected off the Moon. **Total:** The Moon passes completely through the umbra (central dark part) of Earth's shadow. **Partial:** Only part of the Moon passes through the umbra. **Penumbral:** The Moon passes through only the penumbra (area of partial darkness surrounding the umbra). See **page 102** for more information about eclipses.

ECLIPSE, SOLAR: Earth enters the shadow of the new Moon, which cuts off all or part of the Sun's light. **Total:** Earth passes through the umbra (central dark part) of the Moon's shadow, resulting in totality for observers within a narrow band on Earth. **Annular:** The Moon appears silhouetted against the Sun, with a ring of sunlight showing around it. **Partial:** The Moon blocks only part of the Sun.

ECLIPTIC: The apparent annual path of the Sun around the celestial sphere. The plane of the ecliptic is tipped 23½° from the celestial equator.

ELONGATION: The difference in degrees between the celestial longitudes of a planet and the Sun. **Greatest Elongation (Gr. Elong.):** The greatest apparent distance of a planet from the Sun, as seen from Earth.

EPACT: A number from 1 to 30 that indicates the Moon's age on January 1 at Greenwich, England; used in determining the date of Easter.

EQUINOX: When the Sun crosses the celestial equator. This event occurs two times each year: **Vernal** is around March 20 and **Autumnal** is around September 22.

EVENING STAR: A planet that is above the western horizon at sunset and less than 180° east of the Sun in right ascension.

GOLDEN NUMBER: A number in the 19-year Metonic cycle of the Moon, used in determining the date of Easter. See **page 149** for this year's Golden Number.

MAGNITUDE: A measure of a celestial object's brightness. **Apparent magnitude** measures the brightness of an object as seen from Earth. Objects with an apparent magnitude of 6 or less are observable to the naked eye. The lower the magnitude, the greater the brightness; an object with a magnitude of –1, e.g., is brighter than one with a magnitude of +1.

(continued)

New Bladder Control Pill Sales May Surpass Adult Diapers By 2023

Drug-free discovery works, say doctors. Many adults ditching diapers and pads for clinical strength pill that triggers day and night bladder support.

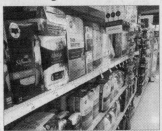

As new pill gains popularity, products like these will become unnecessary.

By J.K. Roberts
Interactive News Media

INM — Over 150,000 doses have shipped to bladder sufferers so far, and sales continue to climb every day for the 'diaper replacing' new pill called BladderMax.

"We knew we had a great product, but it's even exceeded our expectations," said Keith Graham, Manager of Call Center Operations for BladderMax.

"People just keep placing orders, it's pretty amazing," he said.

But a closer look at this new bladder control sensation suggests that maybe the company shouldn't have been caught off guard by its success.

There are very good reasons for BladderMax's surging popularity.

To begin with, clinical studies show BladderMax not only reduces embarrassing bladder leakages quickly, but also works to strengthen and calm the bladder for lasting relief.

Plus, at just $2 per daily dose, it's very affordable.

This may be another reason why American diaper companies are starting to panic over its release.

WHAT SCIENTISTS DISCOVERED

BladderMax contains a proprietary compound with a known ability to reduce stress, urgency, and overflow leakages in seniors suffering from overactive bladder.

This compound is not a drug. It is the active ingredient in BladderMax.

Studies show it naturally strengthens the bladder's muscle tone while relaxing the urination muscles resulting in a decrease in sudden urgency.

Many sufferers enjoy a reduction in bathroom trips both day and night. Others are able to get back to doing the things they love without worrying about embarrassing leakages.

"I couldn't sit through a movie without having to go to the bathroom 3-4 times," says Theresa Johnson of Duluth, GA, "but since using BladderMax I can not only sit through a movie, but I can drive on the freeway to another city without having to immediately go to the bathroom."

With so much positive feedback, it's easy to see why sales for this newly approved bladder pill continue to climb every day.

SLASHES EMBARRASSING LEAKAGES BY 79%

The 6 week clinical study was carried out by scientists in Japan. The results were published in the Journal of Medicine and Pharmaceutical Science in 2001.

The study involved seniors who suffered from frequent and embarrassing bladder leakages. They were not instructed to change their daily routines. They were only told to take BladderMax's active ingredient every day.

The results were incredible.

Taking BladderMax's active ingredient significantly reduced both sudden urges to go and embarrassing urine leakages compared to the placebo.

In fact, many experienced a 79% reduction in embarrassing accidents when coughing, sneezing, laughing or physical activity at 6 weeks.

HOW IT WORKS IS INCREDIBLE

Studies show that as many as one in six adults over age 40 suffers from an overactive bladder and embarrassing leakages.

"Losing control of when and how we go to the bathroom is just an indication of a weakening of the pelvic muscles caused by age-related hormonal changes," says Lewis.

"It happens in both men and women, and it is actually quite common."

The natural compound found in BladderMax contains the necessary ingredients needed to help strengthen bladder muscles to relieve urgency, while reducing frequency.

Plus, it helps relax bladder muscles allowing for complete emptying of the bladder.

This proprietary compound is known as 'EFLA940'®.

And with over 17 years of medical use there have been no adverse side effects reported.

RECOMMENDED BY U.S. MEDICAL DOCTORS

"Many of my patients used to complain that coughing, sneezing or even getting up quickly from a chair results in wetting themselves and they fear becoming a social outcast," reports Dr. Clifford James, M.D. "But BladderMax changes all that."

"BladderMax effectively treats urinary disorders, specifically overactive bladder," said Dr. Christie Wilkins, board certified doctor of natural medicine.

OLD FARMER'S ALMANAC READERS GET SPECIAL DISCOUNT SUPPLY

This is the official release of BladderMax and so for a limited time, the company is offering a special discount supply to our readers. An Order Hotline has been set up for our readers to call, but don't wait. The special offer will not last forever. All you have to do is call TOLL FREE **1-800-615-9302**. The company will do the rest.

These Statements Have Not Been Evaluated By The Food And Drug Administration. This Product Is Not Intended To Diagnose, Treat, Cure Or Prevent Any Disease. All Clinical Studies On BladderMax's Active Ingredient Were Independently Conducted And Were Not Sponsored By The Makers Of BladderMax. Offer Not Available To Iowa Residents.

ASTRONOMICAL GLOSSARY

MIDNIGHT: Astronomically, the time when the Sun is opposite its highest point in the sky. Both 12 hours before and after noon (so, technically, both A.M. and P.M.), midnight in civil time is usually treated as the beginning of the day. It is displayed as 12:00 A.M. on 12-hour digital clocks. On a 24-hour cycle, 00:00, not 24:00, usually indicates midnight.

MOON ON EQUATOR: The Moon is on the celestial equator.

MOON RIDES HIGH/RUNS LOW: The Moon is highest above or farthest below the celestial equator.

MOONRISE/MOONSET: When the Moon rises above or sets below the horizon.

MOON'S PHASES: The changing appearance of the Moon, caused by the different angles at which it is illuminated by the Sun. **First Quarter:** Right half of the Moon is illuminated. **Full:** The Sun and the Moon are in opposition; the entire disk of the Moon is illuminated. **Last Quarter:** Left half of the Moon is illuminated. **New:** The Sun and the Moon are in conjunction; the Moon is darkened because it lines up between Earth and the Sun.

MOON'S PLACE, Astronomical: The position of the Moon within the constellations on the celestial sphere at midnight. **Astrological:** The position of the Moon within the tropical zodiac, whose twelve 30° segments (signs) along the ecliptic were named more than 2,000 years ago after constellations within each area. Because of precession and other factors, the zodiac signs no longer match actual constellation positions.

MORNING STAR: A planet that is above the eastern horizon at sunrise and less than 180° west of the Sun in right ascension.

NODE: Either of the two points where a celestial body's orbit intersects the ecliptic. **Ascending:** When the body is moving from south to north of the ecliptic. **Descending:** When the body is moving from north to south of the ecliptic.

OCCULTATION (OCCN.): When the Moon or a planet eclipses a star or planet.

OPPOSITION: The Moon or a planet appears on the opposite side of the sky from the Sun (elongation 180°).

PERIGEE (PERIG.): The point in the Moon's orbit that is closest to Earth.

PERIHELION (PERIH.): The point in a planet's orbit that is closest to the Sun.

PRECESSION: The slowly changing position of the stars and equinoxes in the sky caused by a slight wobble as Earth rotates around its axis.

RIGHT ASCENSION (R.A.): The celestial longitude of an object in the sky, measured eastward along the celestial equator in hours of time from the vernal equinox; comparable to longitude on Earth.

SOLSTICE, Summer: When the Sun reaches its greatest declination (23½°) north of the celestial equator, around June 21. **Winter:** When the Sun reaches its greatest declination (23½°) south of the celestial equator, around December 21.

STATIONARY (STAT.): The brief period of apparent halted movement of a planet against the background of the stars shortly before it appears to move backward/westward (retrograde motion) or forward/eastward (direct motion).

SUN FAST/SLOW: When a sundial is ahead of (fast) or behind (slow) clock time.

SUNRISE/SUNSET: The visible rising/setting of the upper edge of the Sun's disk across the unobstructed horizon of an observer whose eyes are 15 feet above ground level.

TWILIGHT: See page 106. ■

Note: These definitions apply to the Northern Hemisphere; some do not hold true for locations in the Southern Hemisphere.

RESTORE INTIMACY

Call Now to receive your
FREE INFORMATION KIT:
1-877-266-7699

If your relationship has suffered because of **Erectile Dysfunction (ED)** for any of the following:

Diabetes **High Blood Pressure**
Prostate Cancer **Vascular Disease**
Medications **Aging Process**
Lifestyle Habits **Spinal Cord Injury**

The Vacurect™ offers a solution which is non-invasive and has NO side effects with over a 96% success rate.

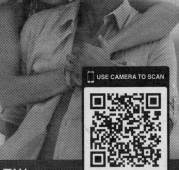

USE CAMERA TO SCAN

THE REVOLUTIONARY NEW
VACURECT™

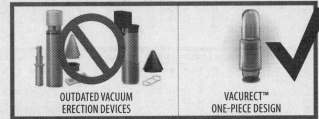

OUTDATED VACUUM
ERECTION DEVICES

VACURECT™
ONE-PIECE DESIGN

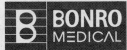

BONRO Medical
205 New Petersburg Dr.
Suite B
Martinez, GA 30907

www.bonro.com
a division of Mainspring Medical, LLC.

YES, I would like to receive a free patient information kit.

Name _____

Address _____

City _____ State ____ Zip _____

Phone _____

Please fax (888) 502-5132 or mail completed coupon to:
Bonro Medical PO Box 1880 Evans, GA 30809   OFA22

2021

JANUARY
S	M	T	W	T	F	S
					1	2
3	4	5	6	7	8	9
10	11	12	13	14	15	16
17	18	19	20	21	22	23
24	25	26	27	28	29	30
31						

FEBRUARY
S	M	T	W	T	F	S
	1	2	3	4	5	6
7	8	9	10	11	12	13
14	15	16	17	18	19	20
21	22	23	24	25	26	27
28						

MARCH
S	M	T	W	T	F	S
	1	2	3	4	5	6
7	8	9	10	11	12	13
14	15	16	17	18	19	20
21	22	23	24	25	26	27
28	29	30	31			

APRIL
S	M	T	W	T	F	S
				1	2	3
4	5	6	7	8	9	10
11	12	13	14	15	16	17
18	19	20	21	22	23	24
25	26	27	28	29	30	

MAY
S	M	T	W	T	F	S
						1
2	3	4	5	6	7	8
9	10	11	12	13	14	15
16	17	18	19	20	21	22
23	24	25	26	27	28	29
30	31					

JUNE
S	M	T	W	T	F	S
		1	2	3	4	5
6	7	8	9	10	11	12
13	14	15	16	17	18	19
20	21	22	23	24	25	26
27	28	29	30			

JULY
S	M	T	W	T	F	S
				1	2	3
4	5	6	7	8	9	10
11	12	13	14	15	16	17
18	19	20	21	22	23	24
25	26	27	28	29	30	31

AUGUST
S	M	T	W	T	F	S
1	2	3	4	5	6	7
8	9	10	11	12	13	14
15	16	17	18	19	20	21
22	23	24	25	26	27	28
29	30	31				

SEPTEMBER
S	M	T	W	T	F	S
			1	2	3	4
5	6	7	8	9	10	11
12	13	14	15	16	17	18
19	20	21	22	23	24	25
26	27	28	29	30		

OCTOBER
S	M	T	W	T	F	S
					1	2
3	4	5	6	7	8	9
10	11	12	13	14	15	16
17	18	19	20	21	22	23
24	25	26	27	28	29	30
31						

NOVEMBER
S	M	T	W	T	F	S
	1	2	3	4	5	6
7	8	9	10	11	12	13
14	15	16	17	18	19	20
21	22	23	24	25	26	27
28	29	30				

DECEMBER
S	M	T	W	T	F	S
			1	2	3	4
5	6	7	8	9	10	11
12	13	14	15	16	17	18
19	20	21	22	23	24	25
26	27	28	29	30	31	

2022

JANUARY
S	M	T	W	T	F	S
						1
2	3	4	5	6	7	8
9	10	11	12	13	14	15
16	17	18	19	20	21	22
23	24	25	26	27	28	29
30	31					

FEBRUARY
S	M	T	W	T	F	S
		1	2	3	4	5
6	7	8	9	10	11	12
13	14	15	16	17	18	19
20	21	22	23	24	25	26
27	28					

MARCH
S	M	T	W	T	F	S
		1	2	3	4	5
6	7	8	9	10	11	12
13	14	15	16	17	18	19
20	21	22	23	24	25	26
27	28	29	30	31		

APRIL
S	M	T	W	T	F	S
					1	2
3	4	5	6	7	8	9
10	11	12	13	14	15	16
17	18	19	20	21	22	23
24	25	26	27	28	29	30

MAY
S	M	T	W	T	F	S
1	2	3	4	5	6	7
8	9	10	11	12	13	14
15	16	17	18	19	20	21
22	23	24	25	26	27	28
29	30	31				

JUNE
S	M	T	W	T	F	S
			1	2	3	4
5	6	7	8	9	10	11
12	13	14	15	16	17	18
19	20	21	22	23	24	25
26	27	28	29	30		

JULY
S	M	T	W	T	F	S
					1	2
3	4	5	6	7	8	9
10	11	12	13	14	15	16
17	18	19	20	21	22	23
24	25	26	27	28	29	30
31						

AUGUST
S	M	T	W	T	F	S
	1	2	3	4	5	6
7	8	9	10	11	12	13
14	15	16	17	18	19	20
21	22	23	24	25	26	27
28	29	30	31			

SEPTEMBER
S	M	T	W	T	F	S
				1	2	3
4	5	6	7	8	9	10
11	12	13	14	15	16	17
18	19	20	21	22	23	24
25	26	27	28	29	30	

OCTOBER
S	M	T	W	T	F	S
						1
2	3	4	5	6	7	8
9	10	11	12	13	14	15
16	17	18	19	20	21	22
23	24	25	26	27	28	29
30	31					

NOVEMBER
S	M	T	W	T	F	S
		1	2	3	4	5
6	7	8	9	10	11	12
13	14	15	16	17	18	19
20	21	22	23	24	25	26
27	28	29	30			

DECEMBER
S	M	T	W	T	F	S
				1	2	3
4	5	6	7	8	9	10
11	12	13	14	15	16	17
18	19	20	21	22	23	24
25	26	27	28	29	30	31

2023

JANUARY
S	M	T	W	T	F	S
1	2	3	4	5	6	7
8	9	10	11	12	13	14
15	16	17	18	19	20	21
22	23	24	25	26	27	28
29	30	31				

FEBRUARY
S	M	T	W	T	F	S
			1	2	3	4
5	6	7	8	9	10	11
12	13	14	15	16	17	18
19	20	21	22	23	24	25
26	27	28				

MARCH
S	M	T	W	T	F	S
			1	2	3	4
5	6	7	8	9	10	11
12	13	14	15	16	17	18
19	20	21	22	23	24	25
26	27	28	29	30	31	

APRIL
S	M	T	W	T	F	S
						1
2	3	4	5	6	7	8
9	10	11	12	13	14	15
16	17	18	19	20	21	22
23	24	25	26	27	28	29
30						

MAY
S	M	T	W	T	F	S
	1	2	3	4	5	6
7	8	9	10	11	12	13
14	15	16	17	18	19	20
21	22	23	24	25	26	27
28	29	30	31			

JUNE
S	M	T	W	T	F	S
				1	2	3
4	5	6	7	8	9	10
11	12	13	14	15	16	17
18	19	20	21	22	23	24
25	26	27	28	29	30	

JULY
S	M	T	W	T	F	S
						1
2	3	4	5	6	7	8
9	10	11	12	13	14	15
16	17	18	19	20	21	22
23	24	25	26	27	28	29
30	31					

AUGUST
S	M	T	W	T	F	S
		1	2	3	4	5
6	7	8	9	10	11	12
13	14	15	16	17	18	19
20	21	22	23	24	25	26
27	28	29	30	31		

SEPTEMBER
S	M	T	W	T	F	S
					1	2
3	4	5	6	7	8	9
10	11	12	13	14	15	16
17	18	19	20	21	22	23
24	25	26	27	28	29	30

OCTOBER
S	M	T	W	T	F	S
1	2	3	4	5	6	7
8	9	10	11	12	13	14
15	16	17	18	19	20	21
22	23	24	25	26	27	28
29	30	31				

NOVEMBER
S	M	T	W	T	F	S
			1	2	3	4
5	6	7	8	9	10	11
12	13	14	15	16	17	18
19	20	21	22	23	24	25
26	27	28	29	30		

DECEMBER
S	M	T	W	T	F	S
					1	2
3	4	5	6	7	8	9
10	11	12	13	14	15	16
17	18	19	20	21	22	23
24	25	26	27	28	29	30
31						

A CALENDAR OF THE HEAVENS FOR 2022

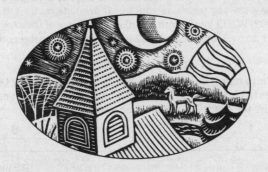

The Calendar Pages (120–147) are the heart of *The Old Farmer's Almanac*. They present sky sightings and astronomical data for the entire year and are what make this book a true almanac, a "calendar of the heavens." In essence, these pages are unchanged since 1792, when Robert B. Thomas published his first edition. The long columns of numbers and symbols reveal all of nature's precision, rhythm, and glory, providing an astronomical look at the year 2022.

HOW TO USE THE CALENDAR PAGES

The astronomical data on the **Calendar Pages (120–147)** are calculated for Ottawa, Ontario. Guidance for calculating the times of these events for your locale appears on **pages 116–117**. Note that the results will be *approximate*. For the *exact* time of any astronomical event at your locale, go to **Almanac.ca/2022** and enter your postal code. While you're there, print the month's "Sky Map," useful for viewing with "Sky Watch" in the Calendar Pages.

For a list of 2022 holidays and observances, see **pages 148–149.** Also check out the **Glossary of Almanac Oddities** on **pages 150–151,** which describes some of the more obscure entries traditionally found on the **Right-Hand Calendar Pages (121–147).**

ABOUT THE TIMES: All times are given in ET (Eastern Time), except where otherwise noted as NT (Newfoundland Time, +1½ hours), AT (Atlantic Time, +1 hour), CT (Central Time, –1), MT (Mountain Time, –2), or PT (Pacific Time, –3). Between 2:00 A.M., March 13, and 2:00 A.M., November 6, Daylight Saving Time is assumed in those locales where it is observed.

ABOUT THE TIDES: For tidal information, see **pages 120–147, 237,** and **238–239.** Tide times and heights also are available via **Almanac.ca/2022.**

The Left-Hand Calendar Pages, 120 to 146

On these pages are the year's astronomical predictions for Ottawa, Ontario (45°25' N, 75°42' W). Learn how to calculate the times of these events for your locale here or go to **Almanac.ca/2022** and enter your postal code.

A SAMPLE MONTH

SKY WATCH: The paragraph at the top of each Left-Hand Calendar Page describes the best times to view conjunctions, meteor showers, planets, and more. (Also see **How to Use the Right-Hand Calendar Pages, page 118.**)

	1		2		3	4	5		6			7	8
DAY OF YEAR	DAY OF MONTH	DAY OF WEEK	☀ RISES	RISE KEY	☀ SETS	SET KEY	LENGTH OF DAY	SUN FAST	SUN DECLINATION	HIGH TIDE TIMES HALIFAX	☽ RISES	RISE KEY	☽ SETS	SET KEY	☽ ASTRON. PLACE	☽ AGE
			H. M.		H. M.		H. M.	M.	° '		H. M.		H. M.			
60	1	Fr.	6:41	D	5:50	B	11 09	*15	7 s. 30	4 5	3:59	E	1:07	A	SAG	25
61	2	Sa.	6:40	D	5:51	B	11 11	*15	7 s. 07	5 6	4:45	E	2:01	A	SAG	26
62	3	F	6:38	D	5:52	C	11 14	*15	6 s. 44	6 6¾	5:24	E	2:58	A	CAP	27
63	4	M.	6:36	D	5:54	C	11 18	*14	6 s. 21	6¾ 7½	5:58	D	3:57	B	CAP	28

1. To calculate the sunrise time in your locale: Choose a day. Note its Sun Rise Key Letter. Find your (nearest) city on **page 240**. Add or subtract the minutes that correspond to the Sun Rise Key Letter to/from the sunrise time for Ottawa.[†]

EXAMPLE:

To calculate the sunrise time in Vancouver, British Columbia, on day 1:

Sunrise, Ottawa, with Key Letter D (above)	6:41 A.M. ET
Value of Key Letter D for Vancouver (p. 240)	+ 17 minutes
Sunrise, Vancouver	6:58 A.M. PT

To calculate your sunset time, repeat, using Ottawa's sunset time and its Sun Set Key Letter value.

2. To calculate the length of day: Choose a day. Note the Sun Rise and Sun Set Key Letters. Find your (nearest) city on **page 240**. Add or subtract the minutes that correspond to the Sun Set Key Letter to/from Ottawa's

length of day. *Reverse* the sign (e.g., minus to plus) of the Sun Rise Key Letter minutes. Add or subtract it to/from the first result.

EXAMPLE:

To calculate the length of day in Brandon, Manitoba, on day 1:

Length of day, Ottawa (above)	11h. 09m.
Sunset Key Letter B for Brandon (p. 240)	+ 28m.
	11h. 37m.
Reverse sunrise Key Letter D for Brandon (p. 240, +46 to -46)	- 46m.
Length of day, Brandon	10h. 51m.

3. Use Sun Fast to change sundial time to clock time. A sundial reads natural (Sun) time, which is neither Standard nor Daylight time. To calculate clock time on a sundial in Ottawa, subtract the minutes given in this column; add the minutes when preceded by an asterisk [*].

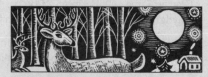

[†]For locations where Daylight Saving Time is never observed, subtract 1 hour from results between the second Sunday of March and first Sunday of November.

To convert the time to your (nearest) city, use Key Letter C on **page 240.**

EXAMPLE:

To change sundial to clock time in Ottawa or Thunder Bay, Ont., on day 1:

Sundial reading (Ottawa or Thunder Bay)	12:00 noon
Add Sun Fast (p. 116)	+ 15 minutes
Clock time, Ottawa	12:15 P.M. ET**
Use Key Letter C for Thunder Bay (p. 241)	+ 53 minutes
Clock time, Thunder Bay	1:08 P.M. ET**

**Note: Add 1 hour to the results in locations where Daylight Saving Time is currently observed.

4. This column gives the degrees and minutes of the Sun from the celestial equator at noon ET.

5. This column gives the approximate times of high tides in Halifax. For example, the first high tide occurs at 4:00 A.M. and the second occurs at 5:00 P.M. the same day. (A dash indicates that high tide occurs on or after midnight and is recorded on the next day.) Because of the great variations in tide times and heights on both the east and west coasts, no one locality can be used as a mean. Twice-weekly times and heights of high tides at Churchill, Manitoba, and Vancouver, British Columbia, are provided on **page 238.**

6. To calculate the moonrise time in your locale: Choose a day. Note the Moon Rise Key Letter. Find your (nearest) city on **page 240.** Add or subtract the minutes that correspond to the Moon Rise

LONGITUDE OF CITY	CORRECTION MINUTES	LONGITUDE OF CITY	CORRECTION MINUTES
58°–76°	0	116°–127°	+4
77°–89°	+1	128°–141°	+5
90°–102°	+2	142°–155°	+6
103°–115°	+3		

Key Letter to/from the moonrise time given for Ottawa. (A dash indicates that the moonrise occurs on/after midnight and is recorded on the next day.) Find the longitude of your (nearest) city on **page 240.** Add a correction in minutes for your city's longitude (see table, bottom left). Use the same procedure with Ottawa's moonset time and the Moon Set Key Letter value to calculate the time of moonset in your locale.[†]

EXAMPLE:

To calculate the time of moonset in Toronto, Ontario, on day 1:

Moonset, Ottawa, with Key Letter A (p. 116)	1:07 P.M. ET
Value of Key Letter A for Toronto (p. 241)	+ 21 minutes
Correction for Toronto longitude, 79°23'	+ 1 minute
Moonset, Toronto	1:29 P.M. ET

7. This column gives the Moon's *astronomical* position among the constellations (not zodiac) at midnight. For *astrological* data, see **pages 224–227.**

Constellations have irregular borders; on successive nights, the midnight Moon may enter one, cross into another, and then move to a new area of the previous. It visits the 12 zodiacal constellations, as well as Auriga **(AUR),** a northern constellation between Perseus and Gemini; Cetus **(CET),** which lies south of the zodiac, just south of Pisces and Aries; Ophiuchus **(OPH),** primarily north of the zodiac but with a small corner between Scorpius and Sagittarius; Orion **(ORI),** whose northern limit first reaches the zodiac between Taurus and Gemini; and Sextans **(SEX),** which lies south of the zodiac except for a corner that just touches it near Leo.

8. This column gives the Moon's age: the number of days since the previous new Moon. (The average length of the lunar month is 29.53 days.) *(continued)*

The Right-Hand Calendar Pages, 121 to 147

The Right-Hand Calendar Pages contain celestial events; religious observances; proverbs and poems; civil holidays; historical events; folklore; tide heights; weather prediction rhymes; Farmer's Calendar essays; and more.

A SAMPLE MONTH

1 2 3 4 5 6 7 8 9 10

1	Fr.	ALL FOOLS' • *If you want to make a fool of yourself, you'll find a lot of people ready to help you.*	*Flakes*	an inch long, who v
2	Sa.	Tap dancer Charles "Honi" Coles born, 1911 • Tides {5.1 / 5.0	*alive!*	in fresh water, pro pond across the r
3	**B**	2nd ☉. of Easter • Writer F. Scott Fitzgerald married Zelda Sayre, 1920	*Spring's*	emerged a month o
4	M.	Annunciation ᵀ • ♂♆☾ • *Ben Hur* won 11 Academy Awards, 1960	*arrived!*	to spend the next 3 on land before ret
5	Tu.	☾ AT ☋ • Blizzard left 27.2" snow, St. John's, Nfld., 1999 • Tides {5.8 / 6.2	*Or is this*	their wet world.
6	W.	☾ ON EQ. • ♂♀☾ • Twin mongoose lemurs born, Busch Gardens, Tampa, Fla., 2012	*warmth*	You can't mis

1. The bold letter is the Dominical Letter (from A to G), a traditional ecclesiastical designation for Sunday determined by the date on which the year's first Sunday falls. For 2022, the Dominical Letter is **B**.

2. Civil holidays and astronomical events.

3. Religious feasts: A ᵀ indicates a major feast that the church has this year temporarily transferred to a date other than its usual one.

4. Sundays and special holy days.

5. Symbols for notable celestial events. For example, ♂♆☾ on the 4th day means that a conjunction (♂) of Neptune (♆) and the Moon (☾) occurs.

6. Proverbs, poems, and adages.

7. Noteworthy historical events, folklore, and legends.

8. High tide heights, in feet, at Halifax, Nova Scotia.

9. Weather prediction rhyme.

10. Farmer's Calendar essay.

Celestial Symbols

☉ Sun	⊕ Earth	♅ Uranus	♂ Conjunction (on the same celestial longitude)	☋ Descending node
○●☾ Moon	♂ Mars	♆ Neptune		☌ Opposition (180 degrees from Sun)
☿ Mercury	♃ Jupiter	♇ Pluto		
♀ Venus	♄ Saturn		☊ Ascending node	

PREDICTING EARTHQUAKES

Note the dates in the Right-Hand Calendar Pages when the Moon rides high or runs low. The date of the high begins the most likely 5-day period of earthquakes in the Northern Hemisphere; the date of the low indicates a similar 5-day period in the Southern Hemisphere. Also noted are the 2 days each month when the Moon is on the celestial equator, indicating the most likely time for earthquakes in either hemisphere.

EARTH AT PERIHELION AND APHELION
Perihelion: January 4, 2022 (EST). Earth will be 91,406,842 miles from the Sun. **Aphelion:** July 4, 2022 (EDT). Earth will be 94,509,598 miles from the Sun.

CALENDAR

Why We Have Seasons

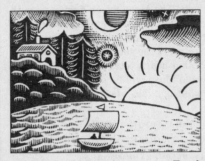

The seasons occur because as Earth revolves around the Sun, its axis remains tilted at 23.5 degrees from the perpendicular. This tilt causes different latitudes on Earth to receive varying amounts of sunlight throughout the year.

In the Northern Hemisphere, the summer solstice marks the beginning of summer and occurs when the North Pole is tilted toward the Sun. The winter solstice marks the beginning of winter and occurs when the North Pole is tilted away from the Sun.

The equinoxes occur when the hemispheres equally face the Sun. At this time, the Sun rises due east and sets due west. The vernal equinox marks the beginning of spring; the autumnal equinox marks the beginning of autumn.

In the Southern Hemisphere, the seasons are the reverse of those in the Northern Hemisphere.

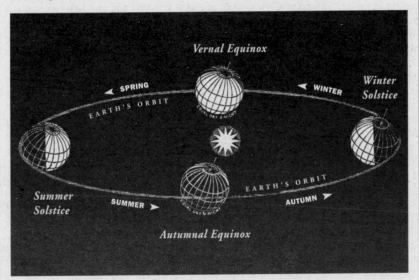

THE FIRST DAYS OF THE 2022 SEASONS

VERNAL (SPRING) EQUINOX:	March 20, 11:33 A.M. EDT
SUMMER SOLSTICE:	June 21, 5:14 A.M. EDT
AUTUMNAL (FALL) EQUINOX:	Sept. 22, 9:04 P.M. EDT
WINTER SOLSTICE:	Dec. 21, 4:48 P.M. EST

NOVEMBER

SKY WATCH: Venus, at a dazzling magnitude –4.33, crosses into Sagittarius and floats directly in front of our galaxy's center, which is off in the far distance. On the 7th, the crescent Moon joins Venus there. The Moon forms a triangle with Jupiter and Saturn on the 10th and then dangles beneath Jupiter on the 11th. Venus reaches its most southerly zodiac position at midmonth. Its declination of –27 degrees makes it set as far left as possible, in the southwest instead of the west. The night of the 18th–19th brings another nearly total lunar eclipse in the hours before dawn. This 98 percent–eclipsed Moon will be a strange, coppery sight—well worth a look by early risers and insomniacs who have unobstructed views of the low western sky.

● **NEW MOON** 4th day 5:15 P.M. ○ **FULL MOON** 19th day 3:57 A.M.

◐ **FIRST QUARTER** 11th day 7:46 A.M. ◑ **LAST QUARTER** 27th day 7:28 A.M.

After 2:00 A.M. on November 7, Eastern Standard Time is given.

GET THESE PAGES WITH TIMES SET TO YOUR POSTAL CODE VIA ALMANAC.CA/2022.

DAY OF YEAR	DAY OF MONTH	DAY OF WEEK	☼ RISES H. M.	RISE KEY	☼ SETS H. M.	SET KEY	LENGTH OF DAY H. M.	SUN FAST M.	SUN DECLINATION ° '	HIGH TIDE TIMES HALIFAX		☾ RISES H. M.	RISE KEY	☾ SETS H. M.	SET KEY	☾ ASTRON. PLACE	☾ AGE
305	1	M.	7:42	D	**5:50**	B	10 08	14	14 s. 39	6	6¼	3:21	B	**4:39**	C	LEO	26
306	2	Tu.	7:44	D	**5:48**	B	10 04	14	14 s. 58	6¾	7	4:36	C	**5:00**	C	VIR	27
307	3	W.	7:45	D	**5:47**	B	10 02	14	15 s. 16	7½	7¾	5:54	C	**5:24**	B	VIR	28
308	4	Th.	7:47	D	**5:45**	B	9 58	14	15 s. 35	8	8½	7:15	D	**5:50**	B	VIR	0
309	5	Fr.	7:48	D	**5:44**	B	9 56	14	15 s. 53	8¾	9¼	8:39	D	**6:21**	A	LIB	1
310	6	Sa.	7:49	D	**5:43**	B	9 54	14	16 s. 11	9½	10¼	10:04	E	**7:01**	A	SCO	2
311	7	**C**	6:51	D	**4:42**	B	9 51	13	16 s. 28	9¼	10	10:24	E	**6:51**	A	OPH	3
312	8	M.	6:52	D	**4:40**	B	9 48	13	16 s. 46	10¼	11	11:34	E	**7:53**	A	SAG	4
313	9	Tu.	6:54	D	**4:39**	B	9 45	13	17 s. 03	11	11¾	12:31	E	**9:03**	A	SAG	5
314	10	W.	6:55	D	**4:38**	B	9 43	13	17 s. 20	12	—	1:14	E	**10:18**	A	CAP	6
315	11	Th.	6:56	E	**4:37**	B	9 41	13	17 s. 36	12¾	1	1:48	E	**11:32**	A	CAP	7
316	12	Fr.	6:58	E	**4:36**	B	9 38	13	17 s. 52	2	2¼	2:14	D	—	-	AQU	8
317	13	Sa.	6:59	E	**4:35**	B	9 36	13	18 s. 08	3¼	3½	2:36	D	12:44	B	AQU	9
318	14	**C**	7:01	E	**4:33**	B	9 32	13	18 s. 24	4½	4½	2:56	C	1:53	B	AQU	10
319	15	M.	7:02	E	**4:32**	B	9 30	13	18 s. 39	5¼	5½	3:14	C	2:59	C	CET	11
320	16	Tu.	7:03	E	**4:31**	A	9 28	12	18 s. 54	6	6¼	3:32	B	4:04	C	PSC	12
321	17	W.	7:05	E	**4:31**	A	9 26	12	19 s. 09	6½	7	3:52	B	5:09	D	PSC	13
322	18	Th.	7:06	E	**4:30**	A	9 24	12	19 s. 23	7¼	7¾	4:15	B	6:14	D	ARI	14
323	19	Fr.	7:07	E	**4:29**	A	9 22	12	19 s. 37	7¾	8¼	4:41	A	7:19	E	TAU	15
324	20	Sa.	7:09	E	**4:28**	A	9 19	11	19 s. 50	8½	9	5:13	A	8:23	E	TAU	16
325	21	**C**	7:10	E	**4:27**	A	9 17	11	20 s. 03	9	9½	5:51	A	9:25	E	TAU	17
326	22	M.	7:11	E	**4:26**	A	9 15	11	20 s. 16	9½	10¼	6:38	A	10:21	E	GEM	18
327	23	Tu.	7:13	E	**4:26**	A	9 13	11	20 s. 29	10¼	11	7:33	A	11:10	E	GEM	19
328	24	W.	7:14	E	**4:25**	A	9 11	10	20 s. 41	10¾	11½	8:35	A	11:52	E	GEM	20
329	25	Th.	7:15	E	**4:24**	A	9 09	10	20 s. 52	11½	—	9:41	A	12:26	E	CAN	21
330	26	Fr.	7:16	E	**4:24**	A	9 08	10	21 s. 03	12¼	12¼	10:50	B	12:54	E	LEO	22
331	27	Sa.	7:18	E	**4:23**	A	9 05	9	21 s. 14	1¼	1	12:00	B	1:19	D	LEO	23
332	28	**C**	7:19	E	**4:23**	A	9 04	9	21 s. 25	2¼	2¼	—	-	1:41	D	LEO	24
333	29	M.	7:20	E	**4:22**	A	9 02	9	21 s. 35	3¼	3½	1:12	B	2:02	C	VIR	25
334	30	Tu.	7:21	E	**4:22**	A	9 01	8	21 s. 45	4¼	4½	2:26	C	2:23	C	VIR	26

To use this page, see p. 116; for Key Letters, see p. 240. LIGHT = A.M. BOLD = P.M. 2022

NOVEMBER

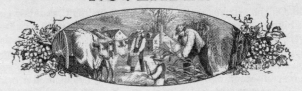

The farmer sat there milking Bess, / A-whistling all the while; /
He was a sunburnt, stalwart man, / And had a kindly smile.
–Mary E. Wilkins

Farmer's Calendar

"Every man looks at his woodpile with a kind of affection," wrote American essayist Henry David Thoreau (1817–62). He's right, too, isn't he? An ample woodpile has a familiar, reassuring presence. It's a satisfactory object in a way that's a little hard to account for. We respond to the sight of a good woodpile with a level of contentment.

What is it that contents us? Not use, or not use alone.

It's not as fuel that a woodpile makes its particular appeal. It's as a symbol. We are cheered and comforted by our woodpile today because a woodpile is one of the stations of the year and expresses the essential ambiguity of all seasonal work. It represents a job that we know we can do well enough but that we also know will never finally be done: Woodpiles are built up that they may be torn down. Massive as they are, they're ephemeral. You'll have to build another next year, which you will then once more throw down. The woodpile reminds us of the fix we're in just by being alive on Earth. It connects us with the years, and so it connects us with one another. We may as well look at our woodpile with affection, then, for it makes us be philosophers.

DAY OF MONTH	DAY OF WEEK	DATES, FEASTS, FASTS, ASPECTS, TIDE HEIGHTS, AND WEATHER	
1	M.	**All Saints'** • Writer Stephen Crane born, 1871 • {5.6 / 5.5	*Bundle*
2	Tu.	All Souls' • **ELECTION DAY (U.S.)** • ☾ON EQ. • Tides {6.0 / 5.8	*up*
3	W.	♂♂☾ • John Adams elected 2nd U.S. president, 1796 • Tides {6.3 / 6.1	*to*
4	Th.	**NEW ●** • ♂♂☾ • ♂ ☿ AT ☍ • Tides {6.7 / 6.3	*your*
5	Fr.	☾AT PERIG. • ☾ AT ☍ • *Better untaught than ill taught.* • Tides {6.9 / 6.3	*necks*
6	Sa.	Sadie Hawkins Day • Basketball-game inventor James Naismith born, 1861 • {6.9 / 6.3	*for*
7	**C**	**24th ☉. af. ℙ.** • **DAYLIGHT SAVING TIME ENDS, 2:00 A.M.** • {6.8 / 6.1	*the*
8	M.	☾RUNS LOW • ♂♀☾ • Astronomer Edmond Halley born, 1656	*polar*
9	Tu.	♂♂♂ • ♂♭☾ • Maj. Robert White flew X-15 rocket plane at Mach 6.04, 1961	*vortex!*
10	W.	♂♭☾ • 70+ tornadoes developed, eastern half of U.S., 2002 • Tides {5.8 / —	*Cold's*
11	Th.	St. Martin of Tours • **REMEMBRANCE DAY** • ♂♃☾ • {5.5 / 5.5	*injurious,*
12	Fr.	Indian Summer • *The wind in the west suits everyone best.* • Tides {5.4 / 5.3	*flurries*
13	Sa.	♂♆☾ • *Mariner 9* became 1st spacecraft to orbit another planet (Mars), 1971 • {5.4 / 5.2	*furious.*
14	**C**	**25th ☉. af. ℙ.** • U.S. first lady Mamie Eisenhower born, 1896 • {5.6 / 5.3	*Hunters*
15	M.	☾ON EQ. • America Recycles Day (U.S.) • {5.7 / 5.4	*find*
16	Tu.	45°F plus 8.4" snow, Anchorage, Alaska, 2019 • Tides {5.9 / 5.5	*plenty*
17	W.	St. Hugh of Lincoln • ♂♂☾ • Social worker Grace Abbott born, 1878 • {5.9 / 5.5	*of*
18	Th.	St. Hilda of Whitby • Standard Railway Time went into effect for most N.Am. railroads, 1883	*snow*
19	Fr.	**FULL BEAVER ○** • **ECLIPSE ☾** • ☾ AT ☍ • Tides {6.0 / 5.6	*for*
20	Sa.	☾ AT APO. • Ballerina Maya Plisetskaya born, 1925 • {6.0 / 5.5	*tracking;*
21	**C**	**26th ☉. af. ℙ.** • H. Truman became 2nd U.S. pres. to dive in sub (T. Roosevelt 1st), 1946	*turkey*
22	M.	☾RIDES HIGH • Agronomist William Evans born, 1786 • Comedian Rodney Dangerfield born, 1921	*roasters,*
23	Tu.	St. Clement • Horseshoe manufacturing machine patented, 1835 • Tides {5.7 / 5.3	*let's*
24	W.	Baseball player Warren Spahn died, 2003 • Tides {5.6 / 5.2	*get*
25	Th.	**THANKSGIVING DAY (U.S.)** • *A good tale is none the worse for being twice told.* • {5.4 / —	*cracking!*
26	Fr.	Buoy recorded 75-foot wave off Cape Mendocino, Calif., 2019 • Tides {5.2 / 5.3	*Woodstove*
27	Sa.	Microsoft's *Internet Explorer 2.0* released, starting 1st "browser war" (with Netscape's *Navigator*), 1995	*owners*
28	**C**	**1st ☉. of Advent** • Chanukah begins at sundown • ☿ IN SUP. ♂	*better*
29	M.	☾ON EQ. • Ensemble of 1,013 cellists played in Kobe, Japan, setting world record, 1998 • {5.5 / 5.2	*start*
30	Tu.	St. Andrew • Welland Canal opened, Ont., 1829 • Tides {5.8 / 5.4	*stacking!*

Find more facts and fun every day at Almanac.ca.

DECEMBER

SKY WATCH: On the 1st, Venus, now at its most brilliant, stands a comfortable 16 degrees high as the constellations emerge in the late evening twilight. On the 6th, it hovers just above the crescent Moon—a lovely sight. Also on the 6th, look for a planet bunch-up in the west after sunset: From lower right to upper left stand Venus, the Moon, Saturn, and Jupiter. The grouping remains on the 8th, with the crescent Moon now second from the top, below Jupiter, which moves back into Aquarius at midmonth. By the holidays, Mercury, at a bright magnitude –0.5, will be visible, too, dangling below Venus from the 24th to the 31st. It will stand left of Venus from the 29th to the 31st. The solstice brings winter to the Northern Hemisphere on the 21st at 10:59 A.M. EST.

● **NEW MOON** 4th day 2:43 A.M.   ○ **FULL MOON** 18th day 11:35 P.M.
◐ **FIRST QUARTER** 10th day 8:36 P.M.   ◑ **LAST QUARTER** 26th day 9:24 P.M.

All times are given in Eastern Standard Time.

GET THESE PAGES WITH TIMES SET TO YOUR POSTAL CODE VIA ALMANAC.CA/2022.

DAY OF YEAR	DAY OF MONTH	DAY OF WEEK	☼ RISES H. M.	RISE KEY	☼ SETS H. M.	SET KEY	LENGTH OF DAY H. M.	SUN FAST M.	SUN DECLINATION ° '	HIGH TIDE TIMES HALIFAX		☾ RISES H. M.	RISE KEY	☾ SETS H. M.	SET KEY	☾ ASTRON. PLACE	☾ AGE
335	1	W.	7:22	E	4:21	A	8 59	8	21 s. 54	5	5½	3:43	D	2:47	B	VIR	27
336	2	Th.	7:24	E	4:21	A	8 57	8	22 s. 03	5¾	6½	5:05	D	3:15	B	LIB	28
337	3	Fr.	7:25	E	4:21	A	8 56	7	22 s. 11	6½	7¼	6:29	E	3:49	A	LIB	29
338	4	Sa.	7:26	E	4:20	A	8 54	7	22 s. 19	7½	8	7:54	E	4:35	A	OPH	0
339	5	**C**	7:27	E	4:20	A	8 53	6	22 s. 27	8¼	9	9:12	E	5:32	A	SAG	1
340	6	M.	7:28	E	4:20	A	8 52	6	22 s. 34	9	9¾	10:18	E	6:42	A	SAG	2
341	7	Tu.	7:29	E	4:20	A	8 51	6	22 s. 40	10	10¾	11:09	E	7:59	A	SAG	3
342	8	W.	7:30	E	4:20	A	8 50	5	22 s. 47	10¾	11½	11:48	E	9:16	A	CAP	4
343	9	Th.	7:31	E	4:20	A	8 49	5	22 s. 52	11¾	—	12:18	D	10:31	B	CAP	5
344	10	Fr.	7:32	E	4:20	A	8 48	4	22 s. 58	12½	12¾	12:41	D	11:43	B	AQU	6
345	11	Sa.	7:33	E	4:20	A	8 47	4	23 s. 03	1½	1¾	1:02	C	—	-	AQU	7
346	12	**C**	7:33	E	4:20	A	8 47	3	23 s. 07	2¾	2¾	1:21	C	12:51	C	PSC	8
347	13	M.	7:34	E	4:20	A	8 46	3	23 s. 11	3¾	4	1:39	C	1:56	C	PSC	9
348	14	Tu.	7:35	E	4:20	A	8 45	2	23 s. 14	4½	5	1:58	B	3:01	D	PSC	10
349	15	W.	7:36	E	4:20	A	8 44	2	23 s. 17	5¼	6	2:19	B	4:06	D	ARI	11
350	16	Th.	7:37	E	4:21	A	8 44	1	23 s. 20	6	6¾	2:44	A	5:10	E	ARI	12
351	17	Fr.	7:37	E	4:21	A	8 44	1	23 s. 22	6¾	7¼	3:14	A	6:15	E	TAU	13
352	18	Sa.	7:38	E	4:21	A	8 43	0	23 s. 24	7¼	8	3:50	A	7:17	E	TAU	14
353	19	**C**	7:38	E	4:21	A	8 43	0	23 s. 25	8	8¾	4:35	A	8:16	E	TAU	15
354	20	M.	7:39	E	4:22	A	8 43	*1	23 s. 26	8½	9¼	5:27	A	9:07	E	GEM	16
355	21	Tu.	7:40	E	4:23	A	8 43	*1	23 s. 26	9¼	10	6:27	A	9:51	E	GEM	17
356	22	W.	7:40	E	4:23	A	8 43	*2	23 s. 25	9¾	10½	7:32	A	10:28	E	CAN	18
357	23	Th.	7:40	E	4:23	A	8 43	*2	23 s. 25	10½	11¼	8:39	A	10:58	E	CAN	19
358	24	Fr.	7:41	E	4:24	A	8 43	*3	23 s. 24	11¼	—	9:48	B	11:23	D	LEO	20
359	25	Sa.	7:41	E	4:25	A	8 44	*3	23 s. 22	12	11¾	10:57	B	11:45	D	LEO	21
360	26	**C**	7:42	E	4:26	A	8 44	*4	23 s. 20	12¾	12¾	—	-	12:05	C	VIR	22
361	27	M.	7:42	E	4:26	A	8 44	*4	23 s. 17	1½	1¾	12:08	C	12:26	C	VIR	23
362	28	Tu.	7:42	E	4:27	A	8 45	*5	23 s. 14	2½	2¾	1:21	C	12:47	B	VIR	24
363	29	W.	7:42	E	4:28	A	8 46	*5	23 s. 11	3½	4	2:37	D	1:12	B	VIR	25
364	30	Th.	7:42	E	4:29	A	8 47	*5	23 s. 07	4¼	5	3:58	D	1:42	A	LIB	26
365	31	Fr.	7:42	E	4:30	A	8 48	*6	23 s. 02	5¼	6	5:20	E	2:20	A	SCO	27

DECEMBER

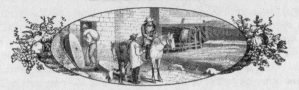

Let Joy light up in every breast, / And brighten every eye,
Distressing Care be lull'd to rest, / And hush'd be every sigh.
—Peter Sherston

DAY OF MONTH	DAY OF WEEK	DATES, FEASTS, FASTS, ASPECTS, TIDE HEIGHTS, AND WEATHER	
1	W.	♅ STAT. • Holography pioneer Stephen Benton born, 1941 • Tides {6.1 {5.7	More
2	Th.	St. Viviana • ♂♂☾ • 1st unmanned landing on Mars, by USSR *Mars 3*, 1971 • {6.5 {5.9	snow
3	Fr.	☾ AT ☋ • 68°F, Portland, Maine, 2009 • Tides {6.7 {6.1	than
4	Sa.	NEW ● • ECLIPSE ☉ • ☾ AT PERIG. • ♂♀☾ • ♀ GR. ILLUM. EXT.	we
5	C	2nd ☉. of Advent • ☾ RUNS LOW • Entrepreneur Walt Disney born, 1901	reckoned
6	M.	St. Nicholas • ♂♀☾ • ♂♇☾ • Tides {6.8 {6.2	for
7	Tu.	St. Ambrose • NATIONAL PEARL HARBOR REMEMBRANCE DAY (U.S.) • ♂♄☾	piles
8	W.	John McCrae's *In Flanders Fields* poem published, 1915 • Tides {6.2 {5.9	up
9	Th.	♂♃☾ • Robert Cushman preached 1st known Christian sermon in America, Plymouth (Mass.), 1621	to
10	Fr.	St. Eulalia • ♂♅☾ • Chemist Alfred Nobel died, 1896 • {5.7 {5.5	the
11	Sa.	♂♀♇ • Statute of Westminster passed, 1931 • Tides {5.6 {5.2	second
12	C	3rd ☉. of Advent • ☾ ON EQ. • Astronomer Henrietta Swan Leavitt died, 1921	floor!
13	M.	St. Lucia • Artist Grandma Moses died, 1961 • {5.5 {5.0	Brief
14	Tu.	Halcyon Days begin. • 5.6-lb. avocado set world record for heaviest, Kahului, Hawaii, 2018 • {5.6 {5.1	relief,
15	W.	Ember Day • ♂♂☾ • U.S. Bill of Rights ratified, 1791 • Tides {5.7 {5.2	then
16	Th.	☾ AT ☋ • *In courtesy, rather pay a penny too much than too little.* • {5.7 {5.2	good
17	Fr.	Ember Day • AT APO. • 1st heart, lung, and liver transplant, 1986 • Tides {5.8 {5.3	grief!
18	Sa.	Ember Day • FULL COLD ○ • ♀ STAT. • Film director Steven Spielberg born, 1946	It's
19	C	4th ☉. of Advent • ☾ RIDES HIGH • Mark Twain rec'd patent for suspenders, 1871	true:
20	M.	Beware the Pogonip. • Astrophysicist Carl Sagan died, 1996 • Tides {5.9 {5.4	Even
21	Tu.	St. Thomas • WINTER SOLSTICE • *After a rainy winter follows a fruitful spring.* • {5.9 {5.4	Santa's
22	W.	Grote Reber, builder of 1st radio telescope, born, 1911 • Tides {5.8 {5.4	checking
23	Th.	♂♀♇ • *Voyager* aircraft completed 1st nonstop flight around world w/o refueling (9 days 4 min.), 1986	real
24	Fr.	Eggnog Riot began, U.S. Military Academy at West Point, N.Y., 1826 • {5.6 {5.5	estate
25	Sa.	Christmas • Poet William Collins born, 1721 • Am. Red Cross founder Clara Barton born, 1821	in
26	C	1st ☉. af. Ch. • BOXING DAY • FIRST DAY OF KWANZAA • {5.5 {5.3	Malibu!
27	M.	St. Stephen[T] • ☾ ON EQ. • Astronomer Johannes Kepler born, 1571 • {5.5 {5.1	Lips
28	Tu.	St. John[T] • ♂♀♇ • Iowa became 29th state, 1846 • 31.5" snow in 24 hrs., Victoria, B.C., 1996	will
29	W.	Holy Innocents[T] • ♂♀♇ • William Lyon Mackenzie King became 10th prime minister of Canada, 1921	be
30	Th.	☾ AT ☋ • ♂♀♇ • *A new broom sweeps clean.* • {6.1 {5.4	blue
31	Fr.	St. Sylvester • ♂♂☾ • Baltimore, Md., incorporated, 1796 • {6.3 {5.7	in '22!

Farmer's Calendar

Now, as the season of storms approaches, a bewildering multiplicity of snow shovels has been on display in practically every store in town. And what snow shovels they are! There are snow shovels with straight handles, snow shovels with bent handles, with fat blades, with thin blades, with D grips, with T grips. Some snow shovels are plastic and cost a couple of bucks; others are so expensive that it seems wrong to expose them to a substance, like snow, that comes for free.

What to do?

It took me a number of winters to discover that very often the best snow shovel is a simple broom, one with long, stiff straw. A broom will take care of better than half the snow you'll get in a winter, and it won't break your back, burst your heart, or dig up your grass by mistake. For cleaning snow off the car, the broom is far superior to the shovel because it can't scratch your paint job. And if you are equipped with a broom and you should, at last, get a fall of snow too deep to overcome, you can fly south until you get to a latitude where snow is unknown and the home centers sell only those shovels that come with pails for use at the beach.

CALENDAR

JANUARY

SKY WATCH: A fine, eclipse-filled year begins with the planets in the evening sky only at the very beginning and then in the final part of 2022. During the rest of the year, the action occurs in the predawn heavens. On the year's first evening, look low in the west 40 minutes after sunset to see Venus, Mercury, Saturn, and Jupiter, with the crescent Moon joining them on the 4th and 5th. Venus becomes too low after that, and the other planets sink lower, too, with only Mercury getting higher and hovering to Saturn's upper left from the 10th to the 14th. In the eastern sky, look for the crescent Moon to the right of Mars during the year's first dawn. By midmonth, Venus is a low morning star, but it rapidly gets higher each morning until easily seen to the left of the Moon and Mars 40 minutes before sunrise on the 29th.

● **NEW MOON** 2nd day 1:33 P.M.   ○ **FULL MOON** 17th day 6:48 P.M.
◐ **FIRST QUARTER** 9th day 1:11 P.M.   ◑ **LAST QUARTER** 25th day 8:41 A.M.

All times are given in Eastern Standard Time.

GET THESE PAGES WITH TIMES SET TO YOUR POSTAL CODE VIA ALMANAC.CA/2022.

DAY OF YEAR	DAY OF MONTH	DAY OF WEEK	☼ RISES H. M.	RISE KEY	☼ SETS H. M.	SET KEY	LENGTH OF DAY H. M.	SUN FAST M.	SUN DECLINATION ° '	HIGH TIDE TIMES HALIFAX		☾ RISES H. M.	RISE KEY	☾ SETS H. M.	SET KEY	☾ ASTRON. PLACE	☾ AGE
1	1	Sa.	7:43	E	4:30	A	8 47	*6	22 s. 57	6¼	7	6:42	E	3:10	A	OPH	28
2	2	**B**	7:43	E	4:31	A	8 48	*7	22 s. 52	7	7¾	7:55	E	4:14	A	SAG	0
3	3	M.	7:42	E	4:32	A	8 50	*7	22 s. 46	8	8¾	8:55	E	5:30	A	SAG	1
4	4	Tu.	7:42	E	4:33	A	8 51	*8	22 s. 40	8¾	9½	9:41	E	6:50	A	CAP	2
5	5	W.	7:42	E	4:34	A	8 52	*8	22 s. 33	9¾	10½	10:16	E	8:09	A	CAP	3
6	6	Th.	7:42	E	4:36	A	8 54	*9	22 s. 26	10½	11¼	10:43	D	9:25	B	AQU	4
7	7	Fr.	7:42	E	4:37	A	8 55	*9	22 s. 18	11½	—	11:05	D	10:37	B	AQU	5
8	8	Sa.	7:42	E	4:38	A	8 56	*10	22 s. 10	12	12¼	11:25	C	11:45	C	PSC	6
9	9	**B**	7:41	E	4:39	A	8 58	*10	22 s. 02	1	1	11:44	C	—	-	CET	7
10	10	M.	7:41	E	4:40	A	8 59	*10	21 s. 53	1¾	2	**12:03**	B	12:51	C	PSC	8
11	11	Tu.	7:41	E	4:41	A	9 00	*11	21 s. 43	2¾	3¼	**12:24**	B	1:56	D	ARI	9
12	12	W.	7:40	E	4:42	A	9 02	*11	21 s. 33	3¾	4½	**12:47**	A	3:01	D	ARI	10
13	13	Th.	7:40	E	4:44	A	9 04	*11	21 s. 23	4½	5½	**1:15**	A	4:06	E	TAU	11
14	14	Fr.	7:39	E	4:45	A	9 06	*12	21 s. 13	5½	6¼	**1:49**	A	5:09	E	TAU	12
15	15	Sa.	7:39	E	4:46	A	9 07	*12	21 s. 02	6¼	7	**2:31**	A	6:09	E	TAU	13
16	16	**B**	7:38	E	4:47	A	9 09	*13	20 s. 50	7	7¾	**3:21**	A	7:03	E	GEM	14
17	17	M.	7:37	E	4:49	A	9 12	*13	20 s. 38	7½	8¼	**4:19**	A	7:50	E	GEM	15
18	18	Tu.	7:37	E	4:50	A	9 13	*13	20 s. 26	8¼	9	**5:24**	A	8:29	E	CAN	16
19	19	W.	7:36	E	4:51	A	9 15	*13	20 s. 14	8¾	9½	**6:31**	A	9:01	E	CAN	17
20	20	Th.	7:35	E	4:53	A	9 18	*14	20 s. 01	9½	10¼	**7:40**	B	9:27	D	LEO	18
21	21	Fr.	7:34	E	4:54	A	9 20	*14	19 s. 47	10	10¾	**8:49**	B	9:50	D	LEO	19
22	22	Sa.	7:34	E	4:56	A	9 22	*14	19 s. 34	10¾	11½	**9:59**	C	10:11	C	LEO	20
23	23	**B**	7:33	E	4:57	A	9 24	*15	19 s. 20	11½	—	**11:10**	C	10:31	C	VIR	21
24	24	M.	7:32	E	4:58	A	9 26	*15	19 s. 05	12	12¼	—		10:51	B	VIR	22
25	25	Tu.	7:31	E	5:00	B	9 29	*15	18 s. 50	12¾	1¼	**12:23**	D	11:13	B	VIR	23
26	26	W.	7:30	E	5:01	B	9 31	*15	18 s. 35	1¾	2¼	**1:39**	D	11:40	A	LIB	24
27	27	Th.	7:29	E	5:03	B	9 34	*15	18 s. 20	2¾	3½	**2:58**	E	**12:13**	A	LIB	25
28	28	Fr.	7:28	E	5:04	B	9 36	*16	18 s. 04	3¾	4¾	**4:17**	E	**12:56**	A	OPH	26
29	29	Sa.	7:27	E	5:05	B	9 38	*16	17 s. 48	4¾	5¾	**5:32**	E	**1:52**	A	SAG	27
30	30	**B**	7:26	E	5:07	B	9 41	*16	17 s. 31	6	6¾	**6:37**	E	**3:01**	A	SAG	28
31	31	M.	7:25	D	5:08	B	9 43	*16	17 s. 15	7	7¾	**7:29**	E	**4:19**	A	SAG	29

To use this page, see p. 116; for Key Letters, see p. 240.   LIGHT = A.M. **BOLD = P.M.**

JANUARY

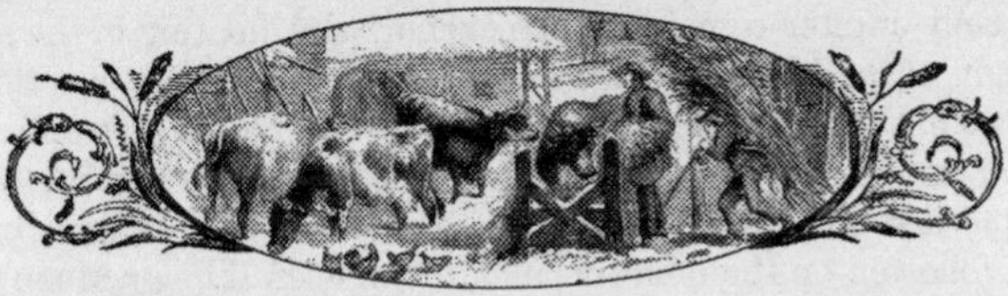

So the bells ring forth with might,
Heralding a future bright.
–G. Weatherly

DAY OF MONTH	DAY OF WEEK	DATES, FEASTS, FASTS, ASPECTS, TIDE HEIGHTS, AND WEATHER	
1	Sa.	Holy Name • NEW YEAR'S DAY • ☾ AT PERIG. • Tides {6.5 5.8	*Solar*
2	**B**	2nd S. af. Ch. • NEW ● • ☾ RUNS LOW • {6.7 6.0	*power!*
3	M.	☌☿☾ • ☌♀☾ • ☌♇☾ • Aretha Franklin 1st woman inducted into Rock & Roll Hall of Fame, 1987	
4	Tu.	St. Elizabeth Ann Seton • ☌♄☾ • ⊕ AT PERIHELION • {6.7 6.2	*An*
5	W.	Twelfth Night • ☌♃☾ • Antarctic explorer Sir Ernest Henry Shackleton died, 1922	*inch*
6	Th.	Epiphany • New Mexico became 47th U.S. state, 1912 • Tides {6.3 6.1	*an*
7	Fr.	Distaff Day • ☌♆☾ • ☿ GR. ELONG. (19° EAST) • Tides {5.9 —	*hour!*
8	Sa.	☾ ON EQ. • ♀ IN INF. ☌ • Entertainer Elvis Presley born, 1935 • {5.9 5.6	*Flurries—*
9	**B**	1st S. af. Ep. • Apple introduced the iPhone, 2007 • Tides {5.7 5.2	*you'll*
10	M.	Plough Monday • *If January calends be summerly gay, It will be winterly weather till the calends of May.*	*need*
11	Tu.	☌♅☾ • 17 lb. 1 oz. ocean whitefish caught, Hurricane Bank, Calif., 2011 • {5.4 4.7	*your*
12	W.	☾ AT ☊ • Fictional Hal 9000 computer in film *2001: A Space Odyssey* became operational, 1992	*furries!*
13	Th.	St. Hilary • ☿ STAT. • Naturalist/artist Maria Sibylla Merian died, 1717 • {5.3 4.8	*Flakes*
14	Fr.	☾ AT APO. • *Jan. 14–15:* –54°F to 49°F in a 24-hour period, setting record, Loma, Mont., 1972	*spittin'—*
15	Sa.	Playwright Molière baptized, 1622 • 1st transpacific hot air balloon flight began, Japan to Canada, 1991	*where*
16	**B**	2nd S. af. Ep. • ☾ RIDES HIGH • ☌♇☉ • Tides {5.6 5.2	*are*
17	M.	MARTIN LUTHER KING JR.'S BIRTHDAY, OBSERVED (U.S.) • FULL WOLF ○ • Ben Franklin born, 1706	*my*
18	Tu.	♅ STAT. • *By going gains the mill, And not by standing still.* • Tides {5.9 5.4	*mittens?*
19	W.	Rare snowfall, Miami, Fla., 1977 • Poet James Dickey died, 1997 • {6.0 5.5	*Mild:*
20	Th.	*Born Free* author Joy Adamson born, 1910 • {8.9 10.2	*Rain and*
21	Fr.	3-day, 81-tornado outbreak in Southeast U.S. began, 2017 • Raccoons mate now. • {5.9 5.7	*snow*
22	Sa.	St. Vincent • Roberta Bondar became 1st Canadian woman in space, 1992 • {5.7 5.7	*blend,*
23	**B**	3rd S. af. Ep. • ☾ ON EQ. • ☿ IN INF. ☌ • {5.6 —	*then*
24	M.	Rover *Opportunity* landed on Mars, 2004 • Tides {5.7 5.3	*it's*
25	Tu.	Conversion of Paul • January thaw traditionally begins about now. • {5.7 5.1	*colder*
26	W.	Sts. Timothy & Titus • Canadian Coast Guard officially established, 1962 • {5.7 4.9	*and*
27	Th.	☾ AT ☋ • ☌☿♇ • *A little stone may upset a large cart.* • Tides {5.7 4.9	*snowy,*
28	Fr.	St. Thomas Aquinas • Scottish-born Canadian statesman Alexander Mackenzie born, 1822	*right*
29	Sa.	☾ RUNS LOW • ☌♂☾ • ☌♀☾ • ♀ STAT. • {5.9 5.3	*to*
30	**B**	☾ AT PERIG. • ☌☿☾ • ☌♇☾ • Yerba Buena renamed San Francisco, 1847	*the*
31	M.	Composer Franz Schubert born, 1797 • Baseball player Nolan Ryan born, 1947 • {6.4 5.9	*end.*

Farmer's Calendar

Dashing through the snow? Check. In a one-horse open sleigh? You betcha—as o'er the fields we rode. Laughing all the way? Well, it was more like speechless awe. Crisp air stung our faces as we hurtled through the winter world in a vehicle without a windshield. Driver Linda Ward held the reins as she guided her Belgian draft horse, Ivy, along a snowy lane while her party of two snuggled under 100-year-old sleigh robes in the seat behind her. For an hour we lived the lyrics of "Jingle Bells" and "Over the River and Through the Woods"—our quiet ride accompanied only by the wooden sleigh's creak as it glided, its runners hissing against the snow and occasionally scrunching on ice—all powered by our equine engine. We watched Ivy's strong haunches as she conveyed as up hills and down them. Perhaps our great-great-grandparents would find our thrill at being pulled by a horse amusing. Our joy ride was their school bus and grocery getter. Yet for the duration of our jaunt, their scenery, what they knew—these arched-over birches, the burly mountain backdrop, the sugar woods, and the snow-smothered field—was our scenery, too. Oh, what fun? Heck, yeah!

FEBRUARY

SKY WATCH: Only Jupiter remains in the evening sky, floating in the southwest to the upper right of the Moon on the 2nd. Besides this, February's action is focused in the predawn east, where Mercury brightens to magnitude zero and ascends a bit higher each morning, hovering to the left of Venus and Mars on the 13th. Look for dazzling Venus just above dim orange Mars and the slender waning crescent Moon on the 27th, followed on the next morning by an even thinner Moon floating just beneath Mercury, with Saturn to its left and the Venus–Mars duo to its right. This planet bunching is very low and challenging but will soon get much easier to see. Venus's supernal brilliance—at its brightest of the year during midmonth, a shadow-casting magnitude –4.9—grabs the attention of anyone gazing east before dawn.

● **NEW MOON** 1st day 12:46 A.M.   ○ **FULL MOON** 16th day 11:56 A.M.
◐ **FIRST QUARTER** 8th day 8:50 A.M.   ◑ **LAST QUARTER** 23rd day 5:32 P.M.

All times are given in Eastern Standard Time.

GET THESE PAGES WITH TIMES SET TO YOUR POSTAL CODE VIA ALMANAC.CA/2022.

Day of Year	Day of Month	Day of Week	☼ Rises H.M.	Rise Key	☼ Sets H.M.	Set Key	Length of Day H.M.	Sun Fast M.	Sun Declination ° '	High Tide Times Halifax	☾ Rises H.M.	Rise Key	☾ Sets H.M.	Set Key	☾ Astron. Place	☾ Age
32	1	Tu.	7:23	D	5:10	B	9 47	*16	16 s. 57	7¾ 8½	8:09	E	5:40	A	CAP	0
33	2	W.	7:22	D	5:11	B	9 49	*16	16 s. 40	8½ 9¼	8:40	D	6:59	B	AQU	1
34	3	Th.	7:21	D	5:13	B	9 52	*17	16 s. 22	9½ 10	9:05	D	8:15	B	AQU	2
35	4	Fr.	7:20	D	5:14	B	9 54	*17	16 s. 05	10¼ 10¾	9:27	C	9:26	C	AQU	3
36	5	Sa.	7:18	D	5:16	B	9 58	*17	15 s. 46	11 11½	9:46	C	10:35	C	CET	4
37	6	**B**	7:17	D	5:17	B	10 00	*17	15 s. 28	11¾ —	10:06	B	11:43	D	PSC	5
38	7	M.	7:16	D	5:19	B	10 03	*17	15 s. 09	12¼ 12½	10:26	B	—	-	CET	6
39	8	Tu.	7:14	D	5:20	B	10 06	*17	14 s. 50	1 1¼	10:49	B	12:49	A	ARI	7
40	9	W.	7:13	D	5:21	B	10 08	*17	14 s. 31	1¾ 2¼	11:15	A	1:55	E	TAU	8
41	10	Th.	7:12	D	5:23	B	10 11	*17	14 s. 11	2¾ 3½	11:46	A	2:59	E	TAU	9
42	11	Fr.	7:10	D	5:24	B	10 14	*17	13 s. 52	3¾ 4¾	12:25	A	4:00	E	TAU	10
43	12	Sa.	7:09	D	5:26	B	10 17	*17	13 s. 32	4¾ 5¾	1:13	A	4:57	E	GEM	11
44	13	**B**	7:07	D	5:27	B	10 20	*17	13 s. 11	5¾ 6½	2:08	A	5:46	E	GEM	12
45	14	M.	7:06	D	5:29	B	10 23	*17	12 s. 51	6½ 7¼	3:11	A	6:28	E	CAN	13
46	15	Tu.	7:04	D	5:30	B	10 26	*17	12 s. 30	7¼ 8	4:19	A	7:02	E	CAN	14
47	16	W.	7:03	D	5:32	B	10 29	*17	12 s. 10	7¾ 8½	5:28	B	7:30	D	LEO	15
48	17	Th.	7:01	D	5:33	B	10 32	*17	11 s. 49	8½ 9	6:39	B	7:54	D	LEO	16
49	18	Fr.	6:59	D	5:34	B	10 35	*17	11 s. 28	9 9¾	7:50	C	8:16	D	LEO	17
50	19	Sa.	6:58	D	5:36	B	10 38	*16	11 s. 06	9¾ 10¼	9:01	C	8:36	C	VIR	18
51	20	**B**	6:56	D	5:37	B	10 41	*16	10 s. 45	10½ 11	10:14	D	8:56	C	VIR	19
52	21	M.	6:55	D	5:39	B	10 44	*16	10 s. 23	11¼ 11½	11:29	D	9:18	B	VIR	20
53	22	Tu.	6:53	D	5:40	B	10 47	*16	10 s. 01	12 —	—	-	9:42	B	LIB	21
54	23	W.	6:51	D	5:42	B	10 51	*16	9 s. 39	12¼ 12¾	12:46	E	10:12	A	LIB	22
55	24	Th.	6:50	D	5:43	B	10 53	*16	9 s. 17	1 1¾	2:04	E	10:51	A	OPH	23
56	25	Fr.	6:48	D	5:44	B	10 56	*16	8 s. 55	2¼ 3¼	3:19	E	11:40	A	OPH	24
57	26	Sa.	6:46	D	5:46	B	11 00	*16	8 s. 32	3½ 4¾	4:26	A	12:42	A	SAG	25
58	27	**B**	6:44	D	5:47	B	11 03	*15	8 s. 10	4¾ 5¾	5:21	E	1:55	A	SAG	26
59	28	M.	6:43	D	5:49	B	11 06	*15	7 s. 47	5¾ 6¾	6:05	E	3:13	A	CAP	27

THE SECOND MONTH · 2022 **FEBRUARY** FEBRUARY HATH 28 DAYS

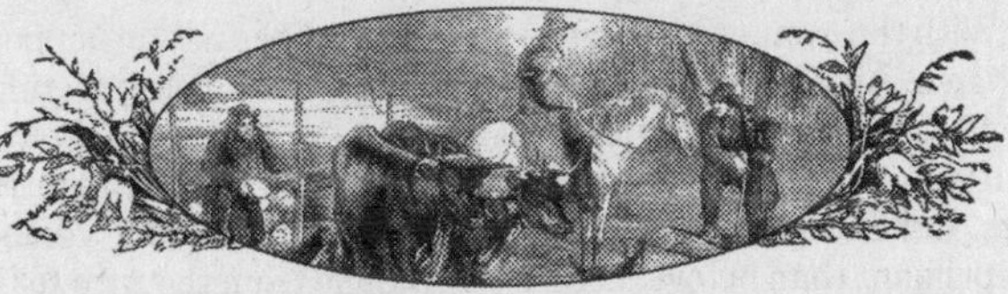

The hoar-frost crackles on the trees,
The rattling brook begins to freeze.
–**James Berry Bensel**

DAY OF MONTH	DAY OF WEEK	DATES, FEASTS, FASTS, ASPECTS, TIDE HEIGHTS, AND WEATHER	
1	Tu.	St. Brigid • LUNAR NEW YEAR (CHINA) • NEW ● • ☌♄☾	*Groundhogs,*
2	W.	Candlemas • Groundhog Day • ☌♃☾ • {6.5 6.2	*mixed up;*
3	Th.	☌♆☾ • ☿ STAT. • Rare Feb. EF1 tornado, Gray/ Roberts/Hemphill Cos., Tex., 2012	*get*
4	Fr.	☌♄☉ • *The Muses love the morning.* • {6.2 6.2	*snowblowers*
5	Sa.	St. Agatha • ☾ ON EQ. • 3.7" snow, San Francisco, Calif., 1887 • {5.9 6.0	*fixed*
6	**B**	Singer Natalie Cole born, 1950 • Tides {5.5 —	*up!*
7	M.	☌⛢☾ • Writer Charles Dickens born, 1812 • Tides {5.7 5.2	*Keep*
8	Tu.	1st radio installed in White House, D.C., 1922 • {5.4 4.8	*them*
9	W.	☾ AT ☊ • "War Time" (yr.-round daylight saving time) began in U.S., 1942 • {5.2 4.6	*humming;*
10	Th.	☾ AT APO. • *When the wind's in the north, You mustn't go forth.* • Tides {5.0 4.5	*another*
11	Fr.	Inventor Thomas Edison born, 1847 • Track and field athlete Abby Hoffman born, 1947	*big*
12	Sa.	☾ RIDES HIGH • ☌☿♇ • ☌♀♂ • ♀ GR. ILLUM. EXT. • Abe Lincoln born, 1809	*one's*
13	**B**	**Septuagesima** • 2nd Hubble Space Telescope tune-up began, 1997	*coming!*
14	M.	Sts. Cyril & Methodius • VALENTINE'S DAY • {5.5 5.2	*Valentine*
15	Tu.	NATIONAL FLAG OF CANADA DAY • Social reformer Susan B. Anthony born, 1820 • {5.7 5.4	*gifts*
16	W.	FULL SNOW ○ • ☿ GR. ELONG. (26° WEST) • Winter's back breaks. • {5.9 5.6	*obscured*
17	Th.	National Congress of Mothers, later known as PTA, founded, 1897 • Tides {6.0 5.8	*by*
18	Fr.	Geochemist Wallace Broecker, who popularized term "global warming," died, 2019 • {6.0 5.9	*drifts.*
19	Sa.	☾ ON EQ. • 1st rescuers reached Donner Party in Sierra Nevada mtns., Calif., 1847 • {6.0 6.0	*Rain and*
20	**B**	**Sexagesima** • Metropolitan Museum of Art opened, N.Y.C., 1872 • {5.8 6.0	*snow*
21	M.	PRESIDENTS' DAY (U.S.) • Polaroid instant camera first demonstrated, 1947 • {5.6 6.0	*alternating,*
22	Tu.	U.S. president George Washington born, 1732 • Tides {5.4 —	*temperature*
23	W.	☾ AT ☋ • 1st powered flight in Canada (by McCurdy in *Silver Dart*), Baddeck, N.S., 1909	*elevating,*
24	Th.	St. Matthias • *Think today and speak tomorrow.* • {5.6 4.8	*which*
25	Fr.	Actor Sean Astin born, 1971 • Tides {5.5 4.7	*is*
26	Sa.	☾ RUNS LOW • ☾ AT PERIG. • Buffalo Creek flood disaster, Logan Co., W.Va, 1972	*well*
27	**B**	**Quinquagesima** • ☌♀☾ • ☌♂☾ • ☌♇☾	*worth*
28	M.	St. Romanus • ☌☿☾ • ☌♄☾ • Skunks mate now. • {5.8 5.6	*celebrating!*

Q: What is smarter than a hummingbird?
A: A spelling bee

CALENDAR

Farmer's Calendar

A homegrown parsnip may take up to 400 days to raise, if you consider that the process begins the moment you place your seed order even as wind scatters more snow. Your single packet, when it arrives, contains plenty. I share my surplus seed with a neighbor because they lose viability if I try to hoard them for another season. Although the packet duly warns that these seeds germinate slowly, you may still lose faith. However, the moment your exasperation wins and you lug a flat of tomatoes over to transplant into the root bed instead, only then will you notice something so faint and delicate, you could mistake it for grass. Your parsnips have emerged; harvest is now merely nine months away. A full winter later, as the last snowbank thaws, and with only sprouting onions and tentacled potatoes remaining from last summer's harvest, you fetch the digging fork and revisit the roots that spent those bitter months buried in your forgotten garden, maturing. When forked loose and yanked free in late April, early May, the pale ivory roots resemble dirty icicles, albino carrots. But their flavor, thanks to the frost, is appreciably sweet—your edible prize for patience.

MARCH

After 2:00 A.M. on March 13, Eastern Daylight Time is given.

GET THESE PAGES WITH TIMES SET TO YOUR POSTAL CODE VIA ALMANAC.CA/2022.

DAY OF YEAR	DAY OF MONTH	DAY OF WEEK	☀ RISES H. M.	RISE KEY	☀ SETS H. M.	SET KEY	LENGTH OF DAY H. M.	SUN FAST M.	SUN DECLINATION ° '	HIGH TIDE TIMES HALIFAX		☾ RISES H. M.	RISE KEY	☾ SETS H. M.	SET KEY	☾ ASTRON. PLACE	☾ AGE
60	1	Tu.	6:41	D	5:50	B	11 09	*15	7 s. 24	6¾	7½	6:38	E	4:33	B	CAP	28
61	2	W.	6:39	D	5:51	B	11 12	*15	7 s. 01	7½	8¼	7:05	D	5:50	B	AQU	0
62	3	Th.	6:37	D	5:53	C	11 16	*15	6 s. 38	8½	9	7:28	C	7:04	C	AQU	1
63	4	Fr.	6:36	D	5:54	C	11 18	*14	6 s. 15	9¼	9½	7:48	C	8:15	D	PSC	2
64	5	Sa.	6:34	C	5:55	C	11 21	*14	5 s. 52	9¾	10¼	8:08	C	9:24	D	PSC	3
65	6	**B**	6:32	C	5:57	C	11 25	*14	5 s. 29	10½	10¾	8:27	B	10:33	D	PSC	4
66	7	M.	6:30	C	5:58	C	11 28	*14	5 s. 05	11¼	11½	8:49	B	11:40	E	ARI	5
67	8	Tu.	6:28	C	5:59	C	11 31	*13	4 s. 42	12	—	9:14	A	—	-	TAU	6
68	9	W.	6:26	C	6:01	C	11 35	*13	4 s. 18	12¼	12¾	9:43	A	12:46	E	TAU	7
69	10	Th.	6:25	C	6:02	C	11 37	*13	3 s. 55	12¾	1½	10:19	A	1:49	E	TAU	8
70	11	Fr.	6:23	C	6:04	C	11 41	*13	3 s. 31	1¾	2¾	11:03	A	2:48	E	TAU	9
71	12	Sa.	6:21	C	6:05	C	11 44	*12	3 s. 08	2¾	4	11:56	A	3:40	E	GEM	10
72	13	**B**	7:19	C	7:06	C	11 47	*12	2 s. 44	5	6¼	1:56	A	5:25	E	GEM	11
73	14	M.	7:17	C	7:08	C	11 51	*12	2 s. 20	6	7	3:02	A	6:01	E	CAN	12
74	15	Tu.	7:15	C	7:09	C	11 54	*12	1 s. 57	7	7¾	4:11	A	6:32	E	LEO	13
75	16	W.	7:13	C	7:10	C	11 57	*11	1 s. 33	7¾	8¼	5:22	B	6:57	D	LEO	14
76	17	Th.	7:11	C	7:11	C	12 00	*11	1 s. 09	8½	9	6:34	B	7:20	D	LEO	15
77	18	Fr.	7:10	C	7:13	C	12 03	*11	0 s. 45	9	9½	7:46	C	7:40	C	VIR	16
78	19	Sa.	7:08	C	7:14	C	12 06	*10	0 s. 22	9¾	10	9:01	C	8:00	C	VIR	17
79	20	**B**	7:06	C	7:15	C	12 09	*10	0 N. 01	10½	10¾	10:17	D	8:22	B	VIR	18
80	21	M.	7:04	C	7:17	C	12 13	*10	0 N. 25	11¼	11½	11:35	D	8:45	B	LIB	19
81	22	Tu.	7:02	C	7:18	C	12 16	*10	0 N. 48	12	—	—	-	9:14	A	LIB	20
82	23	W.	7:00	C	7:19	C	12 19	*9	1 N. 12	12¼	12¾	12:55	E	9:49	A	SCO	21
83	24	Th.	6:58	C	7:21	C	12 23	*9	1 N. 36	1	1½	2:11	E	10:35	A	OPH	22
84	25	Fr.	6:56	C	7:22	C	12 26	*9	1 N. 59	1¾	2¾	3:21	E	11:33	A	SAG	23
85	26	Sa.	6:54	C	7:23	C	12 29	*8	2 N. 23	2¾	4	4:19	E	12:41	A	SAG	24
86	27	**B**	6:52	C	7:25	C	12 33	*8	2 N. 46	4¼	5½	5:04	E	1:57	B	CAP	25
87	28	M.	6:51	C	7:26	C	12 35	*8	3 N. 10	5½	6¾	5:40	E	3:15	B	CAP	26
88	29	Tu.	6:49	C	7:27	C	12 38	*7	3 N. 33	6¾	7½	6:08	D	4:31	B	AQU	27
89	30	W.	6:47	C	7:28	C	12 41	*7	3 N. 56	7½	8¼	6:31	D	5:45	B	AQU	28
90	31	Th.	6:45	C	7:30	C	12 45	*7	4 N. 20	8¼	8¾	6:52	C	6:56	C	PSC	29

MARCH

MARCH HATH 31 DAYS

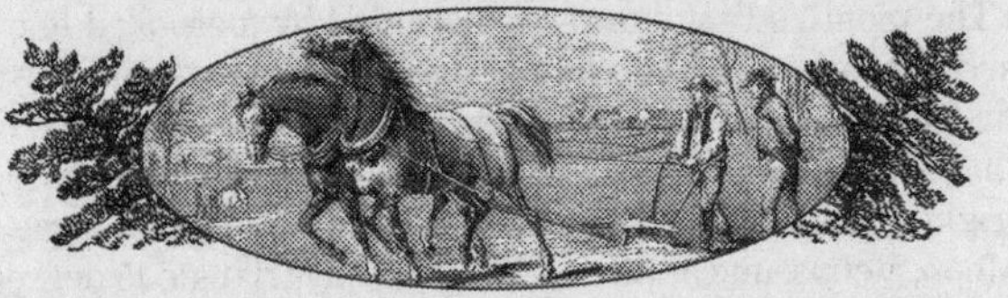

Fled now the sullen murmurs of the North,
The splendid raiment of the Spring peeps forth.
–Robert Bloomfield

DAY OF MONTH	DAY OF WEEK	DATES, FEASTS, FASTS, ASPECTS, TIDE HEIGHTS, AND WEATHER	
1	Tu.	Shrove Tuesday • St. David • 1st U.S. national park (Yellowstone) established, 1872	*Sun-splashed*
2	W.	**Ash Wednesday** • NEW ● • ☌☿♄ • ☌♃☾ • {6.2/6.1	*and*
3	Th.	☌♂♇ • ☌♆☾ • Athlete Jackie Joyner-Kersee born, 1962 • {6.3/6.2	*strangely*
4	Fr.	☾ ON EQ. • ☌♀♇ • Bertha Wilson 1st woman appointed to Supreme Court of Canada, 1982	*vernal;*
5	Sa.	St. Piran • ☌♃☉ • *Many littles make a mickle* [large amount]. • {6.0/6.1	*hopes*
6	**B**	**1st S. in Lent** • Bandmaster John Philip Sousa died, 1932 • Tides {5.7/5.9	*dashed*
7	M.	Orthodox Lent begins • St. Perpetua • ☌⛢☾ • {5.4/5.6	*by*
8	Tu.	☾ AT ☊ • Joseph Lee, father of playground movement, born, 1862 • {5.1/—	*rain*
9	W.	Ember Day • Hummingbirds migrate north now. • Tides {5.3/4.8	*that*
10	Th.	☾ AT APO. • Uranus rings discovered, 1977 • *Pay as you go, And what you have you know.*	*seems*
11	Fr.	Ember Day • ☾ RIDES HIGH • "Faster than it looks" cow wanted by police, Pembroke Pines, Fla., 2020	*eternal.*
12	Sa.	Ember Day • ☌♀♂ • Singer Liza Minnelli born, 1946 • Tides {4.7/4.4	*Saint*
13	**B**	**2nd S. in Lent** • DAYLIGHT SAVING TIME BEGINS, 2:00 A.M. • ☌♆☉	*Patrick's*
14	M.	Gordie Howe 2nd player in NHL history to score 500 career goals, 1962 • Tides {5.0/5.0	*Day*
15	Tu.	Beware the ides of March. • Mi'kmaq poet Rita Joe born, 1932 • Tides {5.3/5.3	*is*
16	W.	United States Military Academy established, West Point, N.Y., 1802 • Tides {5.5/5.6	*damp*
17	Th.	ST. PATRICK'S DAY • 1,263 people dressed as leprechauns (Bandon, Ireland) set world record, 2012	*and*
18	Fr.	FULL WORM ○ • ☾ ON EQ. • Feb. 2019 world's 5th warmest Feb. since 1880, NOAA announced, 2019	*gray.*
19	Sa.	St. Joseph • Elvis Presley paid $1,000 deposit to buy Graceland, Memphis, Tenn., 1957 • {6.0/6.2	*No*
20	**B**	**3rd S. in Lent** • VERNAL EQUINOX • ☌☿♃ • ♀ GR. ELONG. (47° WEST)	*relief;*
21	M.	Twitter founded, 2006 • Astronomer Halton Christian Arp born, 1927 • {5.9/6.2	*the*
22	Tu.	☾ AT ☋ • Animatronic T-rex caught fire, Canon City, Colo., 2018 • Tides {5.7/—	*warmth*
23	W.	☾ AT PERIG. • ☌☿♆ • *Halifax Gazette* became Canada's 1st newspaper, 1752	*is*
24	Th.	Explorer John W. Powell born, 1834 • Tides {5.8/5.1	*brief—*
25	Fr.	**Annunciation** • ☾ RUNS LOW • Musician Elton John born, 1947 • {5.5/4.9	*we*
26	Sa.	☌♇☾ • 12-pound walleye caught with fly tackle, Manistee River, Mich., 1999 • {5.3/4.8	*sing*
27	**B**	**4th S. in Lent** • ☌♂☾ • *March many weathers.* • Tides {5.2/5.0	*of*
28	M.	☌♀☾ • ☌♄☾ • Fireball seen around 6:15 A.M. EDT, northeastern U.S., 2019 • {5.3/5.3	*spring*
29	Tu.	☌♀♄ • Vesta, brightest asteroid known, discovered, 1807 • Tides {5.5/5.7	*through*
30	W.	☌♃☾ • ☌♆☾ • Last rum ration issued in Royal Canadian Navy, 1972	*chattering*
31	Th.	☾ ON EQ. • ☌☿☾ • Chipmunks emerge from hibernation now. • {5.9/6.1	*teeth!*

Farmer's Calendar

Soil is a celebrity at the Main Street Museum in White River Junction, Vermont. The brown powders displayed in clear jars are reminiscent of samples farmers trowel out of their fields and send off to the Extension Service to determine nitrogen and phosphorous levels. This exhibited dirt, however, bears labels that announce: "Silt from the 1927 Flood" and "Sandy Thin Sample from the birthplace of Henry Leland [designer of the Cadillac] near Barton, Vermont." It forces one to consider: What *isn't* sacred, or at least special, ground? A museum in Sidney, Iowa, also possesses an earthly collection, featuring labeled jars filled with two spoonfuls, resembling spices in a pantry. Begun as a farmwife's hobby—gathered in Missouri and Texas, and brought to her from France and the North Pole—they became her legacy. When a museum trustee first unpacked the donation—157 samples—she thought, "Why would we want a bunch of dirt?" Seen as separate from the field, one could forget this humble medium furnishes our food and wood. Or, as the trustee realized, it reminds us the world is bound to the soil. Now, as snow recedes and reveals the long-hidden mud, we might celebrate by the acre and spoonful.

CALENDAR

SKY WATCH: The month's first sunrise is heralded by a crooked line of planets in the predawn southeast, with Mars on the right, Saturn in the middle, and dazzling Venus on the left. On the 4th and 5th, Mars and Saturn come extremely close together. With Venus to their left, they float a comfortable 15 degrees high; Saturn is slightly brighter than orange Mars. On the 27th, the night's three brightest objects—the Moon, Venus, and Jupiter—form a lovely triangle 15 degrees high in the morning twilight. The latter two planets come extremely close together on the 30th in a don't-miss conjunction. Unfortunately, the partial solar eclipse created by the new Moon on the 30th is visible only from southern South America and Antarctica.

- ● NEW MOON 1st day 2:24 A.M.
- ◑ LAST QUARTER 23rd day 7:56 A.M.
- ◐ FIRST QUARTER 9th day 2:48 A.M.
- ● NEW MOON 30th day 4:28 P.M.
- ○ FULL MOON 16th day 2:55 P.M.

All times are given in Eastern Daylight Time.

GET THESE PAGES WITH TIMES SET TO YOUR POSTAL CODE VIA ALMANAC.CA/2022.

DAY OF YEAR	DAY OF MONTH	DAY OF WEEK	☼ RISES H. M.	RISE KEY	☼ SETS H. M.	SET KEY	LENGTH OF DAY H. M.	SUN FAST M.	SUN DECLINATION ° '	HIGH TIDE TIMES HALIFAX		☾ RISES H. M.	RISE KEY	☾ SETS H. M.	SET KEY	☾ ASTRON. PLACE	☾ AGE
91	1	Fr.	6:43	C	7:31	C	12 48	*7	4 N. 43	9	9½	7:11	C	8:06	C	CET	0
92	2	Sa.	6:41	C	7:32	C	12 51	*6	5 N. 06	9¾	10	7:30	B	9:15	D	PSC	1
93	3	**B**	6:39	C	7:34	D	12 55	*6	5 N. 29	10½	10¾	7:51	B	10:24	D	ARI	2
94	4	M.	6:37	B	7:35	D	12 58	*6	5 N. 52	11¼	11¼	8:14	A	11:31	E	ARI	3
95	5	Tu.	6:36	B	7:36	D	13 00	*5	6 N. 15	11¾	—	8:41	A	—	-	TAU	4
96	6	W.	6:34	B	7:37	D	13 03	*5	6 N. 37	12	12½	9:14	A	12:37	E	TAU	5
97	7	Th.	6:32	B	7:39	D	13 07	*5	7 N. 00	12½	1¼	9:55	A	1:38	E	TAU	6
98	8	Fr.	6:30	B	7:40	D	13 10	*5	7 N. 22	1¼	2	10:44	A	2:33	E	GEM	7
99	9	Sa.	6:28	B	7:41	D	13 13	*4	7 N. 45	2	3	11:41	A	3:21	E	GEM	8
100	10	**B**	6:26	B	7:43	D	13 17	*4	8 N. 07	3	4¼	12:44	A	4:00	E	CAN	9
101	11	M.	6:25	B	7:44	D	13 19	*4	8 N. 29	4¼	5½	1:51	A	4:32	E	CAN	10
102	12	Tu.	6:23	B	7:45	D	13 22	*4	8 N. 51	5½	6½	3:01	B	4:59	D	LEO	11
103	13	W.	6:21	B	7:46	D	13 25	*3	9 N. 13	6½	7	4:12	B	5:22	D	LEO	12
104	14	Th.	6:19	B	7:48	D	13 29	*3	9 N. 34	7¼	7¾	5:24	C	5:43	C	LEO	13
105	15	Fr.	6:17	B	7:49	D	13 32	*3	9 N. 56	8	8¼	6:39	C	6:03	C	VIR	14
106	16	Sa.	6:16	B	7:50	D	13 34	*3	10 N. 17	8¾	9	7:56	D	6:24	B	VIR	15
107	17	**B**	6:14	B	7:52	D	13 38	*2	10 N. 38	9½	9½	9:16	D	6:47	B	VIR	16
108	18	M.	6:12	B	7:53	D	13 41	*2	10 N. 59	10¼	10¼	10:38	E	7:13	A	LIB	17
109	19	Tu.	6:10	B	7:54	D	13 44	*2	11 N. 20	11	11	11:59	E	7:47	A	SCO	18
110	20	W.	6:09	B	7:55	D	13 46	*2	11 N. 40	11¾	11¾	—	-	8:30	A	OPH	19
111	21	Th.	6:07	B	7:57	D	13 50	*2	12 N. 01	12½	—	1:13	E	9:25	A	SAG	20
112	22	Fr.	6:05	B	7:58	D	13 53	*1	12 N. 21	12¾	1½	2:16	E	10:32	A	SAG	21
113	23	Sa.	6:04	B	7:59	D	13 55	*1	12 N. 41	1¾	2½	3:06	E	11:46	A	CAP	22
114	24	**B**	6:02	B	8:01	D	13 59	*1	13 N. 01	2¾	4	3:44	E	1:03	A	CAP	23
115	25	M.	6:00	B	8:02	D	14 02	*1	13 N. 20	4	5¼	4:13	D	2:19	B	AQU	24
116	26	Tu.	5:59	B	8:03	D	14 04	*1	13 N. 39	5¼	6¼	4:37	D	3:33	B	AQU	25
117	27	W.	5:57	B	8:04	D	14 07	0	13 N. 59	6½	7	4:57	C	4:43	C	AQU	26
118	28	Th.	5:56	B	8:06	D	14 10	0	14 N. 18	7¼	7¾	5:16	C	5:53	C	CET	27
119	29	Fr.	5:54	B	8:07	D	14 13	0	14 N. 36	8	8¼	5:35	B	7:01	D	PSC	28
120	30	Sa.	5:53	B	8:08	D	14 15	0	14 N. 55	8¾	9	5:55	B	8:09	D	PSC	0

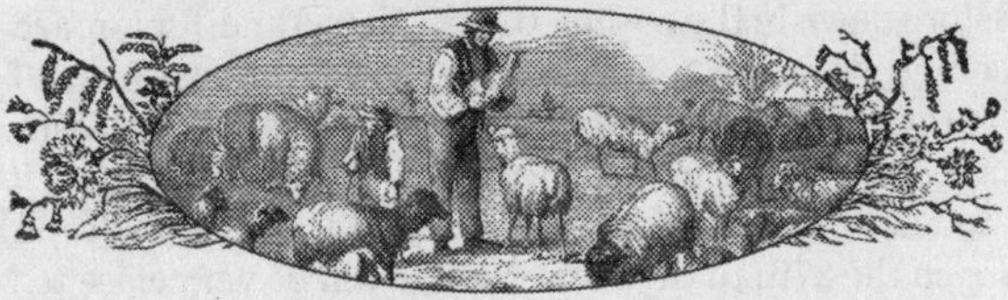

Did you dip your wings in azure dye,
When April began to paint the sky?
–Susan Hartley Swett, of a blue jay

DAY OF MONTH	DAY OF WEEK	DATES, FEASTS, FASTS, ASPECTS, TIDE HEIGHTS, AND WEATHER	
1	Fr.	ALL FOOLS' • NEW ● • *One fool makes a hundred.* • {5.9 6.2	*Cold*
2	Sa.	Ramadan begins at sundown • ☿ IN SUP. ☌ • Inventor Samuel Morse died, 1872	*and*
3	**B**	5th S. in Lent • St. Richard of Chichester • ☌⛢☾ • Actress Doris Day born, 1922	*mucky:*
4	M.	☾ AT ☊ • ☌♂♄ • Astronomer Jérôme Lalande died, 1807 • {5.5 5.7	*yucky!*
5	Tu.	Anne Sullivan conveyed meaning of word "water" to blind/deaf student Helen Keller, 1887	*Thunder's*
6	W.	Vancouver, B.C., incorporated, 1886 • Microsoft released Windows 3.1, 1992 • {5.1 —	*tympani*
7	Th.	☾ AT APO. • NASA's *Mars Odyssey* spacecraft launched, 2001 • Tides {5.2 4.9	*rumbles*
8	Fr.	☾ RIDES HIGH • Honolulu Academy of Arts opened, Hawaii, 1927 • Tides {5.0 4.7	*in*
9	Sa.	Battle of Vimy Ridge (WWI) began, France, 1917 • Tides {4.8 4.5	*a*
10	**B**	**Palm Sunday** • 1st Arbor Day, Nebr., 1872 • Tides {4.7 4.6	*spring*
11	M.	Jackie Robinson became 1st African-American MLB player, 1947 • Tides {4.7 4.8	*symphony,*
12	Tu.	☌♃♆ • Stubbs the Cat, honorary mayor of Talkeetna, Alaska, born, 1997 • {4.8 5.1	*but*
13	W.	U.S. president Thomas Jefferson born, 1743 • Tides {5.1 5.4	*don't*
14	Th.	Maundy Thursday • *April weather, rain and sunshine, both together.* • {5.4 5.7	*put*
15	Fr.	**Good Friday** • Passover begins at sundown • ☾ ON EQ. • {5.6 6.1	*away*
16	Sa.	FULL PINK ○ • Aviator Wilbur Wright born, 1867 • {5.8 6.3	*your*
17	**B**	**Easter** • Writer Thornton Wilder born, 1897 • Tides {6.0 6.4	*galoshes:*
18	M.	Easter Monday • ☾ AT ☋ • ☌☿⛢ • {6.0 6.4	*Everything*
19	Tu.	☾ AT PERIG. • 1st Boston Marathon, 1897 • Tides {5.9 6.3	*sloshes!*
20	W.	54 lb. 8 oz. freshwater drum caught, Nickajack Lake, Tenn., 1972 • Tides {5.7 6.1	*We grope*
21	Th.	☾ RUNS LOW • Environmentalist Aldo Leopold died, 1948 • Tides {5.5 —	*for*
22	Fr.	EARTH DAY • ☌♇☾ • Red River crested at 54.35 ft., Grand Forks, N.Dak., 1997 • {5.8 5.3	*hope:*
23	Sa.	St. George • Canadian prime minister Lester Pearson born, 1897 • Tides {5.5 5.1	*nope.*
24	**B**	2nd S. of Easter • **Orthodox Easter** • ☌♄☾ • *Almanac* founder Robert B. Thomas born, 1766	
25	M.	St. Mark • ☌♂☾ • *Patience wears out stones.* • {5.1 5.3	*Blessed*
26	Tu.	☌♀☾ • ☌♆☾ • Landscape architect Frederick Law Olmsted born, 1822	*sight!*
27	W.	☌♀♆ • ☌♃☾ • U.S. president Ulysses S. Grant born, 1822	*It's*
28	Th.	☾ ON EQ. • Poplars leaf out about now. • Tides {5.4 5.9	*warm*
29	Fr.	☿ GR. ELONG. (21° EAST) • Proposed Nfld. flag design revealed, 1980 • {5.5 6.0	*and*
30	Sa.	NEW ● • ECLIPSE ☉ • ☌♀♃ • ♇ STAT. • {5.6 6.0	*bright!*

Farmer's Calendar

Where the earth produced enough corn to feed a farmer's herd through the winter, a man now wanders, searching for yet another harvest. His boots crunch on thawing stubble and he's wearing headphones as he swings a metal detector, listening for the song of lost things, pieces of the past: treasures. Throughout winter he studies old atlases, town records, and topographical maps to determine the best hunting grounds. Then, in the interval following snowmelt, before the growing season begins, he meanders the grounds of yesteryear's stagecoach stops, boardinghouses, farm dumps, churchyards—places where tools, coins, jewelry, and buttons might still reside. In the decade he's spent hunting Vermont's dirt, he's racked up scores of intriguing finds: a galaxy of buttons, a commissary of soldiers' things, and an exchequer's purse of ancient coins. Now, as he homes in on a signal, he hunches close to the bare soil and remnant stalks. Detaching his microphone-like probe from his detector, he plunges it into the ground. As the beeping grows ever stronger and more constant, he clears away the dirt, searching for the source with tempered optimism, knowing "a diamond ring makes the same sound as a pop-top."

CALENDAR

MAY

SKY WATCH: Before dawn in the east on the 1st, Venus and Jupiter are still wonderfully close together. From the 3rd to the 20th, look for an easy planet lineup featuring, from left to right, Venus, Jupiter, Mars, and Saturn. The crescent Moon serves as an easy guide to all of the planets beginning on the 22nd, when it's just below Saturn. The Moon will dangle below Jupiter and Mars on the 25th and below Venus on the 27th. From the 27th to the 30th, Jupiter will be very close to Mars. A total lunar eclipse appears on the night of the 15th–16th, with the entire eclipse visible from the eastern half of the U.S. and Canada and all of South America. West of the Mississippi, the Moon will rise already eclipsed, offering intriguing photography opportunities.

◐ **FIRST QUARTER** 8th day 8:21 P.M. ◑ **LAST QUARTER** 22nd day 2:43 P.M.
○ **FULL MOON** 16th day 12:14 A.M. ● **NEW MOON** 30th day 7:30 A.M.

All times are given in Eastern Daylight Time.

GET THESE PAGES WITH TIMES SET TO YOUR POSTAL CODE VIA ALMANAC.CA/2022.

DAY OF YEAR	DAY OF MONTH	DAY OF WEEK	☼ RISES H. M.	RISE KEY	☼ SETS H. M.	SET KEY	LENGTH OF DAY H. M.	SUN FAST M.	SUN DECLINATION ° ′	HIGH TIDE TIMES HALIFAX		☾ RISES H. M.	RISE KEY	☾ SETS H. M.	SET KEY	☾ ASTRON. PLACE	☾ AGE
121	1	**B**	5:51	B	**8:10**	D	14 19	0	15 N. 13	9½	9½	6:16	B	**9:17**	E	ARI	1
122	2	M.	5:50	B	**8:11**	D	14 21	0	15 N. 31	10¼	10¼	6:42	A	**10:24**	E	TAU	2
123	3	Tu.	5:48	B	**8:12**	D	14 24	0	15 N. 48	10¾	10¾	7:12	A	**11:27**	E	TAU	3
124	4	W.	5:47	B	**8:13**	D	14 26	0	16 N. 06	11½	11½	7:50	A	—	-	TAU	4
125	5	Th.	5:45	B	**8:15**	D	14 30	0	16 N. 23	12	—	8:35	A	12:25	E	GEM	5
126	6	Fr.	5:44	B	**8:16**	E	14 32	0	16 N. 40	12	12¾	9:29	A	1:16	E	GEM	6
127	7	Sa.	5:42	B	**8:17**	E	14 35	1	16 N. 56	12¾	1½	10:30	A	1:58	E	CAN	7
128	8	**B**	5:41	B	**8:18**	E	14 37	1	17 N. 13	1½	2¼	11:35	A	2:32	E	CAN	8
129	9	M.	5:40	B	**8:19**	E	14 39	1	17 N. 29	2¼	3½	**12:42**	A	3:01	E	LEO	9
130	10	Tu.	5:38	B	**8:21**	E	14 43	1	17 N. 44	3¼	4¾	**1:51**	B	3:25	D	LEO	10
131	11	W.	5:37	A	**8:22**	E	14 45	1	18 N. 00	4½	5½	**3:02**	B	3:46	D	LEO	11
132	12	Th.	5:36	A	**8:23**	E	14 47	1	18 N. 15	5¾	6¼	**4:14**	C	4:06	C	VIR	12
133	13	Fr.	5:35	A	**8:24**	E	14 49	1	18 N. 30	6¾	7	**5:29**	C	4:25	C	VIR	13
134	14	Sa.	5:34	A	**8:25**	E	14 51	1	18 N. 44	7½	7¾	**6:47**	D	4:47	B	VIR	14
135	15	**B**	5:32	A	**8:27**	E	14 55	1	18 N. 58	8¼	8½	**8:10**	E	5:11	B	LIB	15
136	16	M.	5:31	A	**8:28**	E	14 57	1	19 N. 12	9	9¼	**9:34**	E	5:42	A	LIB	16
137	17	Tu.	5:30	A	**8:29**	E	14 59	1	19 N. 26	9¾	10	**10:55**	E	6:21	A	OPH	17
138	18	W.	5:29	A	**8:30**	E	15 01	1	19 N. 39	10¾	10¾	—	-	7:13	A	OPH	18
139	19	Th.	5:28	A	**8:31**	E	15 03	1	19 N. 52	11½	11½	12:06	E	8:17	A	SAG	19
140	20	Fr.	5:27	A	**8:32**	E	15 05	1	20 N. 04	12½	—	1:02	E	9:32	A	SAG	20
141	21	Sa.	5:26	A	**8:33**	E	15 07	0	20 N. 16	12½	1½	1:45	E	10:51	A	CAP	21
142	22	**B**	5:25	A	**8:34**	E	15 09	0	20 N. 28	1½	2½	2:17	E	**12:09**	B	CAP	22
143	23	M.	5:24	A	**8:35**	E	15 11	0	20 N. 40	2½	3½	2:43	D	**1:23**	B	AQU	23
144	24	Tu.	5:23	A	**8:37**	E	15 14	0	20 N. 51	3¾	4¾	3:04	D	**2:35**	C	AQU	24
145	25	W.	5:23	A	**8:38**	E	15 15	0	21 N. 02	5	5¾	3:23	C	**3:44**	C	PSC	25
146	26	Th.	5:22	A	**8:39**	E	15 17	0	21 N. 12	6	6½	3:42	C	**4:52**	C	PSC	26
147	27	Fr.	5:21	A	**8:40**	E	15 19	0	21 N. 22	7	7¼	4:01	B	**5:59**	D	PSC	27
148	28	Sa.	5:20	A	**8:40**	E	15 20	0	21 N. 32	7¾	7¾	4:21	B	**7:06**	D	ARI	28
149	29	**B**	5:20	A	**8:41**	E	15 21	0	21 N. 41	8½	8½	4:45	A	**8:13**	E	TAU	28
150	30	M.	5:19	A	**8:42**	E	15 23	*1	21 N. 50	9¼	9	5:13	A	**9:18**	E	TAU	0
151	31	Tu.	5:18	A	**8:43**	E	15 25	*1	21 N. 58	9¾	9¾	5:48	A	**10:18**	E	TAU	1

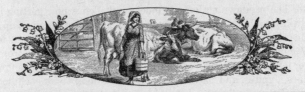

*Now the bright morning star, day's harbinger, / Comes dancing
from the East, and leads with her / The flowery May.*
–John Milton

DAY OF MONTH	DAY OF WEEK	DATES, FEASTS, FASTS, ASPECTS, TIDE HEIGHTS, AND WEATHER		
1	B	3rd ☉. of Easter • **MAY DAY** • ☾ AT ☍ • ☌♂☉ •	{5.5 / 5.9	*Dank,*
2	M.	Sts. Philip & James • ☌♂☾ • 1st FBI director J. Edgar Hoover died, 1972 •	{5.5 / 5.8	*dismal—*
3	Tu.	Magician Doug Henning born, 1947 • Tides	{5.4 / 5.6	*abysmal!*
4	W.	Educator Horace Mann born, 1796 • Damaging windstorm in southern Ont. produced 78-mph gusts in Hamilton, 2018 •		*But*
5	Th.	☾RIDES HIGH • ☾AT APO. • ☌♂☉ • *It rains by planets.* •	{5.1 / —	*never*
6	Fr.	Writer Henry David Thoreau died, 1862 • *Hindenburg disaster, 1937* •	{5.3 / 5.0	*pine—*
7	Sa.	Bigfoot reported seen in Hollis, N.H., 1977 • Tides	{5.1 / 4.9	*now*
8	B	4th ☉. of Easter • **MOTHER'S DAY** • *A mother's love changes never.* •	{4.9 / 4.8	*it's*
9	M.	St. Gregory of Nazianzus • 1st May snow in Boston in 107 years, Mass., 1977 • Tides	{4.8 / 4.8	*fine!*
10	Tu.	☿ STAT. • Victoria Woodhull 1st woman nominated for U.S. president, 1872 •	{4.7 / 5.0	*Summer*
11	W.	20-ton meteor fell to ground near Blackstone, Va., 1922 • Three • Tides	{4.7 / 5.2	*to the*
12	Th.	☾ON EQ. • Susie Maroney swam from Cuba to Fla. in 24.5 hours, 1997 • *Chilly* •	{4.9 / 5.6	*rescue,*
13	Fr.	Cranberries in bud now. • **Saints** • Tides	{5.2 / 5.9	*with*
14	Sa.	Botanist Mikhail Semyonovich Tsvet, inventor of chromatography, born, 1872 • Tides	{5.5 / 6.2	*clover*
15	B	5th ☉. of Easter • ☾ AT ☍ • Writer Emily Dickinson died, 1886		*and*
16	M.	Vesak • **FULL FLOWER** ○ • **ECLIPSE** ☾ • Tides	{5.8 / 6.5	*fescue!*
17	Tu.	☾AT PERIG. • ☌♂♇ • Singer Donna Summer died, 2012 •	{5.9 / 6.5	*Everything's*
18	W.	☾RUNS LOW • Film director Frank Capra born, 1897 • Tides	{5.9 / 6.3	*growing;*
19	Th.	St. Dunstan • Paraplegic Anna Sarol took steps across grad stage to receive H.S. diploma, Kans., 2019		*soon*
20	Fr.	☌♃☾ • 3.5-week study of dust devils began, Eloy, Ariz., 2002 • Tides	{5.6 / —	*you'll*
21	Sa.	☿IN INF. ☌ • Aviator Charles Lindbergh completed 1st nonstop solo flight across Atlantic, N.Y. to Paris, 1927		*be*
22	B	**Rogation Sunday** • ☌♄☾ • Hubble 'scope detected at least two more Saturn moons, 1995		*mowing!*
23	M.	**VICTORIA DAY** • Historian David Ludlum died, 1997 • Tides	{5.2 / 5.3	*Spring*
24	Tu.	☌♂☾ • ☌♃☾ • ☌♇☾ • *Aurora 7 spacecraft launched, 1962* •	{5.0 / 5.4	*has*
25	W.	St. Bede • ☾ON EQ. • Original *Star Wars* released in theaters, 1977		*sprung,*
26	Th.	**Ascension** • ☌♃☾ • Announced: Dumbo octopus sighted 22,825 ft. down, setting record, 2020		
27	Fr.	German ship *Bismarck* sunk, WWII, 1941 • Tides	{5.1 / 5.7	*winter is*
28	Sa.	☾ AT ☍ • ☌♂♃ • ☌♂☾ • Jell-O gelatin introduced, 1897 •	{5.1 / 5.7	*going!*
29	B	1st ☉. af. Asc. • ☌♂☾ • Historian Marcel Trudel born, 1917 •	{5.2 / 5.7	*No*
30	M.	**MEMORIAL DAY (U.S.)** • **NEW** ● • Lincoln Memorial dedicated, D.C., 1922		*more*
31	Tu.	Visit. of Mary • *A good word extinguishes more than a pail full of water.* •	{5.2 / 5.6	*snowing!*

Farmer's Calendar

One spring, a local museum assembled oxen to move its 1823 schoolhouse a third of a mile up the road. The crowd gawked as 22 teams lined up before their 105-ton load. The oxen ranged in size from Jim and John, a diminutive pair of 1-year-olds no bigger than Saint Bernards, to Pick and Axe, 8-year-olds standing as high as the cab on a dump truck, and each weighing more than a ton. At the coordinator's signal, whips swung and oxen pulled; the school inched forward. "A lot of these oxen have never pulled on pavement before," a farmer commented as he hovered by his sons and their straining team. "Oxen need to dig into the ground to really pull a load; they can't do that here." Then he exposed the truth, that theoretically, each ox can pull half its weight. If this building were to be entirely moved by animal power, the farmer calculated, "we'd need about 100 teams." Fortunately, the schoolhouse was on a carriage with hydrostatic drive, so the oxen's success of progressively tugging the building uphill was a mirage. And yet what a sight—the animals' patient, unwavering dedication, I thought, accelerating my car wistfully into this century.

CALENDAR

JUNE

SKY WATCH: The predawn action continues, with Venus now getting low in the east, bright Jupiter above dimmer orange Mars, and Saturn highest up and to the right of the others. From the 16th until month's end, all of the planets form a line like a string of pearls. Moreover, they appear in their true order from the Sun. From lower left to upper right, some 45 minutes before sunrise, look for Mercury, Venus, Mars, Jupiter, and Saturn! The crescent Moon visits each; look for the Moon below Saturn on the 18th, below Jupiter on the 21st, to the right of Mars on the 22nd, above Venus on the 26th, and above Mercury on the 27th. Summer in the Northern Hemisphere begins with the solstice on the 21st at 5:14 A.M. EDT.

| ◑ FIRST QUARTER | 7th day | 10:48 A.M. | ◐ LAST QUARTER | 20th day | 11:11 P.M. |
| ○ FULL MOON | 14th day | 7:52 A.M. | ● NEW MOON | 28th day | 10:52 P.M. |

All times are given in Eastern Daylight Time.

GET THESE PAGES WITH TIMES SET TO YOUR POSTAL CODE VIA ALMANAC.CA/2022.

DAY OF YEAR	DAY OF MONTH	DAY OF WEEK	☼ RISES H.M.	RISE KEY	☼ SETS H.M.	SET KEY	LENGTH OF DAY H.M.	SUN FAST M.	SUN DECLINATION ° '	HIGH TIDE TIMES HALIFAX		☾ RISES H.M.	RISE KEY	☾ SETS H.M.	SET KEY	☾ ASTRON. PLACE	☾ AGE
152	1	W.	5:18	A	8:44	E	15 26	*1	22 N. 07	10½	10½	6:31	A	11:11	E	TAU	2
153	2	Th.	5:17	A	8:45	E	15 28	*1	22 N. 14	11¼	11	7:22	A	11:56	E	GEM	3
154	3	Fr.	5:17	A	8:46	E	15 29	*1	22 N. 22	11¾	11¾	8:20	A	—	-	GEM	4
155	4	Sa.	5:16	A	8:47	E	15 31	*1	22 N. 29	12½	—	9:23	A	12:33	E	CAN	5
156	5	**B**	5:16	A	8:47	E	15 31	*1	22 N. 35	12¼	1	10:29	A	1:03	E	LEO	6
157	6	M.	5:15	A	8:48	E	15 33	*2	22 N. 42	1	1¾	11:36	B	1:28	D	LEO	7
158	7	Tu.	5:15	A	8:49	E	15 34	*2	22 N. 47	1¾	2¾	12:44	B	1:49	D	LEO	8
159	8	W.	5:15	A	8:49	E	15 34	*2	22 N. 53	2¾	3¾	1:54	C	2:09	C	VIR	9
160	9	Th.	5:15	A	8:50	E	15 35	*2	22 N. 58	3¾	4½	3:05	C	2:28	C	VIR	10
161	10	Fr.	5:14	A	8:51	E	15 37	*2	23 N. 02	5	5½	4:20	D	2:48	B	VIR	11
162	11	Sa.	5:14	A	8:51	E	15 37	*3	23 N. 06	6	6¼	5:39	D	3:10	B	VIR	12
163	12	**B**	5:14	A	8:52	E	15 38	*3	23 N. 10	7	7	7:02	E	3:37	A	LIB	13
164	13	M.	5:14	A	8:52	E	15 38	*3	23 N. 14	7¾	8	8:26	E	4:11	A	SCO	14
165	14	Tu.	5:14	A	8:53	E	15 39	*3	23 N. 17	8¾	8¾	9:44	E	4:57	A	OPH	15
166	15	W.	5:14	A	8:53	E	15 39	*3	23 N. 19	9½	9¾	10:49	E	5:56	A	SAG	16
167	16	Th.	5:14	A	8:53	E	15 39	*4	23 N. 21	10½	10½	11:39	E	7:09	A	SAG	17
168	17	Fr.	5:14	A	8:54	E	15 40	*4	23 N. 23	11¼	11½	—	-	8:30	A	CAP	18
169	18	Sa.	5:14	A	8:54	E	15 40	*4	23 N. 24	12¼	—	12:17	E	9:51	A	CAP	19
170	19	**B**	5:14	A	8:54	E	15 40	*4	23 N. 25	12¼	1¼	12:46	D	11:10	B	AQU	20
171	20	M.	5:14	A	8:55	E	15 41	*5	23 N. 26	1¼	2	1:09	D	12:24	B	AQU	21
172	21	Tu.	5:14	A	8:55	E	15 41	*5	23 N. 26	2¼	3	1:29	C	1:35	C	PSC	22
173	22	W.	5:15	A	8:55	E	15 40	*5	23 N. 25	3¼	4	1:48	C	2:44	C	CET	23
174	23	Th.	5:15	A	8:55	E	15 40	*5	23 N. 25	4½	5	2:07	B	3:51	D	PSC	24
175	24	Fr.	5:15	A	8:55	E	15 40	*5	23 N. 23	5½	5¾	2:27	B	4:58	D	ARI	25
176	25	Sa.	5:16	A	8:55	E	15 39	*6	23 N. 22	6½	6½	2:49	A	6:05	E	ARI	26
177	26	**B**	5:16	A	8:55	E	15 39	*6	23 N. 20	7¼	7¼	3:16	A	7:10	E	TAU	27
178	27	M.	5:16	A	8:55	E	15 39	*6	23 N. 18	8¼	8	3:49	A	8:11	E	TAU	28
179	28	Tu.	5:17	A	8:55	E	15 38	*6	23 N. 15	9	8¾	4:29	A	9:07	E	TAU	0
180	29	W.	5:17	A	8:55	E	15 38	*6	23 N. 11	9½	9½	5:17	A	9:54	E	GEM	1
181	30	Th.	5:18	A	8:55	E	15 37	*7	23 N. 08	10¼	10	6:13	A	10:34	E	GEM	2

THE SIXTH MONTH · 2022 **JUNE** JUNE HATH 30 DAYS

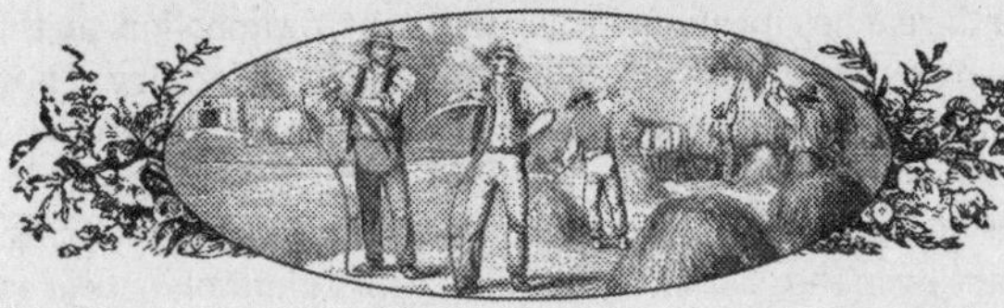

O summer is here with its breezy train
I know by the robin's roundelay.
–**Richard Kendall Munkittrick**

DAY OF MONTH	DAY OF WEEK	DATES, FEASTS, FASTS, ASPECTS, TIDE HEIGHTS, AND WEATHER	
1	W.	☾ RIDES HIGH • ☾ AT APO. • Ky. became 15th U.S. state, 1792 • {5.2 5.5	*Showers*
2	Th.	**Orthodox Ascension** • ☿ STAT. • *Surveyor 1* landed on Moon, 1966 • {5.2 5.4	*are*
3	Fr.	Tenor Roland Hayes born, 1887 • Tides {5.1 5.3	*pattering,*
4	Sa.	Shavuot begins at sundown • Sierra Club incorporated, 1892 • {5.1 —	*not*
5	**B**	**Whit S. • Pentecost** • ♄ STAT. • Tides {5.2 5.0	*so*
6	M.	D-Day, 1944 • Barbara Washburn 1st woman to summit Denali (Mount McKinley), Alaska, 1947	*chilly.*
7	Tu.	Comedian Bill Hader born, 1978 • Extreme Ultraviolet Explorer (EUVE) satellite launched, 1992	*More*
8	W.	Ember Day • Posted: Restaurant rec'd rare blue lobster in seafood shipment, Eastham, Mass., 2019	*showers,*
9	Th.	☾ ON EQ. • *When need is greatest, help is nearest.* • Tides {4.7 5.4	*but*
10	Fr.	Ember Day • Singer Judy Garland born, 1922 • Tides {4.8 5.6	*just*
11	Sa.	St. Barnabas • Ember Day • ☌♀⛢ • Tides {5.0 5.9	*a*
12	**B**	**Trinity** • Orthodox Pentecost • ☾ AT ☋ • {5.3 6.2	*smattering,*
13	M.	Queen Victoria took her 1st train ride, 1842 • {5.5 6.3	*silly.*
14	Tu.	St. Basil • FLAG DAY (U.S.) • FULL STRAWBERRY ○ • ☾ AT PERIG.	*Still*
15	W.	☾ RUNS LOW • *June damp and warm Does the farmer no harm.* • {5.8 6.4	*more showers,*
16	Th.	☌♇☾ • ☿ GR. ELONG. (23° WEST) • Henry Berliner made 1st controlled horizontal helicopter flight in U.S., 1922	
17	Fr.	Double-hulled, 62-ft. Polynesian voyaging canoe *Hōkūle'a* returned to Hawaii after world trip, 2017	*but*
18	Sa.	☌♄☾ • 143-lb. blue catfish caught, Kerr Lake, Buggs Island, Va., 2011 • {5.8 —	*not*
19	**B**	**Corpus Christi** • Orthodox All Saints' • FATHER'S DAY • JUNETEENTH • {5.8 5.7	*a*
20	M.	☌♆☾ • New National Library and Archives building opened, Ottawa, 1967 • {5.5 5.6	*battering.*
21	Tu.	SUMMER SOLSTICE • ☾ ON EQ. • ☌♃☾ • Tides {5.2 5.5	*Glory*
22	W.	St. Alban • ☌♂☾ • 12" rain in 42 mins., Holt, Mo., 1947 • Tides {4.9 5.4	*be!*
23	Th.	From opposite ends, Nik and Lijana Wallenda crossed high wire 25 stories high, N.Y.C., 2019 • {4.8 5.4	*We're*
24	Fr.	Nativ. John the Baptist • MIDSUMMER DAY • ☌⛢☾ • {4.7 5.4	*shower-*
25	Sa.	☾ AT ☊ • Oceanographer Jacques-Yves Cousteau died, 1997 • Tides {4.8 5.4	*free!*
26	**B**	**3rd S. af. P.** • ☌♀☾ • 1st Harry Potter book debuted in UK, 1997	*Sunny,*
27	M.	☌☿☾ • Poet Paul Laurence Dunbar born, 1872 • Tides {4.9 5.4	*cool—*
28	Tu.	St. Irenaeus • NEW ● • ♆ STAT. • *Love makes labor light.* • {5.0 5.5	*no*
29	W.	Sts. Peter & Paul • ☾ RIDES HIGH • ☾ AT APO. • Tides {5.1 5.5	*more*
30	Th.	1st leap second introduced to Coordinated Universal Time (UTC), 1972 • Tides {5.1 5.5	*school!*

Farmer's Calendar

There are many ways to arrive at the magisterial white barn at the University of Vermont's Morgan Horse Farm in Weybridge. If you're a horse, however, you were probably born here, as part of the longest continuous breeding program of Morgans in the nation, one devoted to perpetuating the traits of an extraordinary horse. The breed originated when a Vermont teacher named Justin Morgan accepted a debt repayment in the form of a colt that proved legendary. He grew to clear timber and haul stones; later he raced two horses—one after the other—and won both times. As well, he won a pulling contest. Then, in July 1817, he bore President Monroe through the streets of Montpelier. No wonder the breed became the state's animal, as "it could outdraw, outrun, and out trot any other horse." Mares often deliver their foals in the chilly days of spring. If you find your way to the farm in June, you'll discover those month-old colts in a corral, bumping and nuzzling their mothers, like mischievous shadows. Then, one of the newest progeny, oblivious to both the nearby statue of its famous ancestor and its own storied pedigree, may nibble your bare elbow, sniff opportunistically at your wrist.

CALENDAR

JULY

SKY WATCH: Earth reaches its annual solar far point, or aphelion, on the 4th. In the predawn eastern sky, the lineup is still happening, but Mercury is now lower and harder to see and the other planets are now farther apart and less eye-catching. After the 4th, Mercury is too low to see, but Saturn, rising a half hour earlier each week, now comes up by 11 P.M., with Jupiter, in Pisces, following the Ringed Planet to appear low in the east after midnight. Both giant planets are now at their highest at dawn. Mars, too, is gaining in visibility at a very bright magnitude 0.3, as it rises at 2 A.M. in Aries. Planet viewing has now shifted from the exclusively predawn stage of winter and spring to summer's middle-of-the-night venue.

◐ FIRST QUARTER 6th day 10:14 P.M. ◑ LAST QUARTER 20th day 10:19 A.M.

○ FULL MOON 13th day 2:38 P.M. ● NEW MOON 28th day 1:55 P.M.

All times are given in Eastern Daylight Time.

GET THESE PAGES WITH TIMES SET TO YOUR POSTAL CODE VIA ALMANAC.CA/2022.

DAY OF YEAR	DAY OF MONTH	DAY OF WEEK	☼ RISES H. M.	RISE KEY	☼ SETS H. M.	SET KEY	LENGTH OF DAY H.	LENGTH OF DAY M.	SUN FAST M.	SUN DECLINATION °	SUN DECLINATION '	HIGH TIDE TIMES HALIFAX		☾ RISES H. M.	RISE KEY	☾ SETS H. M.	SET KEY	☾ ASTRON. PLACE	☾ AGE
182	1	Fr.	5:18	A	**8:55**	E	15	37	*7	23 N.	04	10¾	**10¾**	7:15	A	**11:06**	E	CAN	3
183	2	Sa.	5:19	A	**8:55**	E	15	36	*7	22 N.	59	11½	**11¼**	8:20	A	**11:32**	E	CAN	4
184	3	**B**	5:20	A	**8:54**	E	15	34	*7	22 N.	55	**12**	—	9:27	B	**11:54**	D	LEO	5
185	4	M.	5:20	A	**8:54**	E	15	34	*7	22 N.	49	12	**12¾**	10:34	B	—	-	LEO	6
186	5	Tu.	5:21	A	**8:54**	E	15	33	*8	22 N.	44	12¾	**1¼**	11:41	B	12:14	D	LEO	7
187	6	W.	5:22	A	**8:53**	E	15	31	*8	22 N.	38	1½	**2**	**12:50**	C	12:32	C	VIR	8
188	7	Th.	5:22	A	**8:53**	E	15	31	*8	22 N.	31	2¼	**2¾**	**2:01**	D	12:51	C	VIR	9
189	8	Fr.	5:23	A	**8:52**	E	15	29	*8	22 N.	24	3¼	**3¾**	**3:15**	D	1:11	B	VIR	10
190	9	Sa.	5:24	A	**8:52**	E	15	28	*8	22 N.	17	4½	**4¾**	**4:34**	E	1:35	B	LIB	11
191	10	**B**	5:25	A	**8:51**	E	15	26	*8	22 N.	10	5½	**5¾**	**5:56**	E	2:05	A	LIB	12
192	11	M.	5:25	A	**8:51**	E	15	26	*8	22 N.	02	6½	**6½**	**7:16**	E	2:43	A	OPH	13
193	12	Tu.	5:26	A	**8:50**	E	15	24	*9	21 N.	53	7½	**7½**	**8:28**	E	3:35	A	SAG	14
194	13	W.	5:27	A	**8:50**	E	15	23	*9	21 N.	45	8½	**8½**	**9:27**	E	4:41	A	SAG	15
195	14	Th.	5:28	A	**8:49**	E	15	21	*9	21 N.	36	9½	**9½**	**10:11**	E	6:00	A	SAG	16
196	15	Fr.	5:29	A	**8:48**	E	15	19	*9	21 N.	26	10¼	**10¼**	**10:45**	E	7:24	A	CAP	17
197	16	Sa.	5:30	A	**8:47**	E	15	17	*9	21 N.	16	11	**11¼**	**11:11**	D	8:47	B	AQU	18
198	17	**B**	5:31	A	**8:47**	E	15	16	*9	21 N.	06	**12**	—	**11:33**	C	10:06	B	AQU	19
199	18	M.	5:32	A	**8:46**	E	15	14	*9	20 N.	56	12	**12¾**	**11:53**	C	11:20	C	AQU	20
200	19	Tu.	5:33	A	**8:45**	E	15	12	*9	20 N.	45	1	**1½**	—	-	**12:32**	C	CET	21
201	20	W.	5:34	A	**8:44**	E	15	10	*9	20 N.	34	1¾	**2¼**	12:12	B	**1:41**	D	PSC	22
202	21	Th.	5:35	A	**8:43**	E	15	08	*9	20 N.	22	2¾	**3¼**	12:31	B	**2:49**	D	ARI	23
203	22	Fr.	5:36	A	**8:42**	E	15	06	*9	20 N.	10	3¾	**4¼**	12:53	B	**3:56**	E	ARI	24
204	23	Sa.	5:37	A	**8:41**	E	15	04	*9	19 N.	58	5	**5¼**	1:19	A	**5:02**	E	TAU	25
205	24	**B**	5:38	A	**8:40**	E	15	02	*9	19 N.	45	6	**6**	1:49	A	**6:05**	E	TAU	26
206	25	M.	5:39	A	**8:39**	E	15	00	*9	19 N.	32	7	**7**	2:27	A	**7:03**	E	TAU	27
207	26	Tu.	5:40	A	**8:38**	E	14	58	*9	19 N.	19	7¾	**7¾**	3:13	A	**7:53**	E	GEM	28
208	27	W.	5:41	A	**8:37**	E	14	56	*9	19 N.	05	8½	**8½**	4:07	A	**8:34**	E	GEM	29
209	28	Th.	5:42	A	**8:36**	E	14	54	*9	18 N.	52	9¼	**9**	5:08	A	**9:08**	E	CAN	0
210	29	Fr.	5:44	A	**8:34**	E	14	50	*9	18 N.	37	9¾	**9¾**	6:12	A	**9:36**	E	CAN	1
211	30	Sa.	5:45	A	**8:33**	E	14	48	*9	18 N.	23	10½	**10¼**	7:19	A	**9:59**	D	LEO	2
212	31	**B**	5:46	A	**8:32**	E	14	46	*9	18 N.	08	11	**11**	8:26	B	**10:20**	D	LEO	3

To use this page, see p. 116; for Key Letters, see p. 240. LIGHT = A.M. BOLD = P.M.

JULY

JULY HATH 31 DAYS

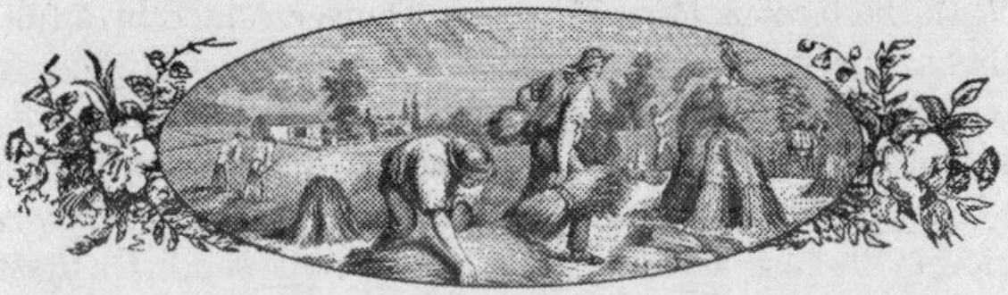

'Tis Summer's noon: High rides the fervid Sun
O'er fresh-mown meads and fields of waving corn.
–John Askham

DAY OF MONTH	DAY OF WEEK	DATES, FEASTS, FASTS, ASPECTS, TIDE HEIGHTS, AND WEATHER	
1	Fr.	CANADA DAY • Dominion of Canada created, 1867 • Tides {5.2 5.5	*Fireworks*
2	Sa.	Aviatrix Amelia Earhart and navigator Fred Noonan disappeared during flight, Pacific Ocean, 1937	*(both*
3	B	4th S. af. P. • Dog Days begin. • *Fruit, Garden and Home* magazine debuted, 1922	*natural*
4	M.	INDEPENDENCE DAY (U.S.) • ⊕ AT APHELION • U.S. president Calvin Coolidge born, 1872	*and*
5	Tu.	110°F, Regina, Sask., 1937 • Burt's Bees cofounder Burt Shavitz died, 2015 • Tides {5.1 5.3	*patriotic)*
6	W.	☾ ON EQ. • Althea Gibson won women's singles title at Wimbledon, 1957 • {5.0 5.3	*amaze*
7	Th.	Sci-fi writer Robert Heinlein born, 1907 • Armadillos mate now. • {4.8 5.4	*our*
8	Fr.	Military press release stated "flying disc" recovered near Roswell, N.Mex., 1947 • Tides {4.7 5.5	*gazes;*
9	Sa.	☾ AT ☋ • 98°F, Buffalo, N.Y., 2020 • Tides {4.7 5.6	*it's*
10	B	5th S. af. P. • Folksinger Arlo Guthrie born, 1947 • Tides {4.8 5.8	*hot*
11	M.	*A heart free from care is better than a full purse.* • {5.1 6.0	*as*
12	Tu.	☾ RUNS LOW • Cornscateous air is everywhere. • {5.3 6.2	*blazes!*
13	W.	FULL BUCK ○ • ☾ AT PERIG. • ☌♇☾ • Tides {5.6 6.4	*Here's*
14	Th.	Bastille Day • Manufacturer Frederick Louis Maytag born, 1857 • Tides {5.8 6.4	*a*
15	Fr.	St. Swithin • ☌♄☾ • Official production of 1958 Edsel began, 1957 • {6.0 6.3	*friendly*
16	Sa.	☿ IN SUP. ☌ • Washington, D.C., became capital of U.S., 1790 • {6.0 6.1	*warning:*
17	B	6th S. af. P. • ☌♆☾ • Mathematician Jules Henri Poincaré died, 1912	*No*
18	M.	☾ ON EQ. • ☌♃☾ • Astrogeologist Eugene Shoemaker died, 1997 • Tides {5.8 5.9	*key,*
19	Tu.	♇ AT ☍ • Horace Tuttle (after Lewis Swift 3 days earlier) discovered what is now Comet 109P/Swift-Tuttle, 1862	
20	W.	78-lb. 14-oz. flathead catfish caught, Neuse River, N.C., 2020 • Tides {5.2 5.5	*no kite,*
21	Th.	☌♂☾ • *If corn is hard to husk, expect a hard winter.* • Tides {4.8 5.3	*stay*
22	Fr.	St. Mary Magdalene • ☾ AT ☊ • ☌♅☾ • Geneticist Gregor Mendel born, 1822 • {4.6 5.2	*in*
23	Sa.	Black-eyed Susans in bloom now. • Tides {4.5 5.1	*at*
24	B	7th S. af. P. • Lightning stroke measured at 345,000 amperes, Pittsburgh, Pa., 1947	*night!*
25	M.	St. James • Moon crater named after scientist Michael Wargo, 2017 • {4.6 5.2	*(Ben*
26	Tu.	St. Anne • ☾ RIDES HIGH • ☾ AT APO. • ☌♀☾ • Tides {4.8 5.3	*Franklin,*
27	W.	Naturalist Thomas Say born, 1787 • Adult gypsy moths emerge. • {4.9 5.4	*though*
28	Th.	NEW ● • 1st U.S. railway post office, Hannibal and St. Joseph Railroad, 1862 • {5.1 5.5	*plucky,*
29	Fr.	St. Martha • First of Muharram begins at sundown • ☌☿☾ • ♃ STAT. • {5.2 5.6	*was*
30	Sa.	Politician/actor Arnold Schwarzenegger born, 1947 • Tides {5.3 5.6	*mighty*
31	B	8th S. af. P. • *Life is half spent before we know what it is.* • Tides {5.4 5.5	*lucky!)*

Farmer's Calendar

You expect tractor pulls, tilt-a-whirls, and prizewinning sows at a county fair. But the "Field Days" in Johnson, Vermont, also host the "Ladies' Underhanded Skillet Toss," wherein females ages 3 to 83 competed in flinging a cast-iron frying pan. This reinforced skillet was manufactured at a local foundry specifically for this opportunity. One year, when the staff couldn't find the special skillet, they destroyed nine regular ones, Jessica, a Field Days board member, informs the crowd, seated safely away from the pitching lane: "Yep, ladies, it's heavier than it looks." As toddlers, then grade schoolers, then preteens, then women all the way up through their golden years each take their turn wielding the skillet and throwing it away, it flies farther and farther across the field, a distance duly noted by Jessica's boyfriend, who uses a measuring wheel. In the last division, "Young at Heart," a first-timer named Vicki steps up. She needs to surpass the current record of 47 feet 9 inches to win. Getting ready, she draws her right hand back like a tennis player readying her serve. Then she sends it hurtling with all her might, tossing that bacon-cooking, egg-scrambling, pancake-flipping pan into the sizzling sky.

AUGUST

SKY WATCH: With the famous Perseid meteor shower ruined by a full Moon, this month's spotlight remains on the planets, with Saturn's earlier 10 P.M. rising offering viewing opportunities to night owls. The Ringed Planet reaches opposition, its closest and brightest of 2022, on the 14th. Still, as morning twilight begins from the 1st to the 3rd, look for bright Mars, now at magnitude 0, halfway between far-apart Venus, low in the east, and Jupiter, nicely up in the south. On these mornings, binocular users can easily see green Uranus next to orange Mars. On the 14th, the Moon is near Jupiter. On the 19th, look for the Moon closely above Mars, a gorgeous conjunction that is at its highest at dawn. On the 25th, the crescent Moon hovers above Venus, with the Moon to the planet's lower left on the next morning.

◐ **FIRST QUARTER** 5th day 7:07 A.M.　　◑ **LAST QUARTER** 19th day 12:36 A.M.
○ **FULL MOON** 11th day 9:36 P.M.　　● **NEW MOON** 27th day 4:17 A.M.

All times are given in Eastern Daylight Time.

GET THESE PAGES WITH TIMES SET TO YOUR POSTAL CODE VIA ALMANAC.CA/2022.

DAY OF YEAR	DAY OF MONTH	DAY OF WEEK	☼ RISES H. M.	RISE KEY	☼ SETS H. M.	SET KEY	LENGTH OF DAY H. M.	SUN FAST M.	SUN DECLINATION ° '	HIGH TIDE TIMES HALIFAX		☾ RISES H. M.	RISE KEY	☾ SETS H. M.	SET KEY	☾ ASTRON. PLACE	☾ AGE
213	1	M.	5:47	A	8:31	E	14 44	*9	17 N. 53	11½	11¾	9:33	B	10:38	C	LEO	4
214	2	Tu.	5:48	A	8:29	E	14 41	*9	17 N. 38	12¼	—	10:41	C	10:56	C	VIR	5
215	3	W.	5:49	B	8:28	E	14 39	*9	17 N. 22	12¼	12¾	11:50	C	11:16	B	VIR	6
216	4	Th.	5:50	B	8:27	E	14 37	*9	17 N. 06	1	1½	1:02	D	11:37	B	VIR	7
217	5	Fr.	5:52	B	8:25	E	14 33	*9	16 N. 50	1¾	2¼	2:17	D	—		LIB	8
218	6	Sa.	5:53	B	8:24	E	14 31	*9	16 N. 33	2¾	3	3:35	E	12:03	A	LIB	9
219	7	**B**	5:54	B	8:22	D	14 28	*9	16 N. 16	4	4¼	4:54	E	12:36	A	SCO	10
220	8	M.	5:55	B	8:21	D	14 26	*8	15 N. 59	5¼	5¼	6:08	E	1:20	A	OPH	11
221	9	Tu.	5:56	B	8:19	D	14 23	*8	15 N. 42	6¼	6¼	7:12	E	2:18	A	SAG	12
222	10	W.	5:58	B	8:18	D	14 20	*8	15 N. 25	7¼	7¼	8:02	E	3:31	A	SAG	13
223	11	Th.	5:59	B	8:16	D	14 17	*8	15 N. 07	8¼	8¼	8:40	E	4:52	A	CAP	14
224	12	Fr.	6:00	B	8:15	D	14 15	*8	14 N. 49	9¼	9¼	9:09	D	6:17	A	CAP	15
225	13	Sa.	6:01	B	8:13	D	14 12	*8	14 N. 31	10	10	9:34	D	7:39	B	AQU	16
226	14	**B**	6:02	B	8:12	D	14 10	*7	14 N. 12	10¾	10¾	9:55	C	8:58	B	AQU	17
227	15	M.	6:04	B	8:10	D	14 06	*7	13 N. 53	11½	11¾	10:14	C	10:13	C	PSC	18
228	16	Tu.	6:05	B	8:08	D	14 03	*7	13 N. 34	12¼	—	10:34	B	11:25	D	PSC	19
229	17	W.	6:06	B	8:07	D	14 01	*7	13 N. 15	12½	1	10:55	B	12:35	D	ARI	20
230	18	Th.	6:07	B	8:05	D	13 58	*7	12 N. 56	1¼	1¾	11:20	A	1:44	E	ARI	21
231	19	Fr.	6:08	B	8:03	D	13 55	*6	12 N. 36	2	2½	11:49	A	2:52	E	TAU	22
232	20	Sa.	6:10	B	8:02	D	13 52	*6	12 N. 17	3	3¼	—		3:57	E	TAU	23
233	21	**B**	6:11	B	8:00	D	13 49	*6	11 N. 57	4¼	4½	12:24	A	4:57	E	TAU	24
234	22	M.	6:12	B	7:58	D	13 46	*6	11 N. 36	5½	5½	1:07	A	5:50	E	GEM	25
235	23	Tu.	6:13	B	7:57	D	13 44	*5	11 N. 16	6½	6½	1:59	A	6:34	E	GEM	26
236	24	W.	6:15	B	7:55	D	13 40	*5	10 N. 56	7½	7¼	2:58	A	7:10	E	GEM	27
237	25	Th.	6:16	B	7:53	D	13 37	*5	10 N. 35	8¼	8	4:02	A	7:40	D	CAN	28
238	26	Fr.	6:17	B	7:51	D	13 34	*5	10 N. 14	8¾	8¾	5:09	B	8:04	D	LEO	29
239	27	Sa.	6:18	B	7:49	D	13 31	*4	9 N. 53	9¼	9¼	6:17	B	8:25	D	LEO	0
240	28	**B**	6:19	B	7:48	D	13 29	*4	9 N. 32	9¾	10	7:25	B	8:44	C	LEO	1
241	29	M.	6:21	B	7:46	D	13 25	*4	9 N. 11	10½	10½	8:33	C	9:03	C	VIR	2
242	30	Tu.	6:22	B	7:44	D	13 22	*3	8 N. 49	11	11¼	9:42	C	9:21	B	VIR	3
243	31	W.	6:23	B	7:42	D	13 19	*3	8 N. 27	11½	12	10:53	D	9:42	B	VIR	4

THE EIGHTH MONTH • 2022 **AUGUST** AUGUST HATH 31 DAYS

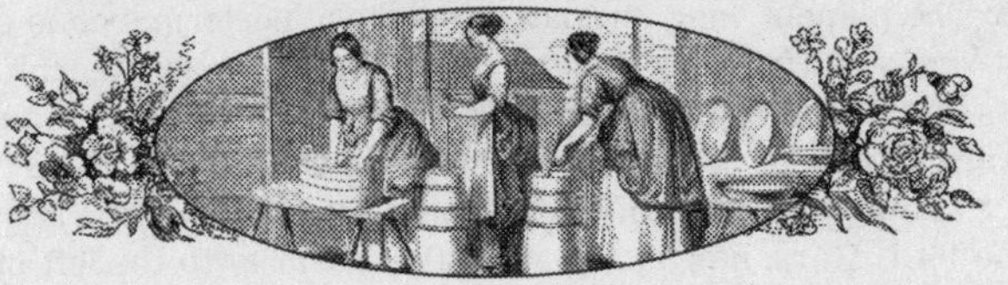

How stealthily the twilight steals around,
Infolding all in the sweet zone of peace!
–J. Dawson

DAY OF MONTH	DAY OF WEEK	DATES, FEASTS, FASTS, ASPECTS, TIDE HEIGHTS, AND WEATHER	
1	M.	Lammas Day • CIVIC HOLIDAY • ☌♂⛢ • Tides {5.5 5.4	*Keep*
2	Tu.	☾ON EQ. • Inventor Alexander Graham Bell died, 1922 • {5.5 —	*an*
3	W.	Canadian governor-general John Campbell Hamilton-Gordon born, 1847 • {5.2 5.5	*eye*
4	Th.	Major geomagnetic storm, 1972 • *Keep some till furthermore come.* • Tides {5.1 5.5	*on*
5	Fr.	☾AT ☋ • NASA's *Juno* spacecraft, to study Jupiter, launched, 2011 • Tides {4.9 5.5	*the*
6	Sa.	Transfiguration • Radio astronomer Sir Bernard Lovell died, 2012 • Tides {4.7 5.5	*sky*
7	**B**	9th S. af. P. • U.S. Badge of Military Merit (succeeded by Purple Heart) established, 1782	*if*
8	M.	St. Dominic • International Cat Day • Paleontologist Henry Fairfield Osborn born, 1857	*you're*
9	Tu.	☾RUNS LOW • For charity, "East Coasters for Kids" group rode 74 roller coasters in 24 hours, setting world record, 2001	
10	W.	St. Lawrence • ☾AT PERIG. • ☌♇☾ • Tides {5.3 6.1	*swimming*
11	Th.	St. Clare • Dog Days end. • FULL STURGEON ○ • ☌♄☾	*or golfing.*
12	Fr.	Botanist Thomas Andrew Knight born, 1759 • Gray squirrels have second litters now.	*Wetter—*
13	Sa.	*If larks fly high and sing long, expect fine weather.* • {6.1 6.3	*you*
14	**B**	10th S. af. P. • ☌♆☾ • ♄ AT ☍ • Tides {6.2 6.1	*might*
15	M.	Assumption • ☾ON EQ. • ☌♃☾ • Tides {6.2 5.8	*need a*
16	Tu.	Battle of Bennington, Vt., 1777 • U.S./Canadian Migratory Bird Treaty signed, 1916	*sweater.*
17	W.	Cat Nights commence. • Asaph Hall discovered Mars's moon Phobos, 1877 • Tides {5.5 5.7	*Dark*
18	Th.	☾AT ☊ • ☌⛢☾ • Ragweed in bloom. • Tides {5.2 5.5	*glasses*
19	Fr.	☌♂☾ • Poet Ogden Nash born, 1902 • Tides {4.8 5.2	*are*
20	Sa.	Damaging widespread early frost, Man. and Sask., 2004 • Tides {4.6 5.0	*wise to*
21	**B**	11th S. af. P. • Total solar eclipse across N.Am. biggest online event yet measured by NASA, 2017	
22	M.	☾RIDES HIGH • ☾AT APO. • Composer Claude Debussy born, 1862 • {4.4 4.9	*protect*
23	Tu.	Fannie Farmer opened cooking school, Boston, Mass., 1902 • Tides {4.6 5.1	*the*
24	W.	St. Bartholomew • ⛢ STAT. • Quebec premier René Lévesque born, 1922 • {4.8 5.3	*eyes;*
25	Th.	☌♀☾ • Astronaut Neil Armstrong died, 2012 • {5.0 5.5	*you'll*
26	Fr.	National Dog Day (U.S.) • Hummingbirds migrate south. • Tides {5.2 5.6	*feel*
27	Sa.	NEW ● • ☿ GR. ELONG. (27° EAST) • Railroad crossing gate patented, 1867 • {5.4 5.7	*bereft*
28	**B**	12th S. af. P. • *Take heed will surely speed.* • Tides {5.6 5.7	*if*
29	M.	St. John the Baptist • ☾ON EQ. • ☌☿☾ • Tides {5.7 5.7	*not*
30	Tu.	Rosemary Brown 1st black woman elected to Canadian provincial legislature, B.C., 1972 • {5.8 5.6	*properly*
31	W.	U.S. Congress authorized what became U.S. Naval Observatory, 1842 • Princess Diana died, 1997	*SPF'd.*

Farmer's Calendar

As Vermont's loon population rebounds from 29 birds in 1983 to an estimated 365 in 2020, Eric Hanson's waking hours, especially between April to November, are preoccupied with the birds' yodeling, mating, nesting, chick-rearing, and migrating. As the state's Loon Biologist, Eric also serves as a public relations director for them, joking that more of his time is spent on people than on the speckled birds with a spooky song. He fields questions, concerns, and sometimes their unfortunate discoveries, such as when a farmer delivers a dead loon he scooped off his manure pit. Nevertheless, sometimes the two species in Eric's work converge beautifully. Twinges of sadness for this recent casualty are replaced with hope when, through Eric's binoculars, he spots the unmistakable profile of a nesting loon jutting from the lake island's edge. Although one has been lost, perhaps one, possibly two, will hatch—that's encouraging math. We paddle his canoe on another lake where Eric spots three mature birds. Two dive below while one remains floating, in a sort of, *"Hey? Guys?"*—then it too dips under. We wait, silent, our paddles hanging, dripping above the water, scanning to discover where they'll bob up next.

SEPTEMBER

SKY WATCH: The planets' long, predawn repertory performance is coming to a close, with Venus getting very low and finishing its run as a morning star. The scene shifts to the evening sky, with Jupiter and Saturn both up in the east after 9 P.M. Saturn hovers to the left of the Moon on the 7th and to its right on the 8th. Jupiter stands to the left of the Moon on the 10th and just above it on the 11th. On the 16th, Mars, now rising at 11:30 P.M., floats to the left of the Moon. Jupiter reaches its opposition on the 26th, when it makes its closest, biggest, and brightest appearance of the year. Autumn begins with the autumnal equinox at 9:04 P.M. EDT on the night of the 22nd.

◑ **FIRST QUARTER** 3rd day 2:08 P.M.   ◐ **LAST QUARTER** 17th day 5:52 P.M.
○ **FULL MOON** 10th day 5:59 A.M.   ● **NEW MOON** 25th day 5:55 P.M.

All times are given in Eastern Daylight Time.

GET THESE PAGES WITH TIMES SET TO YOUR POSTAL CODE VIA ALMANAC.CA/2022.

DAY OF YEAR	DAY OF MONTH	DAY OF WEEK	☼ RISES H. M.	RISE KEY	☼ SETS H. M.	SET KEY	LENGTH OF DAY H. M.	SUN FAST M.	SUN DECLINATION ° ′	HIGH TIDE TIMES HALIFAX		☾ RISES H. M.	RISE KEY	☾ SETS H. M.	SET KEY	☾ ASTRON. PLACE	☾ AGE
244	1	Th.	6:24	B	7:40	D	13 16	*3	8 N. 06	12¼	—	12:07	D	10:06	A	VIR	5
245	2	Fr.	6:26	B	7:38	D	13 12	*2	7 N. 44	12¾	1	1:23	E	10:35	A	LIB	6
246	3	Sa.	6:27	B	7:37	D	13 10	*2	7 N. 22	1½	1¾	2:40	E	11:14	A	SCO	7
247	4	**B**	6:28	B	7:35	D	13 07	*2	7 N. 00	2¼	2½	3:55	E	—	-	OPH	8
248	5	M.	6:29	B	7:33	D	13 04	*1	6 N. 37	3½	3¾	5:01	E	12:05	A	SAG	9
249	6	Tu.	6:30	B	7:31	D	13 01	*1	6 N. 15	5	5	5:54	E	1:10	A	SAG	10
250	7	W.	6:32	C	7:29	D	12 57	*1	5 N. 53	6¼	6¼	6:36	E	2:26	A	CAP	11
251	8	Th.	6:33	C	7:27	D	12 54	0	5 N. 30	7¼	7¼	7:08	D	3:48	A	CAP	12
252	9	Fr.	6:34	C	7:25	C	12 51	0	5 N. 07	8	8¼	7:34	D	5:11	B	AQU	13
253	10	Sa.	6:35	C	7:23	C	12 48	0	4 N. 45	8¾	9	7:56	C	6:31	B	AQU	14
254	11	**B**	6:36	C	7:21	C	12 45	1	4 N. 22	9½	9¾	8:16	C	7:48	C	PSC	15
255	12	M.	6:38	C	7:20	C	12 42	1	3 N. 59	10¼	10½	8:36	B	9:03	C	CET	16
256	13	Tu.	6:39	C	7:18	C	12 39	1	3 N. 36	11	11¼	8:56	B	10:16	D	PSC	17
257	14	W.	6:40	C	7:16	C	12 36	2	3 N. 13	11½	—	9:20	A	11:27	D	ARI	18
258	15	Th.	6:41	C	7:14	C	12 33	2	2 N. 50	12	12¼	9:47	A	12:37	E	ARI	19
259	16	Fr.	6:42	C	7:12	C	12 30	2	2 N. 27	12¾	1	10:20	A	1:45	E	TAU	20
260	17	Sa.	6:44	C	7:10	C	12 26	3	2 N. 04	1½	1¾	11:00	A	2:48	E	TAU	21
261	18	**B**	6:45	C	7:08	C	12 23	3	1 N. 41	2½	2½	11:49	A	3:44	E	TAU	22
262	19	M.	6:46	C	7:06	C	12 20	3	1 N. 17	3½	3¾	—	-	4:31	E	GEM	23
263	20	Tu.	6:47	C	7:04	C	12 17	4	0 N. 54	5	5	12:46	A	5:10	E	GEM	24
264	21	W.	6:49	C	7:02	C	12 13	4	0 N. 31	6	6	1:48	A	5:42	E	CAN	25
265	22	Th.	6:50	C	7:00	C	12 10	5	0 N. 07	7	6¾	2:55	A	6:08	E	LEO	26
266	23	Fr.	6:51	C	6:58	C	12 07	5	0 s. 15	7½	7½	4:03	B	6:30	D	LEO	27
267	24	Sa.	6:52	C	6:56	C	12 04	5	0 s. 38	8¼	8¼	5:11	B	6:50	D	LEO	28
268	25	**B**	6:54	C	6:54	C	12 00	6	1 s. 02	8¾	8¾	6:20	C	7:08	C	VIR	0
269	26	M.	6:55	C	6:53	C	11 58	6	1 s. 25	9¼	9½	7:30	C	7:27	C	VIR	1
270	27	Tu.	6:56	C	6:51	C	11 55	6	1 s. 48	9¾	10	8:42	D	7:47	B	VIR	2
271	28	W.	6:57	C	6:49	C	11 52	7	2 s. 12	10½	10¾	9:56	D	8:09	B	VIR	3
272	29	Th.	6:58	C	6:47	C	11 49	7	2 s. 35	11	11½	11:13	E	8:37	A	LIB	4
273	30	Fr.	7:00	C	6:45	C	11 45	7	2 s. 58	11¾	—	12:31	E	9:13	A	SCO	5

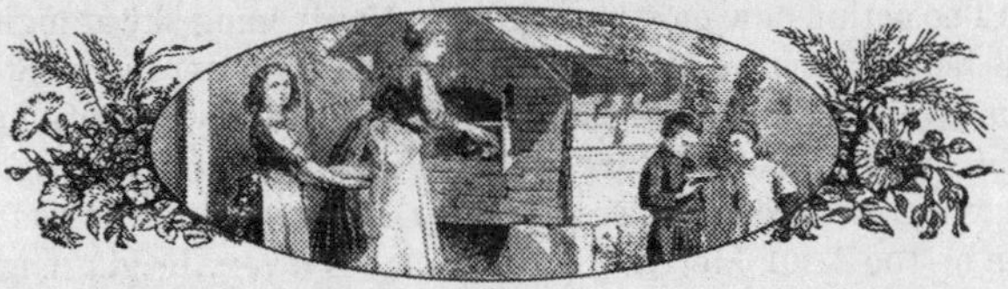

My teacher says, little by little / To the mountaintops we climb,
It isn't all done in a minute, / But only a step at a time.
–Carlotta Perry

DAY OF MONTH	DAY OF WEEK	DATES, FEASTS, FASTS, ASPECTS, TIDE HEIGHTS, AND WEATHER	
1	Th.	☾ AT ☋ • *September rain is much liked by the farmer.* • Tides {5.8 —	*Sunny,*
2	Fr.	Chess rematch between Bobby Fischer and Boris Spassky began, 1992 • Tides {5.2 5.7	*cool, for*
3	Sa.	Poet e. e. cummings died, 1962 • Tides {5.0 5.6	*back to school.*
4	**B**	13th S. af. P. • U.S. swimmer Mark Spitz 1st person to win 7 gold medals in single Olympics, 1972	
5	M.	LABOUR DAY • ☾ RUNS LOW • Saint Teresa of Calcutta died, 1997 • Tides {4.7 5.4	*Apple*
6	Tu.	☌♇☾ • Canadian highway signs converted to metric in many areas, 1977 • {4.8 5.5	*pickers*
7	W.	☾ AT PERIG. • 109°F, Weldon, N.C., 1954 • Tides {5.1 5.7	*gather*
8	Th.	☌♄☾ • Cranberry bog harvest begins, Cape Cod, Mass. • Tides {5.4 6.0	*red*
9	Fr.	☿ STAT. • Montreal founder Paul de Chomedey de Maisonneuve died, 1676 • {5.8 6.2	*fruit*
10	Sa.	FULL HARVEST ○ • ☌♆☾ • New pterosaur species *Cryodrakon boreas,* from Alta., announced, 2019	*in*
11	**B**	14th S. af. P. • PATRIOT DAY (U.S.) • ☾ ON EQ. • ☌♃☾	*yellow*
12	M.	JFK: "*We choose to go to the Moon . . . not because* [it is] *easy, but because* [it is] *hard,*" 1962 • {6.3 6.0	*slickers,*
13	Tu.	Astrophysicist Dilhan Eryurt died, 2012 • Tides {6.2 5.8	*pausing*
14	W.	Holy Cross • ☾ AT ☊ • ☌⛢☾ • First date of Gregorian calendar used by British Empire, 1752	*to*
15	Th.	*Nothing is easy to the unwilling.* • Tides {5.5 5.7	*admire*
16	Fr.	☌♂☾ • ♆ AT ☍ • Botanist Robert Fortune born, 1813 • Tides {5.2 5.4	*the*
17	Sa.	Battle of Antietam, U.S. Civil War, near Sharpsburg, Md., 1862 • Tides {4.9 5.1	*foliage*
18	**B**	15th S. af. P. • ☾ RIDES HIGH • Central Intelligence Agency (CIA) founded, 1947	*fire.*
19	M.	☾ AT APO. • Deadly hurricane made landfall near Chandeleur Islands, La., 1947 • Tides {4.5 4.8	*Only*
20	Tu.	Expectant dog stranded on bridge ledge rescued (and later adopted), Natchez, Miss., 2020 • {4.5 4.8	*thunder*
21	W.	St. Matthew • Ember Day • N.Y. *Sun*'s Frank Church replied, "Yes, Virginia, there is a Santa Claus," 1897	
22	Th.	Harvest Home • AUTUMNAL EQUINOX • Zoologist Victor Ernest Shelford born, 1877	*stops them*
23	Fr.	Ember Day • ☿ IN INF. ☌ • Judy Reed rec'd patent for dough kneader and roller, 1884	*reaping*
24	Sa.	Ember Day • *Least said is soonest mended.* • Tides {5.5 5.7	*crops,*
25	**B**	Rosh Hashanah begins at sundown • NEW ● • ☌☿☾ • ☌♀☾ • ☌☿♀	*while*
26	M.	☾ ON EQ. • ♃ AT ☍ • 1st Shrine Temple organized, N.Y.C., 1872 • Tides {5.9 5.9	*random*
27	Tu.	St. Vincent de Paul • U.S. statesman Samuel Adams born, 1722 • {6.1 5.9	*raindrops*
28	W.	☾ AT ☋ • Woodchucks hibernate now. • Tides {6.2 5.8	*speckle*
29	Th.	St. Michael • Writer Miguel de Cervantes likely born, 1547 • Tides {6.2 5.6	*the*
30	Fr.	St. Gregory the Illuminator • Meteor fireball seen in morning sky, eastern half of U.S., 2020	*treetops.*

Farmer's Calendar

"Excuse me, do you have a white horse?" the man at my door asked one foggy morning. I followed him out, and there, standing in the mists, was a phantom stallion with lustrous eyes and alert ears. Oh, that's Petey, I explained. He belonged to my way-down-the-road neighbor. I'd never seen him roam beyond his ample pasture girded by electrified tape. Yet here he was, looming in a lane trafficked mostly by pickup trucks and tractors, and spooking this driver. Those who tend livestock know: Creatures sometimes go where you least want them. A fencing expert once taught me: An electrical fence is just a psychological boundary. "You've got a 500-pound animal, obeying a 1/16-inch strand of aluminum wire that carries a volt every other second—it's only a discouragement." But, he assured, if the shock carried a strong charge, the fence would be effective. Until it wasn't. Many animal husbands know the phone call, sometimes shrill or gruff, but always urgent: *"Hey! Your animal is out!"* One evening I arrived late for chores at another farm because I'd been rounding up my wayward sheep. I apologized to my boss, but he grinned sympathetically and told me, *"You're farming now."*

OCTOBER

SKY WATCH: The action now mostly remains in the evening sky at nightfall, where the Moon is below Saturn on the 5th, closely below Jupiter on the 8th, and close to Mars on the 14th. All three planets are now worthy targets for backyard telescopes. The Red Planet (Mars), which actually appears orange, reaches a brilliant magnitude –0.86 and rises at 10 P.M. in Taurus. Venus has its superior conjunction on the 22nd. Mercury, which reaches a very bright magnitude –1.0, rises for its best 2022 appearance as a morning star, especially after the 12th. A partial solar eclipse, not visible from the U.S. or Canada, appears over parts of Greenland, Iceland, Europe, northeastern Africa, the Middle East, western Asia, India, and western China on the 25th.

◗ **FIRST QUARTER** 2nd day 8:14 P.M. ◐ **LAST QUARTER** 17th day 1:15 P.M.
○ **FULL MOON** 9th day 4:55 P.M. ● **NEW MOON** 25th day 6:49 A.M.

All times are given in Eastern Daylight Time.

GET THESE PAGES WITH TIMES SET TO YOUR POSTAL CODE VIA ALMANAC.CA/2022.

Day of Year	Day of Month	Day of Week	☀ Rises H. M.	Rise Key	☀ Sets H. M.	Set Key	Length of Day H. M.	Sun Fast M.	Sun Declination ° '	High Tide Times Halifax		☾ Rises H. M.	Rise Key	☾ Sets H. M.	Set Key	☾ Astron. Place	☾ Age
274	1	Sa.	7:01	C	6:43	C	11 42	8	3 s. 22	12¼	12½	1:47	E	10:00	A	OPH	6
275	2	**B**	7:02	C	6:41	C	11 39	8	3 s. 45	1¼	1¼	2:55	E	10:59	A	SAG	7
276	3	M.	7:04	C	6:39	C	11 35	8	4 s. 08	2¼	2¼	3:51	E	—	–	SAG	8
277	4	Tu.	7:05	C	6:37	C	11 32	9	4 s. 31	3½	3½	4:35	E	12:11	A	SAG	9
278	5	W.	7:06	C	6:36	C	11 30	9	4 s. 54	5	5	5:09	E	1:29	A	CAP	10
279	6	Th.	7:07	C	6:34	C	11 27	9	5 s. 17	6	6¼	5:36	D	2:50	A	AQU	11
280	7	Fr.	7:09	C	6:32	C	11 23	9	5 s. 40	7	7	5:59	D	4:09	B	AQU	12
281	8	Sa.	7:10	C	6:30	C	11 20	10	6 s. 03	7¾	8	6:19	C	5:26	B	AQU	13
282	9	**B**	7:11	C	6:28	C	11 17	10	6 s. 26	8½	8¾	6:38	C	6:41	C	CET	14
283	10	M.	7:12	D	6:26	B	11 14	10	6 s. 49	9	9½	6:58	B	7:54	D	PSC	15
284	11	Tu.	7:14	D	6:24	B	11 10	11	7 s. 11	9¾	10¼	7:20	B	9:06	D	ARI	16
285	12	W.	7:15	D	6:23	B	11 08	11	7 s. 34	10¼	10¾	7:45	A	10:18	E	ARI	17
286	13	Th.	7:16	D	6:21	B	11 05	11	7 s. 56	11	11½	8:16	A	11:28	E	TAU	18
287	14	Fr.	7:18	D	6:19	B	11 01	11	8 s. 19	11¾	—	8:53	A	12:35	E	TAU	19
288	15	Sa.	7:19	D	6:17	B	10 58	11	8 s. 41	12¼	12¼	9:39	A	1:35	E	TAU	20
289	16	**B**	7:20	D	6:16	B	10 56	12	9 s. 03	1	1	10:33	A	2:26	E	GEM	21
290	17	M.	7:22	D	6:14	B	10 52	12	9 s. 25	1¾	2	11:33	A	3:09	E	GEM	22
291	18	Tu.	7:23	D	6:12	B	10 49	12	9 s. 47	3	3	—	–	3:43	E	CAN	23
292	19	W.	7:24	D	6:10	B	10 46	12	10 s. 08	4¼	4¼	12:38	A	4:11	E	CAN	24
293	20	Th.	7:26	D	6:09	B	10 43	12	10 s. 30	5½	5¼	1:45	A	4:34	D	LEO	25
294	21	Fr.	7:27	D	6:07	B	10 40	13	10 s. 51	6¼	6¼	2:53	B	4:54	D	LEO	26
295	22	Sa.	7:28	D	6:05	B	10 37	13	11 s. 12	6¾	7	4:02	B	5:13	C	LEO	27
296	23	**B**	7:30	D	6:04	B	10 34	13	11 s. 33	7½	7¾	5:12	C	5:31	C	VIR	28
297	24	M.	7:31	D	6:02	B	10 31	13	11 s. 54	8	8¼	6:23	C	5:50	B	VIR	29
298	25	Tu.	7:32	D	6:01	B	10 29	13	12 s. 15	8½	9	7:38	D	6:12	B	VIR	0
299	26	W.	7:34	D	5:59	B	10 25	13	12 s. 35	9¼	9¾	8:56	D	6:38	A	LIB	1
300	27	Th.	7:35	D	5:57	B	10 22	13	12 s. 56	10	10½	10:16	E	7:11	A	LIB	2
301	28	Fr.	7:37	D	5:56	B	10 19	13	13 s. 16	10½	11¼	11:35	E	7:55	A	OPH	3
302	29	Sa.	7:38	D	5:54	B	10 16	14	13 s. 36	11½	—	12:48	E	8:52	A	OPH	4
303	30	**B**	7:39	D	5:53	B	10 14	14	13 s. 55	12	12¼	1:49	E	10:01	A	SAG	5
304	31	M.	7:41	D	5:51	B	10 10	14	14 s. 15	1	1¼	2:36	E	11:18	A	SAG	6

THE TENTH MONTH · 2022 **OCTOBER** OCTOBER HATH 31 DAYS

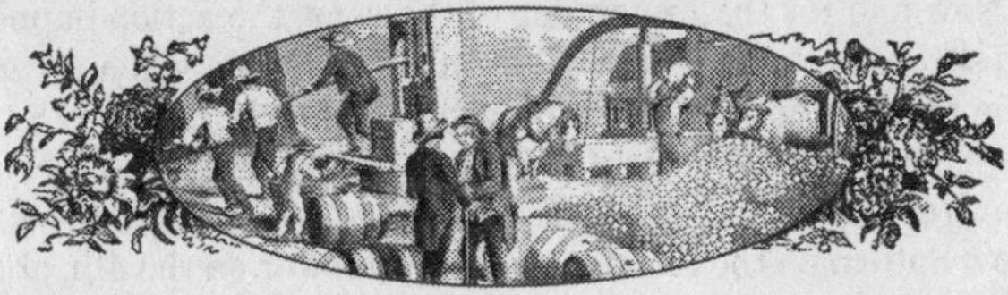

See how the great old forest vies
With all the glory of the skies.
–Alexander M'Lachlan

DAY OF MONTH	DAY OF WEEK	DATES, FEASTS, FASTS, ASPECTS, TIDE HEIGHTS, AND WEATHER	
1	Sa.	☿ STAT. • 1st agricultural fair in U.S. held, Pittsfield, Mass., 1810 • Tides {5.4 5.9	*Light*
2	**B**	**17th S. af. P.** • ☾ RUNS LOW • Tides {5.2 5.6	*rain*
3	M.	☌♇☾ • Watch for banded woolly bear caterpillars now. • Tides {5.0 5.4	*(or*
4	Tu.	St. Francis of Assisi • Yom Kippur begins at sundown • ☾ AT PERIG. • {4.9 5.3	*harder)*
5	W.	☌♄☾ • Businessman Ray Kroc born, 1902 • Professor Robert Goddard born, 1882	*never*
6	Th.	*Respect out of fear is never genuine; reverence out of respect is never false.* • Tides {5.4 5.6	*dampens*
7	Fr.	☌♆☾ • Tornado struck Jenner, Alta., 2017 • {5.7 5.9	*the*
8	Sa.	☌♃☾ • ♇ STAT. • ☿ GR. ELONG. (18° WEST) • Tides {6.1 6.0	*ardor of*
9	**B**	**18th S. af. P.** • Sukkoth begins at sundown • FULL HUNTER'S ○ • ☾ ON EQ.	*the*
10	M.	**Thanksgiving Day** • **Columbus Day, observed (U.S.)** • **Indigenous Peoples' Day (U.S.)**	
11	Tu.	☾ AT ☊ • Little brown bats hibernate now. • Wildlife artist John Ruthven died, 2020	*foliage*
12	W.	**Nat'l Farmer's Day (U.S.)** • OCCN. ♅☾ • Musician John Denver died, 1997	*pilgrims;*
13	Th.	58-lb. muskie caught, Lake Bellaire, Mich., 2012 • Tides {5.9 5.5	*sunny*
14	Fr.	Charles Yeager 1st to break sound barrier, reaching Mach 1.06 in Bell X-1 jet, 1947 • Tides {5.7 —	*skies*
15	Sa.	☌♂☾ • Andy Green 1st to break sound barrier in land-based vehicle, at 763.035 mph, 1997	*couldn't*
16	**B**	**19th S. af. P.** • ☾ RIDES HIGH • 4.0 earthquake occurred near Hollis Center, Maine, 2012	*be*
17	M.	St. Ignatius of Antioch • ☾ AT APO. • Tides {4.8 5.0	*better for*
18	Tu.	St. Luke • St. Luke's little summer. • British Broadcasting Co. (BBC) formed, 1922	*maple-red,*
19	W.	*Blow the wind never so fast, It will lower at last.* • Tides {4.7 4.8	*ash-gold,*
20	Th.	Physicist John Bardeen 1st to win 2nd Nobel Prize in same field (1st, 1956), 1972 • {4.9 5.0	*and*
21	Fr.	Poet Samuel Taylor Coleridge born, 1772 • USS *Constitution* launched, 1797 • {5.2 5.2	*beech-butter;*
22	Sa.	♀ IN SUP. ☌ • At 0.575 mm², OmniVision OV6948 set world record as tiniest commercial image sensor, 2019	
23	**B**	**20th S. af. P.** • ☾ ON EQ. • ♄ STAT. • Tides {5.8 5.7	*dazzled*
24	M.	St. James of Jerusalem[T] • ☌☿☾ • "Father of Microbiology" Antonie van Leeuwenhoek born, 1632	*and*
25	Tu.	NEW ● • ECLIPSE ⊙ • ☌♀☾ • Tides {6.3 6.0	*awed,*
26	W.	☾ AT ☋ • *Pac-Man* arcade game released in U.S., 1980 • Timber rattlesnakes move to winter dens.	*they*
27	Th.	At 16, violinist Jascha Heifetz made his American debut at Carnegie Hall, N.Y., 1917 • {6.5 6.0	*surrender*
28	Fr.	Sts. Simon & Jude • *All is not butter that comes from the cow.* • Tides {6.4 5.8	*to*
29	Sa.	☾ RUNS LOW • ☾ AT PERIG. • Artist Bob Ross born, 1942 • Tides {6.3 —	*the*
30	**B**	**21st S. af. P.** • ♂ STAT. • Bodybuilder Charles Atlas born, 1892	*autumn*
31	M.	All Hallows' Eve • Reformation Day • ☌♇☾ • {5.4 5.7	*splendor.*

Farmer's Calendar

Plenty of people commute *to work,* but our mail lady drives 88 miles a day, over mostly dirt roads, *for work,* delivering letters, catalogs, and rototiller parts on her starfish-shaped circuit around town. As she feeds each of the 350-plus mailboxes on her rural route, she knows the truth: She knows where she'll have to yield for crossing cows, for fawns and does, and for "big old, roly-poly black bears" in the middle of the road. Her Jeep rattles as she zips beneath the canopies of goldening maples. Our town exists thanks to a trail hacked out of wilderness with an ax in 1779—the Bayley-Hazen Military Road—a route that later delivered settlers, including one so determined to get here in 1789 that he took over the yoke when one of his oxen sickened and dragged his sled the last hundred miles. Some 230 years on, this ancient thoroughfare constitutes just one leg of the mail lady's daylong journey to bring us our bills. Her grumbly vehicle pauses at box after box, the way a bee visits each blossom. Here she comes. There she goes—Godspeeding to all the other unpaved places, roads aptly named King Farm, Black River, Auld Lang Syne, and Mud Island.

NOVEMBER

SKY WATCH: Now and for the remainder of the year, the action happens solely in the evening sky, except for on the night of the 7th–8th, when a very nice total eclipse of the Moon is at least partially visible from the entire U.S. and Canada during the second half of the night. West of the Mississippi, the eclipse may be seen in its entirety. The Moon features prominently throughout this month, as it dangles below Saturn on the 1st, closely below Jupiter on the 4th, above Mars on the 10th, below Mars on the 11th, to the left of Virgo's blue star Spica on the 21st, below Saturn again on the 28th, and halfway between Jupiter and Saturn on the 30th.

◑ **FIRST QUARTER** 1st day 2:37 A.M.	● **NEW MOON** 23rd day 5:57 P.M.
○ **FULL MOON** 8th day 6:02 A.M.	◐ **FIRST QUARTER** 30th day 9:37 A.M.
◗ **LAST QUARTER** 16th day 8:27 A.M.	

After 2:00 A.M. on November 6, Eastern Standard Time is given.

GET THESE PAGES WITH TIMES SET TO YOUR POSTAL CODE VIA ALMANAC.CA/2022.

DAY OF YEAR	DAY OF MONTH	DAY OF WEEK	☼ RISES H. M.	RISE KEY	☼ SETS H. M.	SET KEY	LENGTH OF DAY H. M.	SUN FAST M.	SUN DECLINATION ° '	HIGH TIDE TIMES HALIFAX		☽ RISES H. M.	RISE KEY	☽ SETS H. M.	SET KEY	☽ ASTRON. PLACE	☽ AGE
305	1	Tu.	7:42	D	5:50	B	10 08	14	14 s. 34	2	2¼	3:13	E	—	-	CAP	7
306	2	W.	7:44	D	5:49	B	10 05	14	14 s. 53	3¼	3½	3:41	D	12:37	A	CAP	8
307	3	Th.	7:45	D	5:47	B	10 02	14	15 s. 12	4¾	4¾	4:04	D	1:55	B	AQU	9
308	4	Fr.	7:46	D	5:46	B	10 00	14	15 s. 30	5¾	6	4:24	C	3:11	B	AQU	10
309	5	Sa.	7:48	D	5:44	B	9 56	14	15 s. 49	6½	6¾	4:43	C	4:25	C	PSC	11
310	6	**B**	6:49	D	4:43	B	9 54	14	16 s. 07	6¼	6½	4:02	C	4:37	C	PSC	12
311	7	M.	6:51	D	4:42	B	9 51	14	16 s. 24	7	7¼	4:23	B	5:48	D	PSC	13
312	8	Tu.	6:52	D	4:41	B	9 49	13	16 s. 42	7½	8	4:46	A	7:00	D	ARI	14
313	9	W.	6:53	D	4:39	B	9 46	13	16 s. 59	8¼	8¾	5:14	A	8:11	E	TAU	15
314	10	Th.	6:55	D	4:38	B	9 43	13	17 s. 16	9	9½	5:49	A	9:19	E	TAU	16
315	11	Fr.	6:56	D	4:37	B	9 41	13	17 s. 32	9½	10¼	6:31	A	10:23	E	TAU	17
316	12	Sa.	6:57	E	4:36	B	9 39	13	17 s. 48	10¼	11	7:22	A	11:18	E	GEM	18
317	13	**B**	6:59	E	4:35	B	9 36	13	18 s. 04	10¾	11½	8:20	A	12:05	E	GEM	19
318	14	M.	7:00	E	4:34	B	9 34	13	18 s. 20	11½	—	9:23	A	12:42	E	GEM	20
319	15	Tu.	7:02	E	4:33	B	9 31	13	18 s. 35	12¼	12¼	10:29	A	1:12	E	CAN	21
320	16	W.	7:03	E	4:32	B	9 29	12	18 s. 50	1¼	1	11:36	B	1:36	D	LEO	22
321	17	Th.	7:04	E	4:31	B	9 27	12	19 s. 05	2¼	2¼	—	-	1:57	D	LEO	23
322	18	Fr.	7:06	E	4:30	A	9 24	12	19 s. 19	3½	3½	12:43	B	2:16	D	LEO	24
323	19	Sa.	7:07	E	4:29	A	9 22	12	19 s. 33	4¼	4½	1:51	C	2:34	C	VIR	25
324	20	**B**	7:08	E	4:28	A	9 20	12	19 s. 47	5	5¼	3:00	C	2:52	C	VIR	26
325	21	M.	7:10	E	4:27	A	9 17	11	20 s. 00	5¾	6¼	4:13	D	3:13	B	VIR	27
326	22	Tu.	7:11	E	4:26	A	9 15	11	20 s. 13	6¼	6¾	5:29	D	3:37	B	VIR	28
327	23	W.	7:12	E	4:26	A	9 14	11	20 s. 26	7	7½	6:50	E	4:07	A	LIB	0
328	24	Th.	7:14	E	4:25	A	9 11	10	20 s. 38	7¾	8½	8:12	E	4:47	A	SCO	1
329	25	Fr.	7:15	E	4:24	A	9 09	10	20 s. 50	8½	9¼	9:31	E	5:40	A	OPH	2
330	26	Sa.	7:16	E	4:24	A	9 08	10	21 s. 01	9¼	10	10:40	E	6:46	A	SAG	3
331	27	**B**	7:17	E	4:23	A	9 06	9	21 s. 12	10¼	11	11:34	E	8:04	A	SAG	4
332	28	M.	7:19	E	4:23	A	9 04	9	21 s. 22	11	11¾	12:14	E	9:25	A	CAP	5
333	29	Tu.	7:20	E	4:22	A	9 02	8	21 s. 33	12	—	12:45	D	10:45	B	CAP	6
334	30	W.	7:21	E	4:22	A	9 01	8	21 s. 42	1	1	1:10	D	—	-	AQU	7

THE ELEVENTH MONTH • 2022 **NOVEMBER** NOVEMBER HATH 30 DAYS

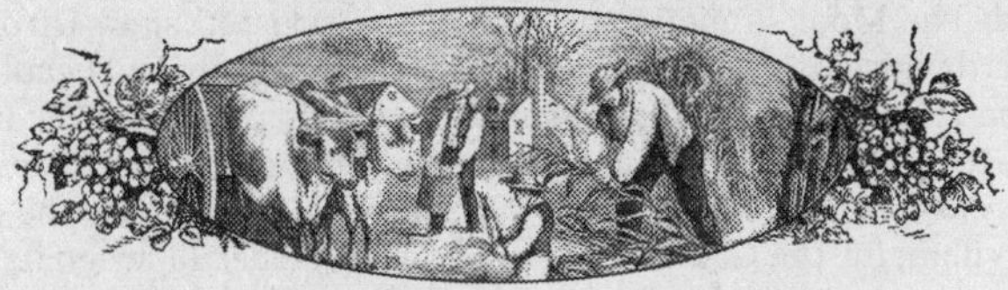

Fill your hearts with old-time cheer:
Heaven be thanked for one more year.
–G. P. Lathrop

DAY OF MONTH	DAY OF WEEK	DATES, FEASTS, FASTS, ASPECTS, TIDE HEIGHTS, AND WEATHER	
1	Tu.	All Saints' • ☌♄☾ • Space Coast's 321 area code went into effect, Brevard Co., Fla., 1999 • {5.3 5.5	*Mild*
2	W.	All Souls' • Howard Hughes's *Hercules* (aka *Spruce Goose*) wooden aircraft flew 1 mile, 1947 • {5.2 5.4	*and*
3	Th.	*Common sense is not always true.* • Tides {5.4 5.4	*drizzly.*
4	Fr.	☌♃☾ • ☌♆☾ • Composer Felix Mendelssohn died, 1847 • {5.7 5.5	*Suddenly*
5	Sa.	Sadie Hawkins Day • ☾ ON EQ. • Susan B. Anthony cast ballot, earning $100 fine, 1872	*grisly:*
6	**B**	**22nd S. af. P.** • DAYLIGHT SAVING TIME ENDS, 2:00 A.M. • {6.2 5.8	*raining*
7	M.	Magnitude 6.3 earthquake struck off coast of Vancouver Island, B.C., 2012 • {6.3 5.8	*and sleeting*
8	Tu.	ELECTION DAY (U.S.) • FULL BEAVER ○ • ECLIPSE ☾ • ☾ AT ☊ • ☌♅☾ • ☿ IN SUP. ☌	
9	W.	♅ AT ☍ • Great Boston fire began, 1872 • 1st launch of NASA's *Saturn V* rocket, 1967 • {6.2 5.7	*and*
10	Th.	Montreal Canadiens' Armand Mondou awarded 1st penalty shot in NHL, 1934 • Tides {6.1 5.6	*freezing,*
11	Fr.	St. Martin of Tours • REMEMBRANCE DAY • ☌♂☾ • {5.9 5.5	*before*
12	Sa.	Indian Summer • ☾ RIDES HIGH • *Rain at seven, fine at eleven.* • {5.7 5.3	*easing.*
13	**B**	**23rd S. af. P.** • Wall of Vietnam Veterans Memorial dedicated, D.C., 1982 • {5.5 5.2	*Don't*
14	M.	☾ AT APO. • Insulin co-discoverer Sir Frederick Banting born, 1891 • Tides {5.3 —	*drop*
15	Tu.	Artist Georgia O'Keeffe born, 1887 • 49 tornadoes tore through Midwest, 2005 • {5.1 5.1	*your*
16	W.	Last Hawaiian king, Kalakaua, born, 1836 • Tides {5.0 5.0	*guard—*
17	Th.	St. Hugh of Lincoln • 1st U.S. patent for clock granted to Eli Terry, 1797 • Tides {5.0 4.9	*snowing*
18	Fr.	St. Hilda of Whitby • 1st dated book printed in England, *Dictes or Sayengis of the Philosophres,* 1477	*hard!*
19	Sa.	☾ ON EQ. • Cat, missing for 3 yrs., reunited w/ owner after walking into hospital, Berlin, N.H., 2020	*You'll*
20	**B**	24th. S. af. P. • Princess Elizabeth (later, Queen Elizabeth II) wed Lt. Philip Mountbatten, 1947	*suffer*
21	M.	"Tweety Bird" cartoon character debuted, 1942 • {5.9 5.6	*without*
22	Tu.	☾ AT ☋ • ☌☿♀ • Filmmaker Gil Cardinal died, 2015 • {6.2 5.8	*a*
23	W.	St. Clement • NEW ● • *Pleasant hours fly fast.* • Tides {6.5 6.0	*muffler!*
24	Th.	THANKSGIVING DAY (U.S.) • ☌☿☾ • ☌♀☾ • ♃ STAT. • {6.6 6.0	*May*
25	Fr.	☾ AT PERIG. • Record 4-min., 17.9-sec. mile run by P. Robinson in Antarctica (–13°F windchill), 2017	*your*
26	Sa.	☾ RUNS LOW • *Peanuts* cartoonist Charles Schulz born, 1922 • Tides {6.6 6.0	*feast*
27	**B**	**1st S. of Advent** • ☌♇☾ • Announced: Britain's Prince Harry engaged to Meghan Markle, 2017	
28	M.	☌♄☾ • 1st ad via skywriting, N.Y.C., 1922 • {6.2 5.7	*be feastly:*
29	Tu.	*Pong* coin-operated video game debuted, 1972 • Tides {5.9 —	*Outside's*
30	W.	St. Andrew • ♂ AT CLOSEST APPROACH • 405-lb. yellowfin tuna caught, Magdalena Bay, Mexico, 2010	*beastly!*

Farmer's Calendar

You can measure a kestrel's life span on one hand. But if you're handy, you can increase the chances that this smallest falcon may have a place to lay its eggs, as my neighbor did some 30 years ago.

In 1989, Dave nailed together boards from rough-cut pine, with a hole big enough for his fist to fit. He stationed the box 16 feet up his telephone pole. The first spring, the place stayed vacant. But the second year and ever since, kestrels have been in residence—arriving as early as March 25 or delayed until April 16—depending on the amount of bare ground nearby. Kestrels need snowless patches to hunt mice and other small rodents, and, as the season warms, insects. In late June, Dave spies the nestlings' faces squeezed into the opening; by mid-July, the box is again hollow. In autumn, Dave fetches a ladder to clean his chimney, then he leans it against the pole and climbs up to rake out old bedding. From his pocket he delivers a fistful of clean shavings. On this dim, chill afternoon, he's preparing for the next handful of kestrels that will perch at this opening, taking their first peek at the world.

SKY WATCH: The Moon is again the star of the celestial show throughout this month, as it dangles below Jupiter on the 1st; floats closely and beautifully above Mars on the 7th, when it is full; dangles below Saturn on the 26th; hangs below Jupiter on the 28th; and stands to the left of Jupiter on the 29th. (It is again beautifully close to Mars on January 3, 2023.) Unfortunately, the Moon plays the role of villain for the Geminid meteors on December 13, when its fat gibbous phase casts unwelcome light. During the final week of the year, Venus may be glimpsed as it returns as an evening star, very low in the southwest. Winter in the Northern Hemisphere begins with the solstice on December 21 at 4:48 P.M. EST.

○ **FULL MOON** 7th day 11:08 P.M. ● **NEW MOON** 23rd day 5:17 A.M.
◐ **LAST QUARTER** 16th day 3:56 A.M. ◑ **FIRST QUARTER** 29th day 8:21 P.M.

All times are given in Eastern Standard Time.

GET THESE PAGES WITH TIMES SET TO YOUR POSTAL CODE VIA ALMANAC.CA/2022.

Day of Year	Day of Month	Day of Week	☼ Rises H.M.	Rise Key	☼ Sets H.M.	Set Key	Length of Day H.M.	Sun Fast M.	Sun Declination ° '	High Tide Times Halifax		☽ Rises H.M.	Rise Key	☽ Sets H.M.	Set Key	☽ Astron. Place	☽ Age
335	1	Th.	7:22	E	4:21	A	8 59	8	21 s. 52	2	2¼	1:31	C	12:01	B	AQU	8
336	2	Fr.	7:23	E	4:21	A	8 58	8	22 s. 01	3¼	3½	1:49	C	1:15	C	PSC	9
337	3	Sa.	7:24	E	4:21	A	8 57	7	22 s. 09	4¼	4½	2:08	B	2:26	C	PSC	10
338	4	**B**	7:25	E	4:20	A	8 55	7	22 s. 17	5	5½	2:27	B	3:37	D	PSC	11
339	5	M.	7:27	E	4:20	A	8 53	6	22 s. 25	5¾	6¼	2:49	B	4:47	D	ARI	12
340	6	Tu.	7:28	E	4:20	A	8 52	6	22 s. 32	6½	7	3:15	A	5:57	E	ARI	13
341	7	W.	7:29	E	4:20	A	8 51	6	22 s. 39	7¼	7¾	3:47	A	7:06	E	TAU	14
342	8	Th.	7:30	E	4:20	A	8 50	5	22 s. 45	7¾	8½	4:26	A	8:11	E	TAU	15
343	9	Fr.	7:31	E	4:20	A	8 49	5	22 s. 51	8½	9¼	5:14	A	9:10	E	TAU	16
344	10	Sa.	7:31	E	4:20	A	8 49	4	22 s. 56	9¼	9¾	6:10	A	10:00	E	GEM	17
345	11	**B**	7:32	E	4:20	A	8 48	4	23 s. 01	9¾	10½	7:12	A	10:41	E	GEM	18
346	12	M.	7:33	E	4:20	A	8 47	3	23 s. 06	10½	11¼	8:16	A	11:13	E	CAN	19
347	13	Tu.	7:34	E	4:20	A	8 46	3	23 s. 10	11	12	9:22	A	11:39	E	LEO	20
348	14	W.	7:35	E	4:20	A	8 45	2	23 s. 14	11¾	—	10:28	B	12:01	D	LEO	21
349	15	Th.	7:36	E	4:20	A	8 44	2	23 s. 17	12½	12½	11:34	B	12:20	D	LEO	22
350	16	Fr.	7:36	E	4:20	A	8 44	1	23 s. 19	1¼	1¼	—	-	12:38	C	VIR	23
351	17	Sa.	7:37	E	4:21	A	8 44	1	23 s. 22	2¼	2½	12:41	C	12:55	C	VIR	24
352	18	**B**	7:38	E	4:21	A	8 43	1	23 s. 23	3¼	3½	1:50	C	1:14	B	VIR	25
353	19	M.	7:38	E	4:21	A	8 43	0	23 s. 25	4	4¾	3:02	D	1:35	B	VIR	26
354	20	Tu.	7:39	E	4:22	A	8 43	0	23 s. 25	5	5½	4:19	D	2:01	A	LIB	27
355	21	W.	7:39	E	4:22	A	8 43	*1	23 s. 26	5¾	6½	5:41	E	2:36	A	LIB	28
356	22	Th.	7:40	E	4:23	A	8 43	*1	23 s. 26	6½	7¼	7:02	E	3:22	A	SCO	29
357	23	Fr.	7:40	E	4:23	A	8 43	*2	23 s. 25	7¼	8	8:18	E	4:24	A	SAG	0
358	24	Sa.	7:41	E	4:24	A	8 43	*2	23 s. 24	8¼	9	9:21	E	5:39	A	SAG	1
359	25	**B**	7:41	E	4:25	A	8 44	*3	23 s. 22	9	9¾	10:09	E	7:02	A	CAP	2
360	26	M.	7:41	E	4:25	A	8 44	*3	23 s. 20	10	10¾	10:45	E	8:27	A	CAP	3
361	27	Tu.	7:42	E	4:26	A	8 44	*4	23 s. 18	10¾	11¾	11:13	D	9:47	B	AQU	4
362	28	W.	7:42	E	4:27	A	8 45	*4	23 s. 15	11¾	—	11:35	D	11:04	B	AQU	5
363	29	Th.	7:42	E	4:28	A	8 46	*5	23 s. 11	12½	12¾	11:55	C	—	-	PSC	6
364	30	Fr.	7:42	E	4:29	A	8 47	*5	23 s. 08	1½	1¾	12:14	C	12:17	C	CET	7
365	31	Sa.	7:42	E	4:29	A	8 47	*6	23 s. 03	2½	2¾	12:33	B	1:28	D	PSC	8

To use this page, see p. 116; for Key Letters, see p. 240. LIGHT = A.M. BOLD = P.M.

CALENDAR

THE TWELFTH MONTH · 2022

DECEMBER

DECEMBER HATH 31 DAYS

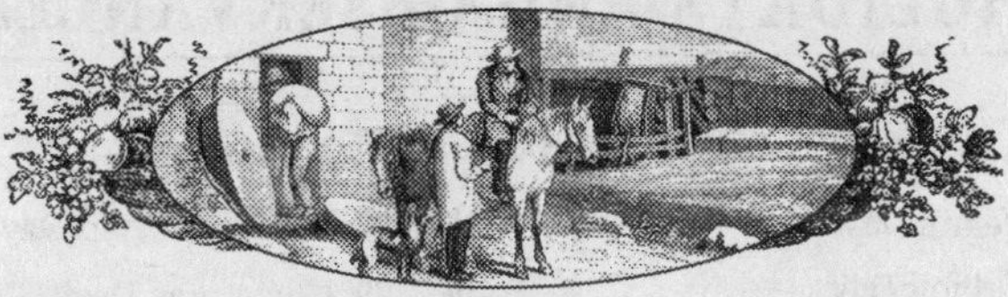

Holly, fir, and spruce boughs / Green upon the wall,
Spotless snow upon the road— / More going to fall.
–Unknown

DAY OF MONTH	DAY OF WEEK	DATES, FEASTS, FASTS, ASPECTS, TIDE HEIGHTS, AND WEATHER	
1	Th.	☌♃☾ • ☌♆☾ • Writer/USN Capt. Edward L. Beach died, 2002 • {5.6 5.3	*Numb*
2	Fr.	St. Viviana • ☾ ON EQ. • 1st pizza party in space, ISS, 2017 • Tides {5.7 5.2	*and*
3	Sa.	*If things were to be done twice, all would be wise.* • {5.8 5.3	*number,*
4	**B**	**2nd S. of Advent** • ♆ STAT. • Tides {5.9 5.4	*with flakes*
5	M.	☾ AT ☊ • ☌⛢☾ • Ship *Mary Celeste* found abandoned, 1872 • {6.0 5.5	*aswirl;*
6	Tu.	St. Nicholas • Everglades Nat'l Park dedicated, Fla., 1947 • Tides {6.0 5.5	*bluster*
7	W.	St. Ambrose • NATIONAL PEARL HARBOR REMEMBRANCE DAY (U.S.) • FULL COLD ○ • OCCN. ♂☾	
8	Th.	♂ AT ☍ • 896 couples in N.H./Mo./Col. kissed under mistletoe, setting world record, 2019	*ceases,*
9	Fr.	☾ RIDES HIGH • Canada's 1st coin club, Numismatic Society of Montreal, formed, 1862 • {6.0 5.5	*sun*
10	Sa.	St. Eulalia • Poet Emily Dickinson born, 1830 • Tides {5.9 5.5	*increases.*
11	**B**	**3rd S. of Advent** • ☾ AT APO. • *Good words cost naught.* • {5.8 5.4	*Hang*
12	M.	OUR LADY OF GUADALUPE • *Apollo 17* astronauts discovered orange soil on Moon, 1972 • {5.7 5.3	*your*
13	Tu.	St. Lucia • National Day of the Horse (U.S.) • {5.5 5.3	*holly:*
14	W.	Ember Day • Halcyon Days begin. • *Mariner 2* passed Venus (1st successful planetary flyby), 1962	*Don't*
15	Th.	Baseball player Dick Stuart died, 2002 • Tides {5.3 5.1	*go*
16	Fr.	Ember Day • Lillian Disney (wife of Walt Disney) died, 1997 • Tides {5.3 5.0	*out*
17	Sa.	Ember Day • ☾ ON EQ. • France formally recognized American independence, 1777	*without*
18	**B**	**4th S. of Advent** • Chanukah begins at sundown • Tides {5.5 4.9	*your*
19	M.	☾ AT ☋ • 1st season of National Hockey League (NHL), 1917 • Tides {5.7 5.1	*brolly!*
20	Tu.	Beware the Pogonip. • J. Russell Coffey, oldest known U.S. WWI veteran at time, died at age 109, 2007	*Leave*
21	W.	St. Thomas • WINTER SOLSTICE • ☿ GR. ELONG. (20° EAST) • Tides {6.2 5.6	*Santa*
22	Th.	U.S. first lady Claudia "Lady Bird" Johnson born, 1912 • Tides {6.5 5.8	*a*
23	Fr.	NEW ● • ☾ RUNS LOW • Saturn's moon Rhea discovered, 1672 • Tides {6.7 6.0	*snack*
24	Sa.	☾ AT PERIG. • ☌☿☾ • ☌♀☾ • ☌♇☾ • Tides {6.8 6.1	*to*
25	**B**	**Christmas** • *If windy on Christmas Day, trees will bring much fruit.* • Tides {6.7 6.1	*be*
26	M.	St. Stephen • BOXING DAY • FIRST DAY OF KWANZAA • ☌♄☾ • {6.6 6.1	*sure*
27	Tu.	St. John • Chemist Louis Pasteur born, 1822 • 141-lb. 8-oz. Pacific sailfish caught on 4# test line, Piñas Bay, Panama, 1992	
28	W.	Holy Innocents • ☌♆☾ • ☿ STAT. • Comic book writer Stan Lee born, 1922	*he comes*
29	Th.	☾ ON EQ. • ☌☿♀ • ☌♃☾ • *Dec. 28–29:* 25.5" snow in 24 hrs., Victoria, B.C., 1996	*back.*
30	Fr.	Samoa skipped this day to move from eastern to western side of International Date Line, 2011 • {5.8 5.2	*Adieu,*
31	Sa.	St. Sylvester • Gymnast Gabby Douglas born, 1995 • Tides {5.7 5.0	*'22!*

Farmer's Calendar

Plowing the roads of Cabot, Vermont, is the second-best job Walter "Rusty" Churchill's ever had. First best? Dairy farming, which he did for 30 years. He didn't know what he'd do after he sold his cows. He thought about taking a shift at the Cabot Creamery; then someone mentioned a job opening at the town garage and encouraged Rusty to throw his name in for it. They hired another guy, but he didn't last. So that's how, for over a decade now, Rusty's knack for spreading lime and manure and tilling soil makes him an ace at scattering salt and sand and plowing for his hometown. The hours are similar—Thanksgiving, Christmas, New Year's, Easter—he works them all. But, he admits, it's satisfying to clear a path after a huge storm: "Then it seems like you're doing something." Rusty's route includes some of the town's 65 miles of blacktop, hilltop, and back roads. "There aren't too many out this early," he says of clearing snow long before sunrise. "You've got Creamery help—they have a shift that starts at 4:00 A.M.—and milk trucks. Otherwise, it's just me. Kinda peaceful. As long as the radio works, I'm all set."

HOLIDAYS AND OBSERVANCES

2022 HOLIDAYS

JAN. 1: New Year's Day*

FEB. 2: Groundhog Day

FEB. 14: Valentine's Day

FEB. 15: National Flag of Canada Day

FEB. 21: Family Day *(Alta., B.C., N.B., Ont., Sask.)*
Louis Riel Day *(Man.)*
Nova Scotia Heritage Day *(N.S.)*
Islander Day *(P.E.I.)*

FEB. 25: Heritage Day *(Y.T.)*

MAR. 8: International Women's Day

MAR. 14: Commonwealth Day

APR. 15: Good Friday

APR. 18: Easter Monday

APR. 22: Earth Day

APR. 25: St. George's Day, observed *(N.L.)*

MAY 8: Mother's Day

MAY 23: Victoria Day

JUNE 5: World Environment Day

JUNE 19: Father's Day

JUNE 21: National Indigenous Peoples Day

JUNE 24: Fête Nationale *(Qué.)*

JUNE 27: June Holiday *(N.L.)*

JULY 1: Canada Day*

JULY 9: Nunavut Day

JULY 11: Orangemen's Day *(N.L.)*

AUG. 1: Civic Holiday *(Alta., B.C., Man., N.B., N.W.T., N.S., Nunavut, Ont., P.E.I., Sask.)*

AUG. 15: Discovery Day *(Y.T.)*

SEPT. 5: Labour Day

OCT. 10: Thanksgiving Day

OCT. 31: Halloween

NOV. 11: Remembrance Day*

NOV. 20: National Child Day

DEC. 25: Christmas Day*

DEC. 26: Boxing Day
First day of Kwanzaa

*When this day falls on a Saturday or Sunday, the following Monday is observed as a holiday.

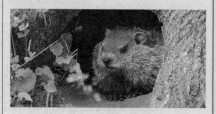

GROUNDHOG DAY

Traditionally, on February 2, farmers looked for signs of what the weather would be for the next 6 weeks. They believed that if an animal came out of hibernation on this day and saw its shadow, winter would continue.

For centuries, farmers in France and England looked to a bear; in Germany, they kept their eye on the badger. In the 1800s, German immigrants to Pennsylvania brought the tradition with them. Finding no badgers there, they adopted the groundhog to fit the lore. Pennsylvania's Punxsutawney Phil has predicted spring's arrival since 1887.

Since 1956, albino groundhogs named Wiarton Willie have made annual weather prognostications in Wiarton, Ontario. Several other groundhogs are employed across the nation, including Nova Scotia's Shubenacadie Sam, who, because of location and special training, has the honor of making the first groundhog end-of-winter prediction for North America.

U.S. FEDERAL HOLIDAYS

JAN. 1: New Year's Day

JAN. 17: Martin Luther King Jr.'s Birthday, observed

FEB. 21: Presidents' Day

MAY 30: Memorial Day

JULY 4: Independence Day

SEPT. 5: Labor Day

OCT. 10: Columbus Day, observed

NOV. 11: Veterans Day

NOV. 24: Thanksgiving Day

DEC. 25: Christmas Day

Movable Religious Observances

FEB. 13: Septuagesima Sunday

MAR. 1: Shrove Tuesday

MAR. 2: Ash Wednesday

APR. 2: Ramadan begins at sundown

APR. 10: Palm Sunday

APR. 15: Good Friday
Passover begins at sundown

APR. 17: Easter

APR. 24: Orthodox Easter

MAY 22: Rogation Sunday

MAY 26: Ascension Day

JUNE 5: Whitsunday–Pentecost

JUNE 12: Trinity Sunday

JUNE 19: Corpus Christi

SEPT. 25: Rosh Hashanah begins at sundown

OCT. 4: Yom Kippur begins at sundown

NOV. 27: First Sunday of Advent

DEC. 18: Chanukah begins at sundown

CHRONOLOGICAL CYCLES

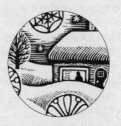

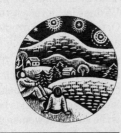

Dominical Letter **B**

Epact **27**

Golden Number (Lunar Cycle) **9**

Roman Indiction **15**

Solar Cycle **15**

Year of Julian Period **6735**

ERAS

ERA	YEAR	BEGINS
Byzantine	7531	September 14
Jewish (A.M.)*	5783	September 25
Chinese (Lunar) [Year of the Tiger]	4720	February 1
Roman (A.U.C.)	2775	January 14
Nabonassar	2771	April 18
Japanese	2682	January 1
Grecian (Seleucidae)	2334	September 14 (or October 14)
Indian (Saka)	1944	March 22
Diocletian	1739	September 11
Islamic (Hegira)*	1444	July 29
Bahá'í*	179	March 20

*Year begins at sundown.

–Beth Krommes

GLOSSARY OF ALMANAC ODDITIES

Many readers have expressed puzzlement over the rather obscure entries that appear on our **Right-Hand Calendar Pages, 121–147.** These "oddities" have long been fixtures in the Almanac, and we are pleased to provide some definitions. Once explained, they may not seem so odd after all!

EMBER DAYS: These are the Wednesdays, Fridays, and Saturdays that occur in succession following (1) the First Sunday in Lent; (2) Whitsunday–Pentecost; (3) the Feast of the Holy Cross, September 14; and (4) the Feast of St. Lucia, December 13. The word *ember* is perhaps a corruption of the Latin *quatuor tempora,* "four times." The four periods are observed by some Christian denominations for prayer, fasting, and the ordination of clergy.

Folklore has it that the weather on each of the 3 days foretells the weather for the next 3 months; that is, in September, the first Ember Day, Wednesday, forecasts the weather for October; Friday predicts November; and Saturday foretells December.

DISTAFF DAY (JANUARY 7): This was the day after Epiphany, when women were expected to return to their spinning following the Christmas holiday. A distaff is the staff that women used for holding the flax or wool in spinning. (Hence the term "distaff" refers to women's work or the maternal side of the family.)

PLOUGH MONDAY (JANUARY): Traditionally, the first Monday after Epiphany was called Plough Monday because it was the day when men returned to their plough, or daily work, following the Christmas holiday. (Every few years, Plough Monday and Distaff Day fall on the same day.) It was customary at this time for farm laborers to draw a plough through the village, soliciting money for a "plough light,"

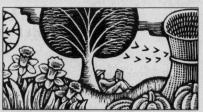

which was kept burning in the parish church all year. This traditional verse captures the spirit of it:

Yule is come and Yule is gone,
and we have feasted well;
so Jack must to his flail again
and Jenny to her wheel.

THREE CHILLY SAINTS (MAY): Mamertus, Pancras, and Gervais were three early Christian saints whose feast days, on May 11, 12, and 13, respectively, are traditionally cold; thus they have come to be known as the Three Chilly Saints. An old French saying translates to "St. Mamertus, St. Pancras, and St. Gervais do not pass without a frost."

MIDSUMMER DAY (JUNE 24): To the farmer, this day is the midpoint of the growing season, halfway between planting and harvest. The Anglican Church considered it a "Quarter Day," one of the four major divisions of the liturgical year. It also marks the feast day of St. John the Baptist. (Midsummer Eve is an occasion for festivity and celebrates fertility.)

CORNSCATEOUS AIR (JULY): First used by early almanac makers, this term signifies warm, damp air. Although it signals ideal climatic conditions for growing corn, warm, damp air poses a danger to those affected by asthma and other respiratory problems.

DOG DAYS (JULY 3–AUGUST 11): These 40 days are traditionally the year's hottest and unhealthiest. They once coincided with the year's heliacal (at sunrise) rising of the Dog Star, Sirius. Ancient folks thought that the "combined heat" of Sirius and the Sun caused summer's swelter.

LAMMAS DAY (AUGUST 1): Derived from the Old English *hlaf maesse,* meaning "loaf mass," Lammas Day marked the beginning of the harvest. Traditionally, loaves of bread were baked from the first-ripened grain and brought to the churches to be consecrated. In Scotland, Lammastide fairs became famous as the time when trial marriages could be made. These marriages could end after a year with no strings attached.

CAT NIGHTS COMMENCE (AUGUST 17): This term harks back to the days when people believed in witches. An Irish legend says that a witch could turn into a cat and regain herself eight times, but on the ninth time (August 17), she couldn't change back and thus began her final life permanently as a cat. Hence the saying "A cat has nine lives."

HARVEST HOME (SEPTEMBER): In Britain and other parts of Europe, this marked the conclusion of the harvest and a period of festivals for feasting and thanksgiving. It was also a time to hold elections, pay workers, and collect rents. These festivals usually took place around the autumnal equinox. Certain groups in the United States, e.g., the Pennsylvania Dutch, have kept the tradition alive.

ST. LUKE'S LITTLE SUMMER (OCTOBER): This is a period of warm weather that occurs on or near St. Luke's feast day (usually October 18) and is sometimes called Indian summer.

INDIAN SUMMER (NOVEMBER): A period of warm weather following a cold spell or a hard frost, Indian summer can occur between St. Martin's Day (November 11) and November 20. Although there are differing dates for its occurrence, for more than 225 years the Almanac has adhered to the saying "If All Saints' [November 1] brings out winter, St. Martin's brings out Indian summer." The term may have come from early Native Americans, some of whom believed that the condition was caused by a warm wind sent from the court of their southwestern god, Cautantowwit.

HALCYON DAYS (DECEMBER): This period of about 2 weeks of calm weather often follows the blustery winds at autumn's end. Ancient Greeks and Romans experienced this weather at around the time of the winter solstice, when the halcyon, or kingfisher, was thought to brood in a nest floating on the sea. The bird was said to have charmed the wind and waves so that waters were especially calm at this time.

BEWARE THE POGONIP (DECEMBER): The word *pogonip* refers to frozen fog and was coined by Native Americans to describe the frozen fogs of fine ice needles that occur in the mountain valleys of the western United States and Canada. According to tradition, breathing the fog is injurious to the lungs. ■

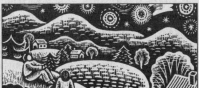

OUR AMAZING
NORTH STAR

The steady sentinel of our northern sky
is more than meets the eye.

BY BOB BERMAN

It's the most famous star. And the most useful. Yet nothing else in the heavens generates as much confusion as Polaris, the North Star.

Go ahead, ask your friends: "What makes the North Star special?" Most will say its brightness. Some will merely shrug. Odds are, none will give the right answer:

It's the only object in the sky that doesn't appear to move—and this is absolutely astounding!

Make no mistake; Polaris's brightness is notable. Of the 6,000 stars visible to the naked eye, it ranks a respectable 45th in brightness. It's bright enough to appear in polluted city skies (on every clear night, it's visible to 88 percent of Earth's humans), but it's not brilliant enough to catch your eye. It is 2nd-magnitude—a medium star, matching those of Orion's Belt and the ones forming the Big Dipper. It's no dim bulb but not a standout, either; its strength is its stability while all else is in perpetual motion.

Thanks to our planet's rotation, the Moon, Sun, and stars rise in the east, cross the sky, and then set in the west. Look up, then an hour later glance skyward again, and you'll notice that nearly everything's shifted rightward (or leftward, for those in the Southern Hemisphere)—except Polaris. It shares this stationary quality with nothing else in the universe. If it's halfway up the sky as you look out your north-facing window, it'll still be there next month, next year, and when your grandchildren are old.

Think of it this way: Imagine you painted hundreds of polka dots on your floor, walls, and ceiling and then performed ballet pirouettes in the middle of the room. As you spun, the dots would seem to whirl around you. Except for one. The polka dot on the ceiling right over your head wouldn't move because your axis of spin points straight up in its direction.

Earth's axis of spin has to point somewhere, too. By chance, it's angled

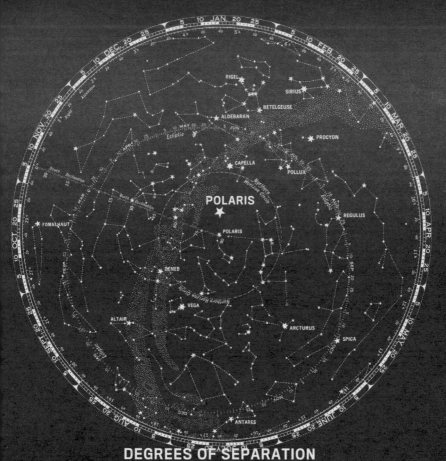

DEGREES OF SEPARATION

As mariners have always known, if you measure the North Star's height in the sky, you'll ascertain your latitude. Latitude is expressed in degrees, with the North Pole at 90°, most U.S. cities at 30° to 40°, and the Equator at 0° latitude. From the North Pole, latitude 90°, Polaris stands almost exactly 90° high—straight up. At the Equator, latitude 0°, Polaris stands 0° high as it hovers atop the horizon. From Denver or New York City, both of which are at approximately latitude 40°, Polaris is 40° high, about halfway up the northern sky.

Measure Polaris's elevation above the horizon and you instantly know your latitude. Here's how to do it: A clenched adult fist held at arm's length blocks 10° of the sky, so, for example, Polaris appears to hover four stacked fists high—approximately 40° up—as seen from Denver. (Longitude is a different matter and requires an onboard clock.)

153

toward Polaris. So, like that one dot on the ceiling, Polaris doesn't seem to move. If you visited the North Pole, you'd see Polaris almost exactly straight overhead. When you moved away from the pole, Polaris would be high overhead but no longer straight up. The farther you traveled from the pole, the lower Polaris would appear, until you reached the Equator, when Polaris would sit on the northern horizon and it wouldn't budge as the hours wore on each night.

If you're south of the Equator, Polaris is below the horizon and invisible. You will find no comparable "South Star" at the south celestial pole—the sky-spot at which the other end of Earth's axis points as our world spins. Serious astronomers can identify 5th-magnitude Sigma Octantis, the very dim southern pole star that hovers over Aussie-land, but it's no standout.

Polaris is unique. The fact that it just happens to sit within a single degree of the celestial pole, the precise motionless spot

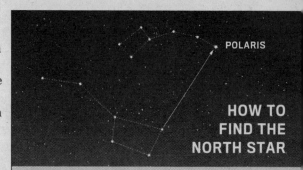

POLARIS

HOW TO FIND THE NORTH STAR

The easiest way to find Polaris is to first locate the Big Dipper. It is visible throughout the year–highest up in spring and quite low in autumn, especially for those in the most southerly states. The Big Dipper has a curved handle and a bowl. Find the two stars at the edge of the bowl that's farthest from the handle. Follow a line from the star at the base of the bowl through the star at the top of that edge onward to a single star that's the same brightness as they are–that's Polaris!

in the sky around which everything pivots, is an unlikely reality. The odds can be easily calculated. There are 41,253 square degrees of sky, and only some 45 stars are as bright or brighter than Polaris. The chance of such a noticeable star occupying the right spot is nearly a thousand to one against. The odds against both poles being occupied by medium-bright stars would be nearly a million to one.

What's more, Polaris is—for all practical purposes—precise. It shows us true north

with far greater accuracy than a compass, which merely follows the magnetic pole and is badly in error from most locations. From Boston, for instance, compasses point a whopping 16 degrees to the left of north, while instruments on the Pacific coast point nearly as erroneously in the other direction. In fact, if we drop an imaginary plumb bob straight down from Polaris, it touches the northern horizon to a precision of better than a degree.

Yet Polaris is not permanent. While our North

Image: ScienceSparks.com

Star appears constant for centuries, it is not in its position for eternity. The wobbly motion of our planet's axis, called precession, gradually creates new stationary sky positions and new north stars over a cycle of 25,780 years. Like a spinning toy top tilting around in a slow drunken circle as its rotation speed decreases, Earth's leisurely wobble once caused our northern axis to point toward a relatively dim star in Draco named Thuban when the Pyramids were being built. And 12,000 years from now, brilliant Vega will be our north star, although it will never be as visually glued in place as our own Polaris.

The north celestial pole, the spot of sky that doesn't move each night, is moving incrementally slowly in Polaris's direction. At present, 2022, Polaris hovers within 1 degree of this pole, but it will stand at less than a half-degree at its closest, an event that is expected to occur within 3 years of 2109 (no one can be more precise on the timing). After that, the celestial pole will start to slowly pull away, and, within a few centuries, Polaris will trace out tiny but noticeable nightly circles. Now, Polaris sits so close to the celestial pole that the circle that it makes each night is too small to notice—but it does show up on long exposure photos. The diameter of Polaris's nocturnal arc will increase over time, and thus will the epoch of Polaris gradually conclude. We'll then have to wait another 260 centuries—a full precessional cycle—before it once again becomes our "North Star."

U sing recent astrophysical discoveries, we know that the distant star to which Earth's axis points is remarkable.
• First, it's no ordinary star; it's a giant. At about 440 light-years distant, it lies some four times farther away than the Big Dipper's two "pointer" stars that guide our eyes to it.
• Being at that distance yet so prominently visible means that it is exceptionally luminous. In fact, Polaris shines with extraordinary brilliance, emitting the light of thousands of Suns.
• Even more remarkable is that Polaris's north rotation pole is located dead center to our observations. This means that we are *its* "north star"!

Viewers using small telescopes with lenses or mirrors at least 3 inches in diameter are encouraged to observe the North Star and see its small companion star. Studies of Polaris's light indicate a second companion star as well.

Or try this more restful exercise: Point your instrument at Polaris and leave it there. Unplug the drive motor. Take a 20-, 30-, or even 40-year sabbatical. When you return, the constant star will still be in the same position, waiting for you. ■

Bob Berman, our astronomy editor, ran the astronomy program at Yellowstone Park for 15 years and was an adjunct professor of astronomy and physics at Marymount College in New York's Westchester County. He writes and hosts the "Strange Universe" show heard weekly during NPR's *Weekend Edition* on Northeast Public Radio.

WHAT, THE HAIL?

TRACKING THE PLAGUE OF "WATERY METEORS"

BY CHRISTOPHER C. BURT

HEAVY WEATHER
Have you experienced a hailstorm?
Share your pics on f @theoldfarmersalmanac

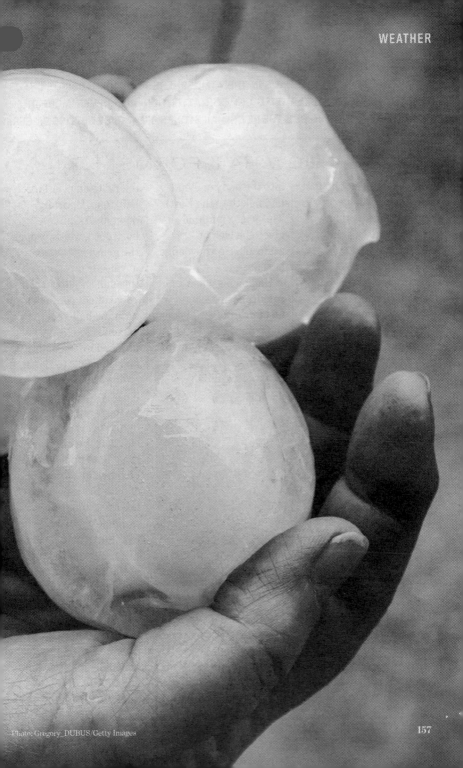

ONE OF NATURE'S MOST FASCINATING AND FEARSOME WEATHER EVENTS IS A HAILSTORM. BORN OF CHAOS IN THE ATMOSPHERE AND THE CAUSE OF CHAOS WHERE THEY FALL, HAILSTONES GET OUR ATTENTION—AND NEVER MORE THAN WHEN THEY ARE BIG. HERE'S THE NEWS: HAILSTONES SEEM TO BE GETTING BIGGER.

HOW HAIL FORMS

The science of hail formation has been understood for a long time. In John Tulley's *Almanac of 1693* (Cambridge, Massachusetts), while speculating on the "Natural Causes of Watery Meteors, such as snow, hail, rain,

into the body of cloud, and falleth to the Earth." This was a fair analysis given the lack of atmospheric knowledge at that time.

Hail forms when raindrops are caught in an updraft of air inside the parent cloud and lifted into the region of

to create an ever larger hailstone. Updrafts, downdrafts, and horizontal winds propel the growing hailstone in various directions through the storm. This yo-yo effect continues until the hailstone becomes too heavy to be lifted by the updrafts and thus falls to Earth.

The size of the hailstone is determined by the strength of the updrafts in the storm cloud. It is estimated that these updrafts can be moving at speeds of over 150 miles per hour and thus can produce grapefruit-size hailstones (5 to 6 inches in diameter). The tops of the cumulonimbus clouds that host large hail can soar as high as 70,000 feet into the atmosphere, well into the stratosphere, which begins at around 35,000 feet in the midlatitudes of the Northern Hemisphere.

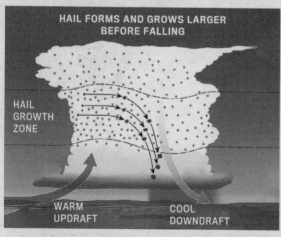

HAIL FORMS AND GROWS LARGER BEFORE FALLING

HAIL GROWTH ZONE

WARM UPDRAFT

COOL DOWNDRAFT

etc.," he wrote "... hail is engendered of rain, congealed into ice, freezing the drops perfectly . . . in the middle region of the air, whereby the extremity of cold, it is thickened

the cloud that is below freezing (which varies depending on what the surface temperature might be). Once frozen, the raindrop can then grow by colliding with still-unfrozen droplets

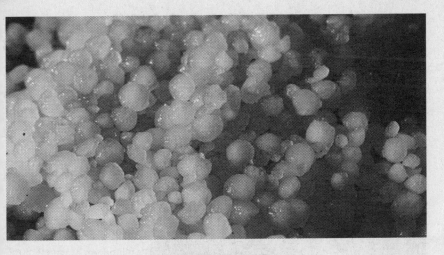

GOING UP

Of course, not every hailstone is citrus-size (the U.S. National Weather Service actually did away with hail descriptions related to food products some time ago). They range from the size of bb's to as big as DVDs. Weak thunderstorms normally produce smaller hailstones and powerful ones larger ones, but in recent years there has been an apparent increase in the frequency of large-hail (2-inch or greater diameter) events, the kind that can put dents in a car's hood and roof—especially if you're foolish enough to drive through a storm producing hail that size, as I once did on I-80 over the Donner Summit in the Sierra Nevada.

Why this increase in hail size? The science is still unclear, but it appears that the most

HAIL SIZE DESCRIPTION		
Hailstone Size	Diameter in.	cm
BB	<1/4	<0.64
PEA	1/4	0.64
DIME	7/10	1.8
PENNY	3/4	1.9
NICKEL	7/8	2.2
QUARTER	1	2.5
HALF-DOLLAR	1 1/4	3.2
GOLF BALL	1 3/4	4.4
BILLIARD BALL	2 1/8	5.4
TENNIS BALL	2 1/2	6.4
BASEBALL	2 3/4	7.0
SOFTBALL	3.8	9.7
CD/DVD	4 3/4	12.1

-Hendricks County (Ind.) Radio Amateur Civil Emergency Service

extreme hail days now tend to have greater instability (the contrast between warm, moist air near Earth's surface and cold air aloft), perhaps as a result of long-term warming. (This is happening in hail-prone areas around the world.)

Curiously, however, some studies suggest that the actual number of hail events (not just large-hail ones) is decreasing. We do not fully understand why, but comparisons of the number of hail days and average hailstone sizes reported from before and after the year 2000 have shown this to be true. *(continued)*

MATTERS OF SIZE

Hail occurs at some time everywhere in the U.S. and Canada south of the Arctic Circle, but the majority of hail reports emanate from the Plains/Prairies regions because it is here where the most severe across and 18.5 inches around, with a weight of almost 2 pounds—was collected by Lee Scott near Vivian, South Dakota, on July 23, 2010. Scott claims that it actually measured close to 11 inches across when he picked it up largest hailstone on record was a 4.5-inch–diameter head-knocker that was measured in Cedoux, Saskatchewan, on August 27, 1973.

Very large hail (4-inch or greater diameter) is rare outside of the U.S. Midwest and Plains states, but it can occur—-even in Hawaii: At Kailua on Oahu Island, on March 9, 2012, hailstones measuring 4.25 inches in diameter pummeled the ground.

Even larger hailstones have been reported from other places. On February 8, 2018, a thunderstorm in Cordoba province, Argentina, produced a stone collected and measured at 7.1 inches in diameter. Video taken of the stones falling through the air has been analyzed by meteorologists who estimated that some of them were as large as 9.3 inches in diameter. The experts even proposed a new size category— "gargantuan"—for hailstones that are at least 6 inches in diameter.

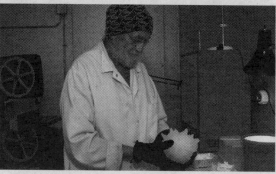

A SCIENTIST PREPARES TO MAKE A THREE-DIMENSIONAL MODEL OF THE VIVIAN HAILSTONE, THE LARGEST EVER RECORDED IN THE U.S.

thunderstorms and—not coincidentally—the most tornadoes occur.

Large hail and tornadoes go together. The months of May through August account for 85 percent of all annual hailstorm reports in the U.S. and Canada, with June being the peak month. It's perhaps no surprise, then, that the largest hailstone ever recorded in the U.S.—8 inches and placed it in his freezer. This was before a power outage (a result of the storm), during which the stone melted to *only* 8 inches before it refroze when the power returned. Scott eventually turned the stone over to the NWS for preservation and analysis. Vermont's record hailstone measured 3.3 inches in diameter in Westford on July 16, 2009. Canada's

HAILING A STORM TRAIN

That's big, but it pales when compared to the glacial effect: Training thunderstorms, a series of storms passing over the same location, can dump hail for hours and result in massive accumulations of it. Such an event took place in Selden, Kansas, on June 3, 1959, when, during an 85-minute storm, hailstones piled up to 18 inches deep. Often, rainfall accompanying such events will wash the

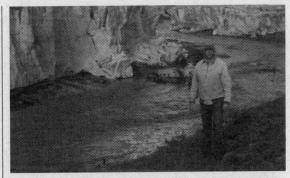

HAIL CLIFFS IN CLAYTON, NEW MEXICO, 2004

hail to a low point in the terrain and pile it up into fantastic heaps. This occurred near Clayton, New Mexico, on August 13, 2004, when an accumulation of hail washed into a creek bed and backed up behind a clogged culvert. Hail cliffs resembling the edge of a glacier rose some 15 feet high and took weeks to melt.

UNDERRATED IMPACT

Although the vast majority of hailstorms cause no significant damage, hail is an underrated economic hazard in the U.S. In most years, it causes more damage than tornadoes—and its havoc can rival that of hurricanes. Canada is not immune to its impact, as evidenced in the Calgary, Alberta, area on June 13, 2020, when a massive hailstorm became the fourth costliest natural disaster in that country's history. Just as they were in 1693 and before, "watery meteors" are but one more awesome example of Mother Nature's powerful potential. *(continued)*

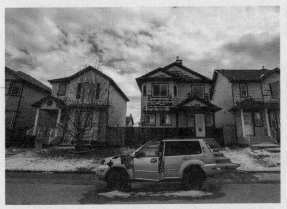

HAIL DAMAGE IN CALGARY, ALBERTA, 2020

Photos, from top: National Weather Service; NOAA

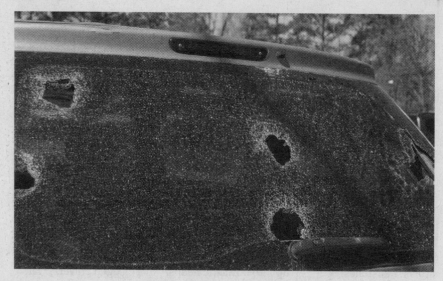

THE COLD REALITY: HAILSTONE DAMAGE

Hailstones can hurt or even kill randomly. Only a few documented human fatalities as a result of being struck have been recorded in modern U.S. history; Canada has experienced none. Fatalities to animals are more numerous, and injuries to both people and animals caught in hailstorms are relatively common—and can be painful. Dollar costs based on structural damage are well documented and can run into the billions for a single event.

Take these precautions if you are caught in a "watery meteor" barrage:

• Indoors—Close curtains, blinds, and shades to prevent injury from glass broken by hailstones. Remain indoors until the storm passes and the hailstones melt; they can be slippery underfoot.

• Outdoors—Seek shelter, but not under trees; lightning, which often accompanies hailstorms, can strike a tree—and thus you. Tree limbs can break and also strike you. Protect your head while moving to safety.

• In a car or other vehicle—Pull off the road. Remain inside. Instruct passengers to turn away from the windows and cover their eyes and head (with a sweatshirt, jacket, etc.) to protect against any glass broken by hailstones. If possible before the storm, seek safety nearby—for example, under an overpass or service station awning or in a garage. ■

Christopher C. Burt is the weather historian for Weather Underground, an IBM Company, and author of *Extreme Weather: A Guide and Record Book* (W. W. Norton & Co., 2007).

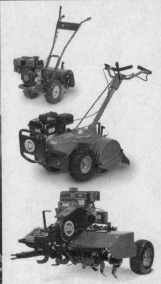
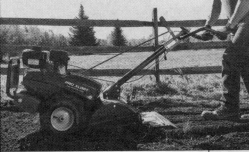
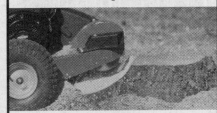

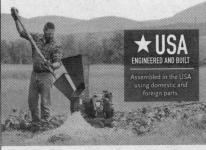

163

THE TOOTH,
THE WHOLE TOOTH,
AND NOTHING BUT THE TOOTH

AN EXAMINATION OF TEETH,
FROM CRADLE TO GRAVE

BY TIM CLARK

NATAL TEETH

About 1 in 1,000 babies is born with teeth. Some cultures celebrate the "natal teeth," as they are called. Ancient Romans considered such babies lucky, and they were often named "Dentatus." However, other cultures considered natal teeth as a bad omen. The children were thought likely to become vampires. Some were killed.

MILK TEETH

Most babies are born with 20 milk teeth, which usually erupt (appear in the mouth) within the first 3 years after birth. They start to get pushed out of the jaw at around age 5 by adult teeth growing in. The Vikings paid children for their milk teeth, which warriors wore around their necks in battle, believing that they would bring good luck.

Many cultures have strong beliefs about the disposal of these teeth. The most common practice involves offering the tooth to rodents like mice, rats, or even beavers. Known for their strong teeth, rodents were thought to give the child's succeeding teeth strength and beauty in return.

Rodents appeared in a book called *The Tooth Fairy,* written by Lee Rogow in 1949, which popularized the custom (already old by then) of putting a child's lost tooth under his or her pillow, to be miraculously replaced by money—perhaps a penny in colonial days but rising with inflation to an average of $3.19 these days, according to researchers at Visa.

PROPHETIC TEETH

While the baby teeth are falling out, a child starts growing his or her 32 adult teeth. Once the complete set has formed, several long-held superstitions take over.

Teeth set close together mean that a girl will live near her parents, while a space between the two front upper incisors means that she will make her eventual home far away—and she'll live a long life, be lucky, make a lot of money and, oddly enough, marry twice.

If a young man loses his teeth before he is 21, he won't live long; if after 21, he will live to be 100.

WISDOM TEETH

The last teeth to emerge, usually between the ages of 17 and 21, are called "wisdom teeth." This third pair of molars, at the back of the mouth, are surrounded by folklore, including the belief that a child will never gain any knowledge or be wise until his wisdom teeth appear—an observation upheld by science, which has found that the part of the brain responsible for decision-making and judgment is not completely developed until the early 20s.

The Romani people of central Europe deeply respect wisdom teeth and believe that those who have all four of them are spiritually strong. To keep wisdom teeth healthy, they may cast a spell on them by using water that reflects a full Moon as a mouthwash, while saying, "Wisdom is mine, protection is mine, but pain and diseases are not mine."

TOOTHACHE CURES

Sumerians living 7,000 years ago frequently complained of "tooth worms" drilling into their teeth and causing toothaches. This was not such a crazy idea at the time. Cavities produced holes that looked like the ones tiny worms made when digging into the ground or fruit.

The belief in tooth worms persisted well into the 18th century. The English thought that the worms looked like eels, while Germans favored something more like maggots. People suffering from toothaches would inhale smoke or spread honey on their teeth to persuade the worms to come out.

Weird, you say? Here are five of the strangest toothache cures suggested by American folklore:
• Run three times around a church without thinking of a fox.
• Cook earthworms in oil, then place them in the ear opposite the toothache.
• Plug the cavity with your own earwax.
• Chase a cat across a plowed field (perpendicular to the furrows) until it sweats, then rub the sweat on the aching tooth.
• Eat the eyes of a vulture.

MISSING TEETH

The most common cure for a toothache in years past was to pull the tooth. Then you had to dispose of the pulled tooth properly, and folk wisdom has plenty of suggestions on how to do it:
• Put the tooth in a glass of water, and in 24 hours, it will become money.
• Throw the tooth over your left shoulder, and you'll have good luck.
• Carry a wisdom tooth on your person for luck.
• After a tooth is pulled, if you swallow a bubble from milk, a gold tooth will come into your mouth to replace it.

• If you throw away your first tooth and a chicken picks it up, you will get chicken teeth.

> ## UNHELPFUL HYGIENE
> If you've heard it, don't believe it:
> • Chew tobacco to preserve your teeth.
> • Clean your teeth with cigar ashes to preserve them and make them white.
> • Eat bread crusts to make teeth white.

WATERLOO TEETH

Long ago, the best source of replacement teeth was corpses. The demand was so great that dentists and doctors employed men called "resurrectionists" to dig up graves and remove teeth from dead bodies.

But this was slow and inefficient. The best source of vast numbers of teeth—and teeth from young, healthy men—was the battlefield. Such teeth came to be called "Waterloo teeth" after the 1815 showdown that ended Napoleon's reign. More than 50,000 men died there, and a British resurrectionist named Butler was ready. "There'll be no want of teeth," he boasted before the fight. "I'll draw them as fast as the men are knocked down."

Dentists cheerfully advertised their dentures as "Waterloo teeth" or "Waterloo ivory." Fifty years later, dental catalogs still advertised the teeth of freshly killed soldiers. But these came from the casualties of the American Civil War (1861–65) and were shipped across the Atlantic. ∎

Tim Clark still has all four of his wisdom teeth.

Top Digestive Aid Pill Quietly Slows Premature Aging, Users Report Big Health Boost

Clinical research shows how a gastrointestinal "tonic" can restore GI health and slow an accelerated aging process; studies find the pill helps protect users from metabolic decline, cardiovascular issues, and serious conditions that accompany premature aging

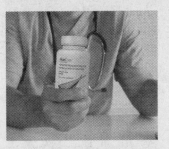

Seattle, WA – A published study on a leading acid buffer shows that its key ingredient improves digestive health while supporting healthy inflammation response that slows down signs of premature aging in men and women.

And, if consumer sales are any indication of a product's effectiveness, this 'GI-tonic turned anti-aging phenomenon' is nothing short of a miracle.

Sold under the brand name AloeCure®, its ingredient was already backed by research showing its ability to neutralize acid levels and improve gastric discomfort.

But soon doctors started reporting some incredible results...

"With AloeCure, my patients started reporting better sleep, more energy, stronger immune systems... even less stress and better skin, hair, and nails," explains Dr. Liza Leal, a leading integrative health specialist and company spokesperson.

AloeCure contains an active ingredient that helps optimize the pH balance of your stomach.

Scientists now believe that having optimal acid levels could be a major contributing factor to a healthy immune system.

The daily allowance of AloeCure has been shown to optimize the acid levels needed to manage healthy immune function which is why AloeCure is so effective.

It relieves other stressful issues related to GI health like discomfort, excess gas and bloating, and bathroom stress.

Now, backed with new scientific studies, AloeCure is being doctor-recommended to help improve digestive function, help build better bones, support healthy joint function.

FIX YOUR GUT & SUPPORT HEALTHY INFLAMMATION

Since hitting the market, sales for AloeCure have taken off and there are some very good reasons why. To start, the clinical studies have been impressive.

Virtually all participants reported stunning improvement in digestive symptoms including gastric discomfort.

Users can also experience higher energy levels and endurance, less discomfort and better sleep,.

An unhealthy gut can wreak havoc on the human body. Doctors say this is why AloeCure works on so many aspects of your health.

EXCITING USER REPORTS

To date millions of bottles of AloeCure have been sold, and the community seeking non-pharma therapy for their GI health continues to grow.

According to Dr. Leal, her patients are absolutely thrilled with their results and are often shocked by how fast it works.

"I recommend it to everyone who wants to improve GI health."

"All the problems with my stomach are gone. Completely gone. I can say AloeCure is a miracle. It's a miracle." Another user turned spokesperson said, "I started to notice a difference because I was sleeping through the night and that was great. AloeCure does work for me. It's made a huge difference."

With so much positive feedback, it's easy to see why the community of believers is growing and sales for the new pill are soaring.

THE SCIENCE BEHIND ALOECURE

AloeCure is a gastric and digestive tonic.

The active ingredient is a compound only found in Aloe Vera called Acemannan.

Millions spent in developing a proprietary process for extracting acemannan resulted in the highest quality, most bio-available levels of acemannan known to exist, and it's made from organic aloe.

According to Dr. Leal and leading experts, improving the pH balance of your stomach and restoring gut health is the key to revitalizing your entire body.

When your digestive system isn't healthy, it causes unwanted stress on your immune system and that might lead to unhealthy inflammation.

The recommended daily allowance of AloeCure has been proven to support digestive health, manage healthy immune function, and promote healthy inflammation response without side effects or drugs.

This would explain why so many users are experiencing impressive results so quickly.

AloeCure Taken Daily

- Helps End Digestion Nightmares
- Reduces appearance of Wrinkles & Increases Elasticity
- Supports Healthy Immune System
- Supports Joint Health
- Promotes Healthy Inflammation Response
- Supports Bowel Health & Regularity

REVITALIZE YOUR ENTIRE BODY

With daily use, AloeCure helps users look and feel decades younger and defend against premature aging that can make life hard.

By helping acid levels stay optimal and promoting gut health, AloeCure's ingredient supports joint health...helps skin appear smooth...maintains healthy cholesterol and oxidative stress...improves sleep and associated weight loss....and supports brain function by way of gut biome...without side effects or expense.

Readers can now support their energy, vitality, and youth regardless of age.

HOW TO CLAIM A FREE SUPPLY TODAY

This is an exclusive offer for our readers. And so, AloeCure is offering up to 3 FREE bottles and FREE S&H with their order. While supplies last you may also receive a FREE book on Aloe Vera health benefits.

A special hotline number has been created. All you have to do is call **TOLL-FREE 1-800-561-6637**, and the special promotion will be automatically applied. This is the best way to try AloeCure with their 100% satisfaction guarantee, and any free gifts are yours to keep no matter what.

Important: Due to a surge in sales supplies are not guaranteed. Call now to not lose out on this offer.

THE ART AND SCIENCE OF ANIMAL TRACKING

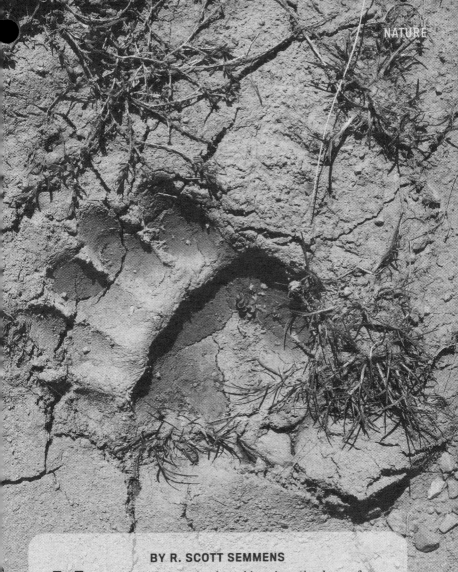

BY R. SCOTT SEMMENS

Humans have been animal tracking since the dawn of our species. The ancient art and science of animal tracking has its practical uses even today. There are two aspects of animal tracking: (1) studying the tracks and signs that animals leave behind, which is like reading the headlines about an animal, and (2) trailing an animal with the hope of seeing it while you remain undetected. *(continued)*

Photo: habrda/Getty Images

NATURE

"Track and sign" is a basic skill that helps you to recognize little scenes from the lives of animals. If there is snow on the ground, you can find tracks everywhere. Otherwise, they appear in sandy, dusty, or muddy areas.

"Trailing" builds on tracks and signs to reveal a more comprehensive story. It is more complex and requires more skills, such as knowledge of how to "age" a trail and of the animal's ecology and seasonal behavior, which helps to predict where an animal may go when you lose the trail. Familiarity with the topography and an ability to move stealthily through it also help.

Animals seldom leave perfect tracks. Those of some species overlap in size and shape, making them difficult to identify. Through practice, your observation skills will be sharpened. By identifying some key features, you will be able to place the tracks within a family or order and then narrow them down to species, usually with the aid of animal track guidebooks.

THE FINE POINTS OF THE FOOT

Learning about foot morphology can help you to understand how the foot leaves the tracks behind.

A TRACKER'S TECHNIQUE

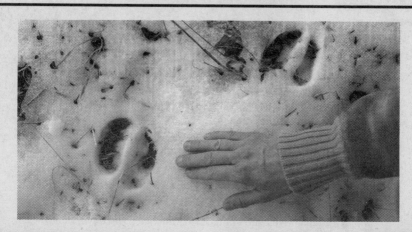

Before I identify a track, I look for similar tracks in the vicinity to ascertain the morphology, or form. I count the number of toes, examine their shapes and relationship to the pads, and determine whether they are front or hind feet. This can help to identify the family or order of the animal. I try to find associative signs (scats, scrapes, etc.) and evaluate the animal's gait, if possible, to understand its behavior. I note the context, such as habitat, ground, season, and specific location. Then I mentally match the evidence collected to a master list of possible animals that may reside in the area.

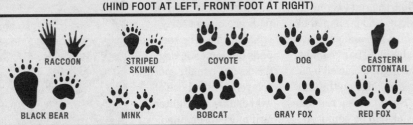

TREAD MARKS
(HIND FOOT AT LEFT, FRONT FOOT AT RIGHT)

RACCOON

STRIPED SKUNK

COYOTE

DOG

EASTERN COTTONTAIL

BLACK BEAR

MINK

BOBCAT

GRAY FOX

RED FOX

Mammals in the same order or family group often have similar foot morphology. Take the gray squirrel: Its front feet have four toes, plus one vestigial toe (toe #1, equivalent to our thumb). The hind feet have five toes. These toe patterns—especially the arrangement of toes #2, #3, and #4 in the hind feet—and the number of toes are characteristics of most members of the Sciuridae family. Similar patterns exist in the tracks of the squirrel's cousins, the chipmunk and the woodchuck.

The foot patterns of the canids (the dog family, which includes coyotes, foxes, wolves, and domestic dogs) are also similar to each other.

Measuring the size of the tracks can give some clue as to "owner"—but often not enough for identification. Consider that gray fox and red fox tracks can be similar in size; to know which is which, you have to examine the overall shapes of the tracks, the clarity of the toe pads, and the shapes of the metacarpal (front paw) pads. (Canids, unlike members of the

squirrel family, have no heel pads.)

Here is how they differ:

• Overall, the gray fox print shape is round; that of the red fox is oval.

• The nails of the gray fox often do not show up on their tracks because their claws are semi-retractable; not so for the red fox, whose claws do appear.

• The toe pads in the gray fox show up clear and defined, while those of the red fox appear fuzzy—and that's a clue: The red fox's foot is furrier, thus blurring

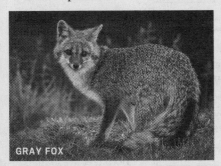

GRAY FOX

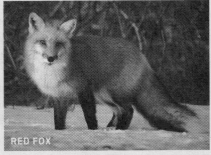

RED FOX

Photos, clockwise from top: klerik78/Getty Images; OliverChilds/Getty Images; Johnpane/Getty Images the overall appearance. Plus, the red fox metacarpal pad is shaped like a chevron and can have a distinct "bar" running through it, caused by a raised ridge on the pad.

Sometimes a red fox track can be confused with a small coyote track because both are oval. But look again: The pads on coyote tracks are well defined, unlike those of the red fox, which are blurred because of the fur on the bottom of its feet.

Domestic dog tracks can also be confused with coyote tracks—even though dog tracks vary considerably in shape and size. However, there are some commonalities that distinguish domestic dog tracks from those of wild canids.

Domestic dog tracks usually have clear pads.

The metacarpal (front) and metatarsal (hind) pads are often nearly equal in size. The toe pads on domestic dog tracks are usually more splayed, while those of wild canids are tighter, as if more disciplined. Also, the nails of the domestic dog are blunt and large, whereas the nails of wild canids are sharp and fine.

Here are a few more commonly found animal families and the characteristics of their tracks:

FELIDAE FAMILY
E.G., BOBCAT

• Four toes front and hind. (A fifth toe is in the front but too high to register on the track.)
• Toes are asymmetrical. Note leading toe #3. (Only in the dog family are they symmetrical on both feet.)
• Large pads when

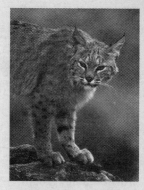

compared to toe size
• Three lobes (bumps) on the posterior edge of the pads
• The front and hind feet are round. The hind foot may be a little longer than it is wide.

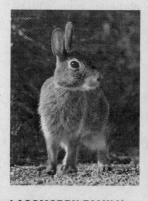

LAGOMORPH FAMILY
E.G., EASTERN COTTONTAIL

• Five toes in the front foot and four toes in the hind foot
• Toe #1 is not always present. If present, it drops very low on the inside of the foot.
• Both feet are J-shape

WHEN IN THE WILD . . .

When you first encounter a set of tracks, look at them as if it's your first time tracking. Notice the details without bias or expectations. Take measurements. Make notes on the texture, overall shape, color, and shading. Draw the tracks; this forces you to notice even more details. Any photos that you take should have some scale (e.g., a measuring tape) associated with them.

(especially the hind)
• Metacarpal and metatarsal pads rarely show up.

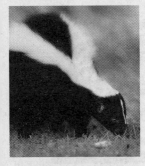

MEPHITIDAE FAMILY
E.G., STRIPED SKUNK

• Five toes front and hind
• Nails in the front foot are longer than those in the hind foot.
• Toes are partially fused in the front and hind feet.
• Toe #1 is the smallest and lowest on both feet.

MUSTELIDAE FAMILY
E.G., MINK

• Five toes front and hind
• Pads are arch-shape, with a relatively large

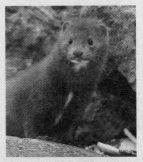

amount of space between pads and toes.
• Toe #1 is small on front and hind feet. All toes are distinct. In mink and otter, the hind foot toe #1 drops lower than toe #5.

PROCYONIDAE FAMILY
E.G., RACCOON

• Five toes front and hind
• Long, fingerlike toes, especially in the front feet
• Toe #1 is the lowest and smallest on front and hind.

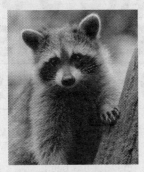

• The front is distinguished by an abrupt anterior ridge of the metacarpal pad leading toward the toes in the front foot, as opposed to the more tapering anterior edge of the metatarsal pad transitioning to the toes in the hind foot.

URSIDAE FAMILY
E.G., BLACK BEAR

• Five toes front and hind
• Toe #1 is the smallest

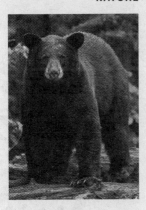

and lowest on both feet.
• In the front foot, the inside lobe of the metacarpal pad is narrower and forms a distinct arch around toe #5.
• The hind foot has a continuous pad leading to the heel.

Animal tracking is a great way to enjoy the great outdoors. Now that you've learned the steps and acquired some skills in track identification, go outside and track! ◼

R. Scott Semmens of Stoddard, New Hampshire, tracks animals around the world and teaches animal tracking to people of all ages—especially children—to get them excited about learning biology, ecology, and other sciences. He recommends that enthusiasts read Mark Elbroch's *Mammal Tracks & Sign: A Guide to North American Species,* 2nd ed. (Stackpole Books, 2019).

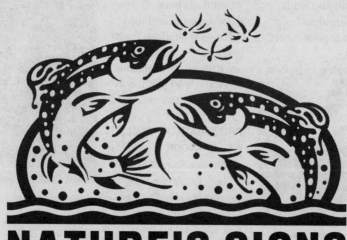

NATURE'S SIGNS
MEAN FISH
ON LINES

BY GLENN SAPIR • ILLUSTRATIONS BY TIM ROBINSON

When the telephone rang, the screen showed that it was my old fishing buddy, Ray Goodson, calling.

"The shadbushes are flowering," he said excitedly. "You know what *that* means!"

The Caller ID feature on my phone may have been newfangled when he made that call decades ago, but the message was one that has been repeated by shad fishermen all along the Delaware River year after year since people first figured out how to catch these anadromous fish on artificial lures. The American shad, prized for its fight in the water and its roe on the table, makes its annual spawning run every spring from the Atlantic Ocean through Delaware Bay and then along the Pennsylvania–New Jersey and then Pennsylvania–New York borders, which the river defines.

You could never be sure when the first shad might find their way into the commercial fishing nets, but you knew that when the shadbush was in bloom, it was time to go fishing.

Scientists call this

174

"phenology," the study of cyclic and seasonal natural phenomena. Anglers across the continent, in both the United States and Canada, however, simply call it Mother Nature. These fishermen believe that her plants and wildlife—even tiny insects—can tell them when to grab their rods and reels.

Fly-fishers seeking trout, especially in streams, base their strategy on the somewhat predictable timing of the emergence of aquatic insects that hatch in the water, sometimes fly into the air and then, often, lay their eggs before their brief life ends. During this time, these insects provide trout with a feast and fishermen

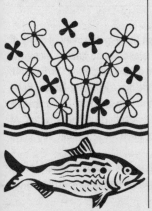

with obvious clues as to what to tie to their leaders. Simply put, it's called "matching the hatch," and those anglers who can tie on convincing imitations when they are in the right place at the right time—that is, when these insects are hatching, emerging, and falling back to the surface—might have fishing action that they will never forget.

What other natural indicators signal good fishing? One inquiry posted on Facebook and an email to several in-the-know anglers drew a variety of examples for both fresh and salt waters.

SIGNS IN SPRING

Shad enthusiasts in Quebec know that when the yellow flowers of dandelions are replaced by wispy white tufts, typically in mid-May, it's time to head for the Rivière des Prairies, which flows into the St. Lawrence River, to cash in on the run.

The shadbush that flowers along the Delaware telling fishermen to get to the river sends a

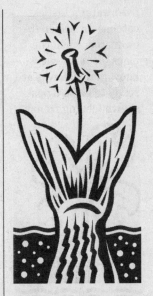

different message when it blooms on Martha's Vineyard in Massachusetts. There, fishermen then know to head for the salt ponds and estuaries because the striped bass have arrived.

Lilacs are another of nature's indicators that deliver a message to fishermen on various parts of the continent. Their blooming on Long Island, New York, is a welcome sign, hinting at the arrival of weakfish. In Great Lakes country, fishermen know that when that bush produces its fragrant flowers, it's time to hit Lake Erie for walleyes, one of

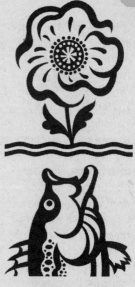

freshwater's tastiest catches. In Saskatchewan, too, when the lilacs bloom, anglers know that walleyes are ready to go on a post-spawn feeding frenzy.

Some fishermen attentively watch for dogwood blossoms. One angler swears that when dogwood blossoms are the size of a squirrel's ear, bass are ready for the taking.

This same fisherman, who grew up in the Chicago area, notes another cyclical activity that suggests good bass fishing. "When you see people collecting young dandelion leaves from plants, the bass are on the beds."

Another flower sends the same signal on the West Coast.

"When the poppies start blooming, the bass are heading into the shallows for the spawn," says one Californian, a veteran fisherman.

He's observed another of nature's indicators in the Southwest: When the yuccas start blooming, the bluegills move into the shallows to spawn, he reports.

Why is such information important?

First, it's a clue that fish have moved from the deep area of a body of water to its shallows. Second, when fish head for the spawning beds, the males—loaded with milt (semen)—and the females—laden with roe (eggs)—are at their heaviest weight. Third, the fish are in a protective mode, guarding the area that they have

SIGNS OF CHANGE

Climate change–specifically, water temperature–may threaten the dependability of some of these observations in coming years. For example, the Long Island Sound habitat along the New York and Connecticut coasts has warmed by 3 degrees in a 38-year period (1976-2014), changing the area from one characteristic of New England to one more like New Jersey, Delaware, and Maryland. This has triggered a northward migration of two-thirds of 82 northeastern marine species, according to the National Oceanic and Atmospheric Administration. At least two warm-water species, black sea bass and red hake, have moved about 200 miles north, according to the the Environmental Protection Agency.

Scientists can only watch and wonder how quickly fish will evolve or adapt, while fishermen keep an eye out for new signs. In parts of the U.S. Northeast, spring now arrives a full week earlier than it did a few decades ago.

staked out as a nursery and likely to attack anything, including your bait, that threatens their territory.

Bass and bluegill aren't the only species for which nature drops clues that fish are on their spawning beds.

In the Ozarks, it's said that there are often a few days when the redbud blooms start to fade and the dogwoods begin flowering simultaneously. When this happens, the crappie are shallow and spawning.

In central Missouri, when the black locusts are in bloom, the walleye spawning run is in full swing.

AUTUMNAL INDICATORS

Not all of nature's indicators arrive in spring and summer.

In the Rocky Mountain states and provinces, when the aspens turn yellow in the fall, the lake brown trout are moving into stream mouths for their spawning run. This is when they are aggressive and vulnerable.

In coastal New England, anglers believe that when apples fall from the trees in October, the false albacore, a prized gamefish, migrate. This indicator has earned the species a nickname of "apple-knockers."

FEATHERED FORECASTERS

Year after year, birds, too, serve as a seasonal signal corps for anglers.

In mid-Atlantic region coastal waters, laughing gulls arrive at

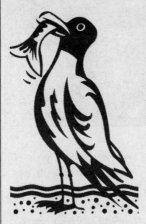

the same time that summer flounder, aka fluke, make their appearance.

When New Englanders see flocks of night herons standing watch on the shoreline of a river, they know that the alewife and herring spawning run is under way and large striped

bass will be close to shore, eager to attack anything that disturbs the surface along the bank. This presents fishermen with a perfect opportunity for action on topwater plugs.

I t is not serendipity that lends validity to all of these observations. The day length and angle of sunlight and the rising and lowering of water and air temperatures are key factors that trigger these coincidental occurrences in nature that repeat themselves year after year. Successful anglers have long known that following the weather and nature's signs are surefire keys to a great catch. ∎

Glenn Sapir of Putnam County, New York, is an award-winning writer and editor who has devoted his 50-plus-year career to communicating about the outdoors. He has served on the editorial staffs of major outdoors publications and is the author and/or editor of several books, including *A Sapir Sampler: Favorites by an Outdoor Writer* (Ashmark Communications, 2018).

10 THINGS YOU (PROBABLY) DIDN'T KNOW ABOUT ALBERT JACKSON

Enjoy this special delivery of
facts about our first black postman.

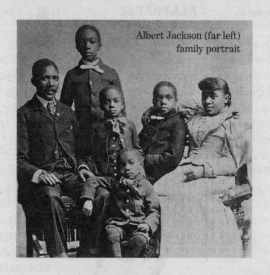

Albert Jackson (far left)
family portrait

1. He was born into a struggling family in Delaware in 1856, the youngest of nine children. Soon after, two of his brothers, James and Richard, were sold into slavery, and his father, John, died from grief. In 1858, Ann Maria Jackson, fearing that more of her children were to be sold, bundled them up and fled. Hiding and traveling with 2-year-old Albert was difficult, as his occasional crying put them at risk. Luckily, antislavery agents smuggled them by carriage through Pennsylvania and then eventually into Toronto.

2. He was reunited with James, who had escaped captivity at about the same time his mother and siblings fled. The family settled together in an area of Toronto known as "St. John's Ward" in 1859.

3. Jackson received a full public school education—the only one of his family to do so. Most of his siblings could not read or write and would never learn how. His older siblings and their mother worked as linen washers, waiters, and barbers to enable Jackson to attend school. He graduated in 1882 and immediately applied for the job of postman.

4. He was appointed a letter carrier on May 12, 1882, but his first day ended before lunch: None of his colleagues would train or work with him. His family could not bear the injustice. Two of his brothers, John Jr. and Robert, organized the black community to protest.

5. Jackson's plight sparked a national debate about racism. On May 17, 1882, *The Evening Telegram* published "The Objectionable African," an article in which Jackson was described as "the obnoxious coloured man" and post office employees were quoted as being "disgusted" by his appointment to a higher position than that of some of their white colleagues. Newspapers grabbed on to the story, publishing arguments both against and in support of Jackson.

The issue was in the headlines for weeks.

6. The postmaster reassigned Jackson as a porter in an attempt to defuse the situation, but this only further enraged the black community. The reassignment was withdrawn.

> **Jackson received a full public school education— the only one of his family to do so.**

7. The prime minister intervened to resolve the matter. The postmaster was a friend of John A. MacDonald and asked him for help. As the incumbent in the 1882 election, MacDonald realized how important the matter was to the black community and how their votes could affect his candidacy. Two days after MacDonald stepped in, Jackson began training as a

letter carrier, and there were no more objections.

8. A postman's minimum annual salary in 1882 was $600–enough to support a family. Jackson married Canadian-born Henrietta Jones in 1883, and they eventually had four children: Alfred, Bruce, Richard, and Harold. Jackson worked as a letter carrier for 36 years, until his death at age 62 on January 14, 1918.

9. Jackson's descendants live in Toronto today. Shortly after his death, Henrietta and their sons bought houses in Harbord Village. Several generations of Jacksons continued to be raised there.

10. Jackson's story was not well known until 2007, when Karolyn Smardz Frost's book *I've Got a Home in Glory Land: A Lost Tale of the Underground Railroad* was published. In 2013, a Toronto laneway was named for him. Two years later, his story came to life in a play called "The Postman." ■

–compiled by Benjamin Kilbride

BEYOND THE

WHAT HAPPENED ON THE ICE WAS ONLY PART

PHIL ESPOSITO (7) OF TEAM CANADA
PLAYS AGAINST TEAM USSR
DURING THE 1972 SUMMIT SERIES

BOARDS

OF THE 1972 CANADA-SOVIET HOCKEY SUMMIT. BY PAT HICKEY

This year marks the 50th anniversary of the eight-game clash of hockey and political ideologies between Canada and the Soviet Union known as the Summit Series. Stats and stories of the games, the first ever between Canadian pros and the Soviet national team, are legendary; less well known are some of these off-ice incidents.

THE GOLDEN JET IS GROUNDED

There was controversy over the roster before the series. High-scoring winger Bobby Hull, aka The Golden Jet, was named to the team but later dropped because the competition was limited to National Hockey League players and he had signed a contract with the Winnipeg Jets of the rival World Hockey Association. Prime Minister Pierre Trudeau joined fans and the media to protest Hull's exclusion, but their pleas fell on deaf ears. Derek Sanderson, Gerry Cheevers, and J. C. Tremblay were also excluded after signing with the WHA.

ORR CASHES IN

Bobby Orr, who was the top defenseman in the NHL, was named to the team but unable to play because he was recovering from knee surgery. However, he was a big winner financially. With some help from agent Alan Eagleson, who also served as the main organizer of the series, Orr and Toronto Maple Leafs owner Harold Ballard secured the TV rights for the series for $750,000. They later walked away with a profit of $1.2 million.

TROUBLE WITH SHOTS?

When Team Canada scouts Bob David-son and John McLellan saw Soviet goaltender Vladislav Tretiak give up eight goals in an intrasquad game, they weren't impressed. What they didn't know was that the 20-year-old was playing on the night before he got married and—perhaps more important—the night after his bachelor party.

READY TO FIGHT

Soviet coach Vsevolod Bobrov recalled being roughed up by the Penticton Vees when he was playing in the 1955 world championships, so he added boxing lessons to his team's training program.

COSTLY FENDER BENDER

When the Soviets arrived in Montreal for Game 1 of the series, their equipment was seized at the airport after a Montreal resident filed a suit claiming that his car had been damaged by Soviet tanks during the invasion of Prague in 1968. The equipment was released after Eagleson wrote a check to cover the damages.

SHOCKER AT THE FORUM

When Phil Esposito scored 30 seconds into the opening game and then Paul Henderson scored to make it 2–0, fans were expecting a high-scoring romp

BOXING LESSONS WERE ADDED TO TEAM USSR'S TRAINING PROGRAM.

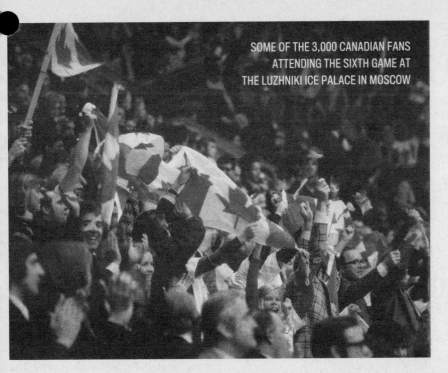

SOME OF THE 3,000 CANADIAN FANS ATTENDING THE SIXTH GAME AT THE LUZHNIKI ICE PALACE IN MOSCOW

for Canada on the Montreal Forum ice. In the end, the Soviets proved to be a better-conditioned team that baffled the Canadians with their precision passing. The visitors led 3–2 after the first period and went on to win 7–3.

TO BOO OR NOT TO BOO

Canada rebounded for a 4–1 win in Toronto and had to settle for a 4–4 tie in Game 3 in Winnipeg, but the final home contest in Vancouver was a disaster. The crowd at the PNE Coliseum booed the Canadian players as they stumbled to a 5–3 loss. The Soviets dominated the game, and only a late goal by Dennis Hull made the final score respectable. Phil Esposito, who was named the player of the game for Canada, was interviewed on television after the game and expressed the players' frustration

at being booed. He assured fans that the players were giving 150 percent against a very good team and ended with the promise: "We're gonna get better." The Canadian portion of the series ended with one win, two losses and a tie.

THE BIG M'S PARANOIA

As the series shifted to the Soviet Union, Frank Mahovlich, whose parents had emigrated to Canada from Yugoslavia, was deeply suspicious of the Soviets, who were the de facto rulers of the Balkan country—and he may have been right to suspect that the Canadians' hotel rooms were bugged. Wayne Cashman believed that the Russians were using two-way mirrors to monitor the players, so he threw any reflective items in his room into the hallway. One story that was never verified concerned

IT WAS US VERSUS THEM. AND KHARLAMOV WAS KILLING US.

players who discovered a suspicious metal plate under a carpet. When they unscrewed the plate, a lighting fixture in the room below crashed to the floor.

THE CASE OF THE SHRINKING STEAKS

The Canadians brought their own food to Moscow, including a supply of inch-thick steaks. When the steaks were served, they were found to have been cut in half diagonally. After the players complained, at their next steak dinner they were properly served their full-size steaks—but the pieces had been cut down to ½ inch in thickness. Team Canada also brought its own beer, which disappeared on the tarmac at the Moscow airport.

KEEPING THE WIVES HAPPY

While the Canadian players were experiencing frustration on and off the ice, the situation was no better for the wives who accompanied them to Moscow. They were originally booked into a second-class hotel, but Eagleson pulled strings to move them into the Intourist hotel, which housed the players. The wives also complained about the quality of the available food and received handouts from their husbands.

THE FERGY FACTOR

Canada lost the first game in Moscow, 5–4, but there were no boos, as nearly 3,000 visiting Canadian fans showed their support. Canada was on the verge of defeat in the series, but the fans and a controversial incident in Game 6

changed the momentum. Bobby Clarke took a two-handed swipe at Soviet star Valeri Kharlamov's ankle. Assistant coach John Ferguson, who had been a hard-nosed enforcer in his playing days, later recalled: "I told Clarke, 'I think he needs a tap on the ankle.' I didn't think twice about it. It was Us versus Them. And Kharlamov was killing us. I mean, somebody had to do it." Kharlamov missed Game 7 and was not at his best in the final game.

A HALL OF FAME PERFORMANCE?

Paul Henderson, who almost skipped the series because he and his wife had planned a European vacation, became a national hero when he scored the winning goal with 34 seconds remaining in Game 8, the final. Many fans believe that the goal, which was watched by an estimated 4.26 million television viewers, should have earned Henderson a place in the Hockey Hall of Fame. The selection committee hasn't shared that view, deciding that Henderson's career fell short of recognition. In a 2019 interview with CTV, Henderson said: "The worst thing they could do would be to put me in the Hall of Fame, because people get ticked off all the time, saying, 'You should be in the Hall of Fame!' and they talk about it. If I get put in, they'll forget all about me." ∎

Pat Hickey has been writing about sports for 55 years. He covered the opening games of the 1972 Summit Series and is currently a hockey columnist and beat writer for the *Montreal Gazette*.

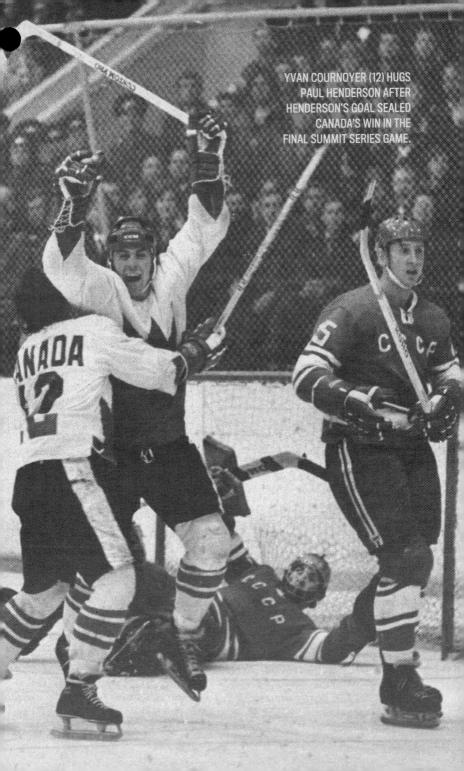

YVAN COURNOYER (12) HUGS PAUL HENDERSON AFTER HENDERSON'S GOAL SEALED CANADA'S WIN IN THE FINAL SUMMIT SERIES GAME.

REMAINS to BE SEEN

BY TIM CLARK

From earliest human times, the bodies of deceased dictators, saints, philosophers, criminals, eccentrics, and beloved animals have been preserved often for the edification of future generations. Here are a few that are still on display.

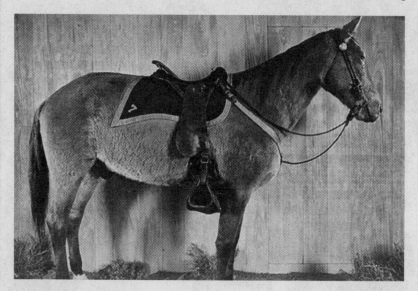

Sole Survivor

Comanche, a horse belonging to an officer of the U.S. 7th Cavalry—the unit that was wiped out at the Little Bighorn in 1876—is often described as the sole survivor of Custer's Last Stand. It's now clear that other horses were captured or scattered by the victorious Lakota Sioux and Cheyenne warriors. But Comanche's story is the only one we know. Suffering from seven bullet wounds, he was found by U.S. troops who arrived too late to save Custer and his 210 soldiers. Nursed back to health at Ft. Abraham Lincoln in the Dakota Territory, Comanche was given the honorary title of "second-in-command" of the 7th Cavalry. Upon his death in 1890, he was given a funeral with full military honors, and his body was sent to the University of Kansas to be stuffed. It is currently on display there.

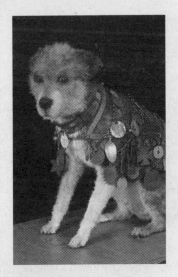

POSTAL PUP

At the end of the 19th century, a terrier named Owney was informally adopted by the post office in Albany, New York. The employees declared him an official mail dog and let him ride the trains that delivered it across the nation. He is said to have visited all 48 contiguous states and made a 'round-the-world trip in 1895—to deliver the mail, of course. After his death in 1897, he was stuffed and displayed at the 1904 World's Fair as the mascot of the U.S. Post Office. He's still on display at the Smithsonian National Postal Museum in Washington, D.C.

Trigger Happy

When the Roy Rogers and Dale Evans Museum closed in 2009, many of its fans wondered, "What will happen to Trigger?" Trigger, of course, was the name of several golden palomino horses that Roy Rogers (1911-98) rode in nearly 100 cowboy films and two TV series. When the original Trigger died in 1965, Rogers had him stuffed, and eventually he went on display in the museum, along with Buttermilk, the horse that his wife and co-star Dale rode, and Bullet, a German shepherd that also appeared in the films. The contents of the museum were auctioned off in 2010. The rural cable network WRFD-TV paid $266,500 for Trigger and $35,000 for Bullet. In 2019, Trigger and Bullet made their way to The Cowboy Channel TV and Live Recording Studio in the Fort Worth Stockyards, Texas.   *(continued)*

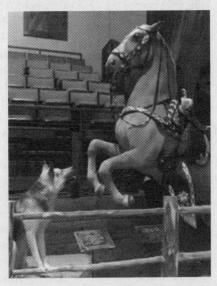

Goofy Gophers

In the mid-1990s, folks in Torrington, Alberta (pop. approx. 200), sought to attract visitors. It was a challenge: Torrington is on the prairie, 90 minutes from Calgary. It has no hotels and only two restaurants, one a gas station that sells pizza. What Torrington had was gophers–Richardson's Ground Squirrels–that hibernate 7 months of the year and are only sporadically active when they're awake. Hearing opportunity knock, in 1996, folks opened the Gopher Hole Museum. It houses 47 dioramas of stuffed, costumed, posed gophers. Want to see gophers at the beauty parlor? This is the place.

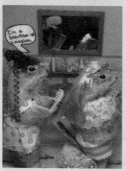

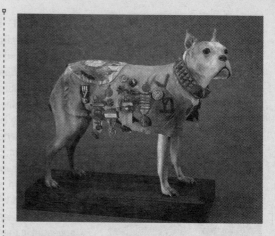

WAR HERO

In 1917, Pvt. J. Robert Conroy found a brindle puppy on the playing fields at Yale University, where his unit, part of the 26th "Yankee" Division, was training to be deployed in World War I. Although animals were not allowed in camp, officers let "Stubby" stay and even taught him to salute. When the 26th shipped out, Stubby (named for his short tail) was smuggled on board and served as mascot for the 102nd Infantry Regiment. Stubby recognized the scent of poisonous gas and barked when he detected it. He found lost or wounded men between the lines and led them back or barked until medics arrived. After capturing a German infiltrator by biting his leg and holding on, Stubby was promoted to sergeant. Wounded by shrapnel, he visited other patients in the hospital while convalescing. He served in 17 battles, won medals for bravery, and met three presidents. When Conroy went to law school at Georgetown after the war, Stubby came along to become the university's mascot. He died in 1926, and his preserved body is in the National Museum of American History in Washington, D.C.

Photos, from left: Gopher Hole Museum; National Museum of American History

Political Posers

Vladimir Ilich Lenin, father of the Soviet Revolution, died in 1924. His embalmed body rests under glass in a tomb in Moscow's Red Square, where scientists continue to work to halt its deterioration. According to Alexei Yurchak, a professor of social anthropology at the University of California-Berkeley, the Russians focus not on preserving the original body, but "substitute occasional parts of skin and flesh with plastics and other materials . . . so the body is less and less of what it used to be."

Soviet experts were also called in to preserve the bodies of Vietnam's Ho Chi Minh (d. 1969), who rests in a mausoleum in Hanoi, and father-and-son North Korean dictators Kim Il-Sung (d. 1994) and Kim Jong-Il (d. 2011) in Pyongyang.

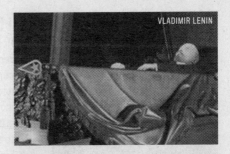

VLADIMIR LENIN

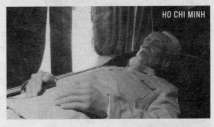

HO CHI MINH

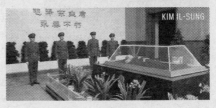

KIM IL-SUNG

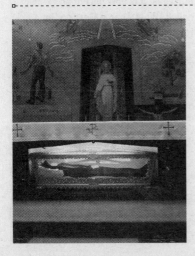

WHOLLY DEVOTED

For centuries, devout Catholics have believed that God has preserved unchanged the bodies of saints. One "incorruptible saint" is Mother Cabrini, the first American saint. Born in Italy, Sister Frances Cabrini (1850–1917) emigrated to America and worked tirelessly in the United States on behalf of her countrymen and -women who were struggling to assimilate. Her mummified remains are visible at her chapel in Manhattan (N.Y.). *(continued)*

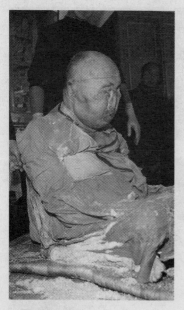

STILL LIFE

Dashi-Dorzho Itigilov, a Russian Buddhist monk who died in 1927, had ordered his followers to bury him exactly as he was found. They followed his instructions and interred him sitting up in the lotus position of meditation. When he was exhumed 30 years later, his body was still soft and flexible. Reinterred, his body was re-exhumed in 1973, with no changes evident. After extensive study, in 2002 his body was declared a Buddhist relic and placed in Russia's Ivolginsky monastery, where it may be seen seven times a year on Buddhist holidays.

Headmaster

Political philosopher and reformer Jeremy Bentham showed his commitment to Utilitarianism (a doctrine best summarized by his motto, "The greatest good for the greatest number") by leaving his body to the University of Edinburgh, where he taught. It can be seen today at University College London's student center, in a glass cabinet, stuffed with straw and clothed in 18th-century garments. The head on the body is not Bentham's; he had asked that it be removed from his body and mummified, but the result was so terrifying that it was replaced with a wax replica. The mummified head was placed in a box between his feet. Student pranksters once stole it and held it for ransom, which was duly paid and donated to charity, but the head was hidden away to prevent further outrages. It is now part of an exhibit called "What Does It Mean to Be Human? Curating Heads at UCL."

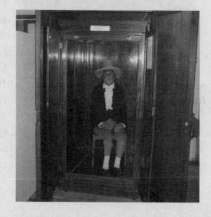

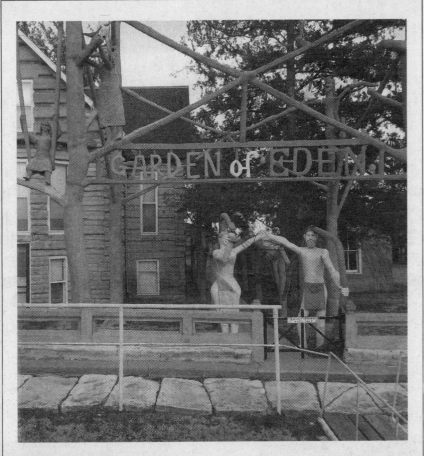

HOME AT LAST

Samuel P. Dinsmoor started building his "cabin home" in Lucas, Kansas, in 1907. After construction was done, he began developing his yard into a "Garden of Eden" full of unique sculptures. The project's *pièce de résistance* was a Dinsmoor-designed concrete coffin with glass top to be placed inside the house as the permanent resting place for his remains after his demise—which occurred in 1932. After the death of his wife Emilie in 1967, the site was opened to the public as a tourist attraction. It's now on the National Register of Historic Places and receives some 10,000 visitors a year who can meet the architect of the "Garden of Eden" face to face. ■

Tim Clark lives in Dublin, New Hampshire, with his wife and two dogs.

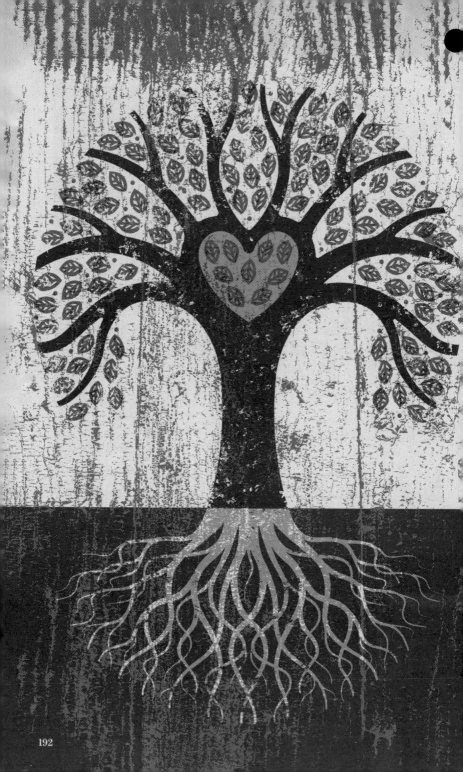

FINE-TUNE
YOUR FAMILY TREE

10 SIMPLE TIPS FOR DIGGING DOWN DEEP TO REACH ALL OF YOUR ROOTS

by the editors of *Family Tree* magazine

Whether you're an experienced genealogist or someone whose family tree still grows only in the imagination, these techniques for researching your past will ensure that your search is thorough and fun!

1. GATHER WHAT YOU ALREADY KNOW ABOUT YOUR FAMILY. Scour your basement, attic, and closets (and those of your family members!) and collect family records, old photos, letters, diaries, photocopies from family Bibles and religious books, even newspaper clippings.

2. TALK TO YOUR RELATIVES. Ask your parents, grandparents, aunts, and uncles about their memories. Don't ask just about facts and dates; get the stories of their growing up and of the ancestors whom they remember. Try to phrase questions with "why?," "how?," and "what?" Reach out to far-flung relatives to ask whether they have records that may be of help in your genealogy quest.

BEST CONVERSATION STARTERS:
Familytreemagazine.com/interviews

3. PUT IT ON "PAPER." Write down (physically or digitally) what you know so that you can decide what you don't yet know.

BEST WORKSHEETS:
Familytreemagazine.com/freeforms

4. FOCUS YOUR SEARCH. What are the blanks in your family tree? Don't try to fill them in all at once; focus on someone from the most recent generation where your chart is missing information. Try to answer that "mystery" first, then work backward in time.

BEST SEARCH TIPS:
Familytreemagazine.com/google

5. SEARCH THE INTERNET. The Internet is a terrific place to find leads and share information, but don't expect to "find your whole family tree" online. Check on whether your local library offers an Ancestry.com subscription free on its computers. You can also search many of the Web's biggest databases of names with one click by using "One-Step Webpages by Stephen Morse."

BEST DATABASE FOR ANCESTRY.COM OR FAMILYSEARCH.ORG:
stevemorse.org/ *(continued)*

6. EXPLORE SPECIFIC WEB SITES. Once you've searched for the surnames in your family, try Web sites specifically about your ethnic heritage or parts of the country where your relatives lived. You may even find Web sites about your family created by distant relatives researching the same family tree. A good place to start is with *Family Tree*'s international directory of more than 100 sources.

BEST DIRECTORY: Familytreemagazine.com/101websites

7. DISCOVER YOUR LOCAL FAMILY HISTORY CENTER. The Church of Jesus Christ of Latter-day Saints has more than 4,000 Family History Centers where anyone can tap the world's largest collection of genealogical information. Using your local center, you can view microfilm of records such as the birth, marriage, or death certificates of your ancestors. More than 2 million rolls of microfilmed records from all over the world are available. Compare the information in these sources with what you already know, fill in the blanks in your family tree, and look for clues to more answers to the puzzles of your past.

BEST FAMILY HISTORY CENTER SOURCE: Familysearch.org/locations/

8. ORGANIZE YOUR NEW INFORMATION. Enter your findings in family tree software programs or on paper charts. (Make sure that you note your sources!) File photocopies and notes by family, geography, or source so that you can refer to them easily. Decide what you want to focus on next.

BEST WAYS TO CITE SOURCES: Familytreemagazine.com/sources

9. PLAN YOUR NEXT STEP. Once you've exhausted your family sources, the Internet, and your Family History Center, you may want to travel to places where your ancestors lived to visit courthouses, churches, cemeteries, and other places where old records are kept. This is also a rewarding way to walk in the footsteps of your ancestors and bring your heritage to life. You'll find that the quest to discover where you came from is fun, as exciting as a detective story, and never-ending.

BEST SOURCE FOR DIGGING DEEPER: Pinterest.com/familytreemagazine/genealogy-for-beginners/

10. SHARE YOUR RESEARCH. Now that you've planted your family tree, show it off! Print family trees or start a family history Web site to share your research with loved ones. Looping others into your genealogy can help you to add more stories and family members to your research—not to mention that it's always exciting to learn more!

BEST PLACE TO PRINT FAMILY TREES: Familytreemagazine.com/print

Using the tips and links in this article should bring you not just a host of information, but also a great deal of satisfaction. Plus, your ancestors will be proud of you! ■

For more information about *Family Tree* magazine and all things genealogical, go to Familytreemagazine.com.

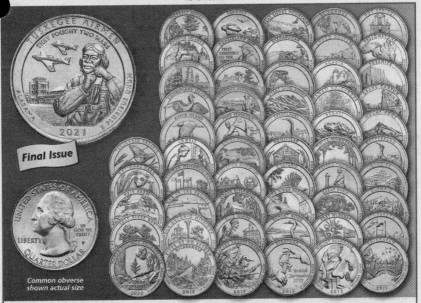
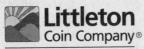

(continued from page 56)

PUT UP YOUR POTPOURRI

Use the ingredients in one of the recipes here while following these basic directions: Measure and gently mix all of the dry ingredients in a large, nonmetallic bowl (or paper bag). Scatter drops of essential oil(s) over the mixture, stirring (or shaking) gently until thoroughly blended. Fill a widemouthed glass or ceramic jar ¾ full, cover tightly, and store in a cool, dark place. Gently shake the jar every day to distribute the fragrance throughout the mixture. Check the fragrance after several days and add more oil(s), if desired. Let your nose be your guide. Cure for 2 to 6 weeks, then place the mixture in glass bowls or candy dishes.

After about 3 months, the scent of the potpourri will start to diminish. Revive it by adding small amounts of essential oil, as needed. Dry potpourri seldom keeps its true scent for longer than 2 years.

DRYING TIPS

All ingredients in a potpourri must be thoroughly dried. You don't need any fancy equipment—just air!

The secret to successfully air-drying *flowers and herbs* for maximum color retention is to dry them as quickly as possible. Gather bunches of flowers and herbs, tie them together with string in small bundles, and hang them upside down in a warm, dry, dark area—in an attic or empty closet or from the ceiling of an unused room. Air-drying times vary with the humidity, but most flowers and herbs will be dry enough to use within 7 to 15 days.

To prepare *citrus peels,* cut long, thin spirals of peel from whole fruit. Air-dry them on a baking sheet or inside a paper-towel–lined gift box for 10 to 15 days.

Using small *pinecones and evergreen sprigs?* Lay them flat on a baking sheet and dry them until the evergreen needles are brittle and the sap on the cones is dry to the touch—usually 2 to 3 weeks.

Essential Advice

Avoid essential oils sold in clear glass or plastic bottles; buy only those in amber or other dark glass bottles. Store them in a cool, dark place, well out of the reach of children.

Before using oils from already open bottles, place a drop on a paper towel, wait a minute or two, and then sniff to evaluate. As oils age, they lose their fragrance, generally in 1 to 3 years.

Never use powdered spices in your potpourri mixtures. They quickly lose their scent and stick to glass containers.

ESSENCE-OF-ROSE POTPOURRI

3 cups mixed rose petals (pink, yellow, rose, lavender, red)

1 cup small rose blossoms

1 cup small rose leaves

½ cup statice blossoms (white)

½ cup globe amaranth blossoms (white or pale pink)

¼ cup cut orrisroot*

10 drops rose oil*

MIXED FLOWER POTPOURRI

2 cups mixed rose petals

2 cups mixed herbs

1 cup lavender

2 cups mixed colorful blossoms

1 stick cinnamon, broken into small pieces

½ vanilla bean, chopped into small pieces

½ cup rosemary

½ cup cut orrisroot*

6 drops rose oil*

2 drops lavender oil*

2 drops carnation oil*

2 drops nutmeg oil*

1 drop lemon oil*

1 drop frankincense oil*

SPICY BLEND POTPOURRI

½ cup orange peel

½ cup lemon peel

2 cups mixed marigold petals, chamomile flowers, scented geranium leaves (lemon and orange), globe amaranth blossoms

¼ cup broken cinnamon sticks

¼ cup whole cloves

¼ cup whole allspice

¼ cup cut orrisroot*

8 to 10 drops orange oil*

WOODLAND POTPOURRI

½ cup bayberry leaves

½ cup globe amaranth blossoms

½ cup snipped balsam needles

½ cup miniature pinecones

½ cup rose hips

½ cup lemon verbena leaves

½ cup broken cinnamon sticks

¼ cup whole coriander

¼ cup juniper berries

¼ cup cut orrisroot*

8 to 10 drops evergreen oil*

YOUR OWN BLEND POTPOURRI

Create your own bewitching blends using almost anything from your flower or herb garden. Use this formula as a starting point:

4 cups mixed flower petals

2 cups herbs

1 cup whole or broken spices or citrus peel

¼ cup cut orrisroot*

10 to 15 drops essential oil* ∎

Orris Origins

Orrisroot is the dried and ground rhizome of several iris species, including *Iris pallida,* an eastern Mediterranean native (also known as zebra, sweet, or Dalmatian iris) that bears an especially fragrant flower. Dried orrisroot has been used since medieval times as a fragrance fixative as well as a perceived magical medicinal. Its oil is used as a flavoring agent.

Betty Earl is an author, photographer, and speaker. Her books include *Fairy Gardens: A Guide to Growing an Enchanted Miniature World* (B. B. Mackey, 2012) and the forthcoming *Enchanting Miniature Gardens: Captivating Ideas for Special Occasions* (B. B. Mackey).

(continued from page 72)

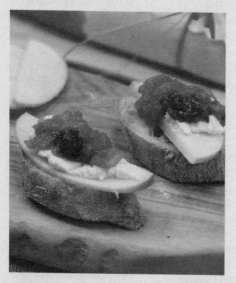

SPRING
RHUBARB CHUTNEY

Serve this tangy chutney alongside chicken or pork or as an appetizer with goat cheese and apples.

2 cups diced rhubarb
1 tart apple, peeled and chopped
½ cup raisins
½ cup brown sugar
¼ cup apple cider vinegar
1 tablespoon lemon juice
1 teaspoon ground ginger
½ teaspoon ground cumin

Combine all of the ingredients in a heavy, nonaluminum saucepan. Bring slowly to a boil, then reduce heat and simmer for 10 minutes, or until the rhubarb and apple are very soft but still hold their shape. Do not allow them to turn into mush. Taste and adjust seasonings. Cool and chill before serving.

Makes about 2½ cups.

SUMMER
TOMATO AND STRAWBERRY SALSA

Serve with tortilla chips or as an accompaniment to grilled fish, chicken, or pork.

1 pint (about 12 ounces) fresh strawberries, diced
1 pint (about 10 ounces) ripe cherry or grape tomatoes, diced
1 small or medium-size jalapeño pepper, seeded and minced
1 clove garlic, minced
½ cup diced red onion
½ cup loosely packed cilantro leaves, roughly chopped
¼ cup freshly squeezed lime juice
2 tablespoons honey
½ teaspoon kosher salt

In a bowl, combine all of the ingredients. Chill in the refrigerator before serving.

Makes about 3 cups.

(continued)

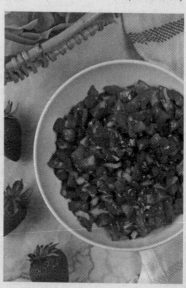

Photos: Samantha Jones/Quinn Brein Communications

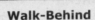
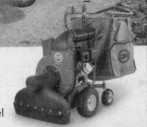
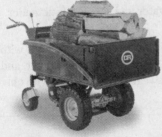

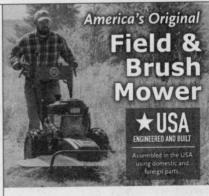
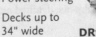

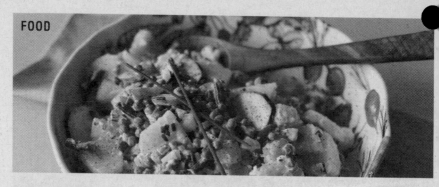

GARDEN PATCH POTATO SALAD

Serve this salad at room temperature or after chilling in the refrigerator.

1 cup fresh green
 beans, trimmed
5 small potatoes,
 peeled
1 cup fresh or frozen
 green peas
½ cup thinly sliced
 zucchini
½ cup thinly sliced
 carrot
¼ cup finely chopped
 onion
¾ cup mayonnaise
1½ teaspoons salt
⅛ teaspoon freshly
 ground black pepper
chives, for garnish

In a pot of salted water, simmer green beans until just tender and bright green, about 3 to 5 minutes. Reserving the cooking liquid, remove beans and transfer to a bowl of ice water to stop cooking, then drain.

Add potatoes to cooking water and simmer until tender, about 12 minutes. Remove potatoes with a slotted spoon, then slice them.

Add peas to cooking water and simmer until tender, about 2 to 3 minutes.

In a bowl, combine zucchini, carrots, and onions with beans, potatoes, and peas. Add mayonnaise, salt, and pepper and stir to coat vegetables. Garnish with chives.

Makes 8 servings. ■

(continued from page 78)

HONORABLE MENTION
CHICKPEA, ORZO, RAISIN, AND CARROT SALAD IN FIG BALSAMIC VINEGAR

1 can (15 ounces) chickpeas, drained and rinsed
1 cup cooked orzo
1 cup freshly grated carrots
⅓ cup fig balsamic vinegar
¼ cup raisins (softened in warm water if hard)
2 grinds fresh black pepper
¼ teaspoon salt

In a large bowl, combine all ingredients.

Place in the refrigerator and chill for at least 1 hour.

Makes 4 to 6 servings.

*–Susan Skrtich,
Hamilton, Ontario* ■

Photo: Samantha Jones/Quinn Brein Communications

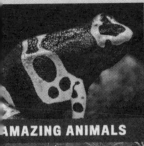

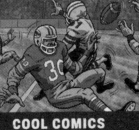
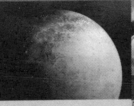
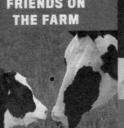
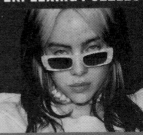

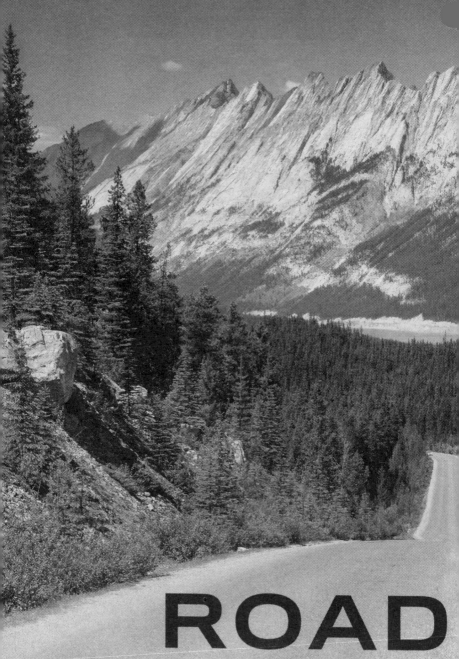

ROAD

Our Trans-Canada Highway is long not just in kilometers but

TRIP

also in fun trivia and fascinating facts. • *by Sandy Newton*

P eople say that our national road is not celebrated quite as romantically as our great Canadian Pacific Railway; with no last spike to drive, the route just had a patch of asphalt to roll. Nevertheless, the highway has an undeniable pull. If you've got the urge for going but not the time, you can be "Goin' Down the Road" right here—even if you weren't a part of that famous 1970 film.

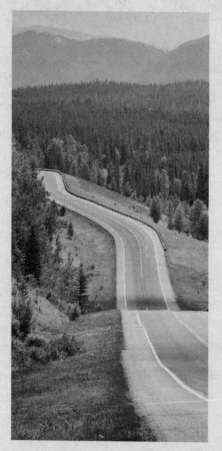

WHEN "IT" IS NOT AN "IT"

The first thing to know about the TCH is that "it" is not an "it." Ours is not a single national highway but a network of bits and strips. Nor is "Canada's Main Street" overseen by a national department. Instead, each province takes care of the pieces inside its borders.

Completing the highway— which meant connecting existing roads to purpose-built sections— did require federal legislation (Trans-Canada Highway Act, 1949) and financing. After construction began in 1950, the highway grew organically before opening in 1962, as it branched out with this-way-or-that-way choices (there are southern and northern Ontario routes, for example) to eventually become a network.

In 1970, it connected to the northwest as well, when the Yellowhead Highway (Highway 16, between Portage la Prairie and Prince Rupert) was added.

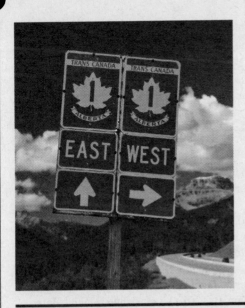

ROUTE WORDS

Because of how it was made, the TCH is not known by the same name all across the country. Depending on where you are, you might hear (or read) Highway Number One, Highway 17 or 69 or 401 (or more), the TCH, the Island Highway, the T CAN, Autoroute 20 or 85. Where the route still runs through a downtown, most locals probably use a street name for it—New Gower in St. John's, for example, or Portage Avenue in Winnipeg.

JUST PASSING THROUGH

Why did the wolf and the elk cross the road? Because they could do it without getting killed, thanks to overpasses and underpasses built specifically for wildlife where the Trans-Canada runs through two national parks (Banff and Yoho). Parks Canada has built 42 underpasses and seven overpasses in these two western parks, which have drastically reduced wildlife deaths on the highway. Some spots have protective fencing, as well. *(continued)*

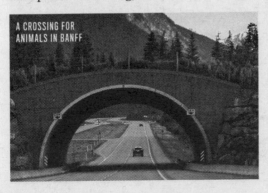

A CROSSING FOR ANIMALS IN BANFF

HIGHWAY 1 BY THE NUMBERS

6: number of time zones spanned

10: number of provinces passed through

1962: year the road was finished, east coast to west coast

1971: year the road was all paved, coast to coast

7,821: number of kilometers in the east-west portion

12,800: total kilometers for the whole network

S'NO JOKE

In the snowiest mountain passes, how do you protect a national artery from an avalanche blockage? By building "snow sheds" over the road where avalanches occur, so that the white torrents can flow harmlessly over the top. Sometimes the action is proactive, too—with an explosion to trigger the big event.

FROM ZERO TO ZERO

Both ends of the highway—one in St. John's, the other in Victoria—claim a "Mile 0," which is how the starts were styled before Canada went metric.

On the island of Newfoundland, the official spot is noted outside the St. John's city hall with a sign that is mere steps from Mile One Centre, the stadium named for the first stretch of highway. In B.C., there is a Mile Zero monument in Beacon Hill Park, at the foot of Douglas Street.

But wait! There's also a sign announcing the "Pacific Terminus of the Trans-Canada Highway" in Tofino, B.C. This bit of wishful thinking dates in concept to 1912, when the town dreamed that it would be the western terminus of a future highway (the first sign went up in the 1950s). Decades later, more isolated Tofino lost out to the better connected Victoria.

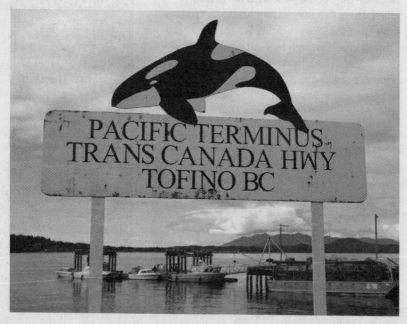

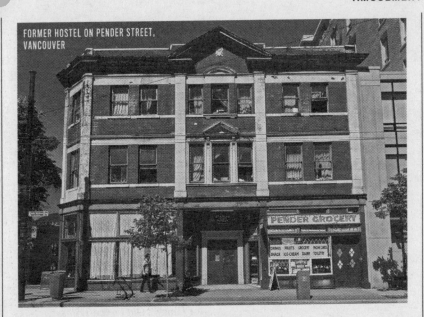

FORMER HOSTEL ON PENDER STREET, VANCOUVER

HITCHHIKING'S HEYDAYS

In the late 1960s, many young people found the lure of our new coast-to-coast road irresistible. Summertime hitchhiking flourished, so the government, led by erstwhile hitchhiker PM Pierre Elliott Trudeau, created a chain of hostels (some in empty military barracks) across the country to provide youthful wanderers with cheap and safe places to sleep.

Ottawa also printed *On the Road,* a brochure filled with tips such as "Don't hitchhike on a bridge" and "Carry a large sign." The government even erected a series of kiosks shaped like tepees along the highway's edge to offer the explorers advice, water, and free phone calls.

THE HIGHS AND LOWS

The highest point in the TCH is at Alberta's Kicking Horse Pass: 1,627 meters above sea level. And as you might expect of a coast-to-coast highway, the pavement ends within a few meters of sea level on each coast.

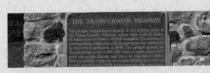

ARE WE THERE YET?

The midpoint of the original east–west Trans-Canada route is marked on Highway 17, north of Sault Ste. Marie near Chippewa Falls, Ontario. A historic plaque notes the spot. *(continued)*

Photos, from top: Michael Wels/Getty Images; OntarioPlaques.com

FOR THE RECORD BOOKS

The Trans-Canada Highway itself claims many honors, including:

WORLD'S LONGEST BRIDGE OVER ICY WATERS: The Confederation Bridge connects New Brunswick and Prince Edward Island across 12.9 kilometers of Canada's sometimes ice-covered Northumberland Strait.

CANADA'S LONGEST BRIDGE-TUNNEL: The Louis-Hippolyte Lafontaine Tunnel-Bridge traverses the St. Lawrence River at Montreal/Longueuil. Its underwater portion is about 1.4 kilometers long.

SECOND LONGEST NATIONAL HIGHWAY: We finish behind Australia, whose Highway 1 stretches 14,500 kilometers.

Many have claimed their own TCH fame for feats such as:

FASTEST BIKE TRIP: Arvid Loewen, a grandfather from Winnipeg, set the Guinness Book of Records mark in 2011 when he pedaled the TCH from Halifax to Vancouver in 13 days, 6 hours, 13 minutes. He has tried to beat this record three times—unsuccessfully.

FEWEST FILL-UPS: In 2012, to celebrate the highway's 50th birthday, one car drove from St. John's to Victoria on no gas. It was an electric car, of course—and the team claimed that it was the first to cross the country via the TCH using only public charging stations.

MAKING "REAL" RECORDS: A few songsters have worked the TCH into their lyrics (notably our own Neil Young in 1985 with "Bound for Glory": *Out on the Trans-Canada Highway / There was a girl / hitchhiking with her dog / Fireflies buzzin' 'round her head / like candles in the fog*), but we can thank American Gene Pitney for recording the rockin' "Trans-Canada Highway" in 1974. ∎

ROAD TEST

1. Long before the official TCH was complete, Brigadier R. A. Macfarlane drove from Louisburg (NS) to Victoria (BC) in 9 days. In what year?

2. Name the causeway that joins Cape Breton to mainland Nova Scotia and was created as part of the TCH project. It opened in 1955.

3. What percentage of the TCH was gravel when it officially opened in 1962?

4. Why is TCH signage on a green (not red) maple leaf?

ANSWERS: **1.** 1946, in a Chevrolet Stylemaster sedan. **2.** Canso Causeway. **3.** 50 percent. **4.** The green maple leaf was chosen before the red one showed up on our national flag.

Sandy Newton is a regular contributor to the Almanac who lives on the island of Newfoundland, the eastern terminus of the Trans-Canada Highway.

HOW WE PREDICT THE WEATHER

We derive our weather forecasts from a secret formula that was devised by the founder of this Almanac, Robert B. Thomas, in 1792. Thomas believed that weather on Earth was influenced by sunspots, which are magnetic storms on the surface of the Sun.

Over the years, we have refined and enhanced this formula with state-of-the-art technology and modern scientific calculations. We employ three scientific disciplines to make our long-range predictions: solar science, the study of sunspots and other solar activity; climatology, the study of prevailing weather patterns; and meteorology, the study of the atmosphere. We predict weather trends and events by comparing solar patterns and historical weather conditions with current solar activity.

Our forecasts emphasize temperature and precipitation deviations from averages, or normals. These are based on 30-year statistical averages prepared by government meteorological agencies and updated every 10 years. Our forecasts are based on the tabulations that span the period 1981 through 2010.

The borders of the provincial weather regions (page 210) are based primarily on climatology and the movement of weather systems. For example, while both Ottawa and Toronto are in Ontario, we place Ottawa in Region 2 rather than Region 3 (Toronto) because its weather trends more closely resemble those of other locales in Region 2.

We believe that nothing in the universe happens haphazardly, that there is a cause-and-effect pattern to all phenomena.

However, although neither we nor any other forecasters have as yet gained sufficient insight into the mysteries of the universe to predict the weather with total accuracy, our results are almost always very close to our traditional claim of 80%.

WEATHER

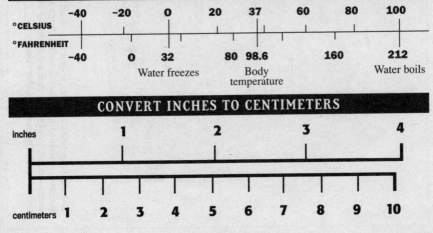

CONVERT FAHRENHEIT TO CELSIUS

°CELSIUS: −40, −20, 0, 20, 37, 60, 80, 100
°FAHRENHEIT: −40, 0, 32, 80, 98.6, 160, 212

32 Water freezes 98.6 Body temperature 212 Water boils

CONVERT INCHES TO CENTIMETERS

inches: 1, 2, 3, 4
centimeters: 1, 2, 3, 4, 5, 6, 7, 8, 9, 10

WEATHER REGIONS

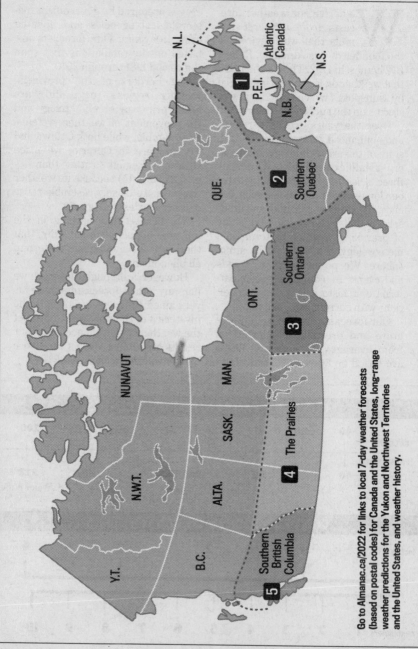

N.L.

Atlantic Canada

N.S.

1

P.E.I.

N.B.

QUE.

2

Southern Quebec

Southern Ontario

ONT.

3

NUNAVUT

MAN.

The Prairies

SASK.

4

N.W.T.

ALTA.

Southern British Columbia

B.C.

Y.T.

5

Go to Almanac.ca/2022 for links to local 7-day weather forecasts (based on postal codes) for Canada and the United States, long-range weather predictions for the Yukon and Northwest Territories and the United States, and weather history.

WEATHER

Illustrations of Canadian map and regional maps 1-5: Rob Schuster

ATLANTIC CANADA

SUMMARY: Winter temperatures will be above normal in the north and near normal in the south, with the coldest periods in early to mid- and late January and early to mid- and late February. Precipitation will be below normal in the north and above in the south. Snowfall will be below normal in the east and above in the west, with the snowiest periods in early and mid-December, early to mid- and mid- to late January, and mid-March. **April** and **May** will have near-normal temperatures and be drier than normal. **Summer** will be warmer and rainier than normal. The hottest periods will be in late July and mid- to late August. **September** and **October** will have near-normal temperatures and be rainier than normal. Watch for hurricane threats in early and mid-October.

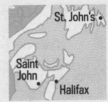

NOV. 2021: Temp. 1°C (2°C below avg.); precip. 80mm (60mm below avg.). 1–4 Rainy periods, mild. 5–12 Snow showers, cold. 13–20 Rain, then sunny north; sunny south; mild, then cold. 21–27 Rainy, mild, then snow showers, cold. 28–30 Sunny, cold.

DEC. 2021: Temp. –3°C (avg.); precip. 120mm (10mm below avg.). 1–4 Heavy rain to snow. 5–10 Rain and snow showers. 11–14 Rain to snow, then flurries, cold. 15–19 Heavy rain to snow, then flurries. 20–24 Heavy rain to wet snow. 25–29 Snow showers, cold. 30–31 Rainy north, flurries south.

JAN. 2022: Temp. –6.5°C (1°C above avg. north, 2°C below south); precip. 150mm (30mm below avg. north, 90mm above south). 1–4 Heavy rain north, snow south. 5–9 Rain, then flurries, cold. 10–13 Flurries north, snowstorm south. 14–18 Rain to snow north, sunny south. 19–23 Snowstorm. 24–31 Flurries east, snowy periods west; cold.

FEB. 2022: Temp. –4.5°C (2°C above avg.); precip. 75mm (25mm below avg.). 1–5 Flurries, milder. 6–13 Snowy periods, cold. 14–18 Rain and wet snow, then sunny, cold. 19–22 Rain and snow south, flurries north. 23–28 Snow showers, turning cold.

MAR. 2022: Temp. –1°C (2°C above avg.); precip. 130mm (20mm below avg. north, 40mm above south). 1–6 Sunny, turning mild. 7–12 Rain and snow showers. 13–19 Snowy periods, some heavy. 20–24 Showers, mild. 25–31 Rainy periods, cool.

APR. 2022: Temp. 4°C (avg.); precip. 50mm (60mm below avg.). 1–8 Rain and snow showers, cold. 9–10 Showers north, snowy periods south; cool. 11–16 Showers north, sunny south; turning warm. 17–20 Rain and snow showers, cool. 21–30 A few showers, cool.

MAY 2022: Temp. 9.5°C (avg.); precip. 100mm (10mm above avg.). 1–10 Rainy periods, cool. 11–15 Sunny, warm. 16–23 Showers, turning cool. 24–31 Showers; warm, then cool.

JUNE 2022: Temp. 14.5°C (avg.); precip. 120mm (10mm below avg. northwest, 50mm above southeast). 1–7 Showers; turning hot north, cool south. 8–18 Scattered showers, cool. 19–26 Isolated showers, warm. 27–30 Showers, cool.

JULY 2022: Temp. 19°C (1°C above avg.); precip. 185mm (40mm above avg.). 1–6 Sunny, cool. 7–12 Scattered showers, warm. 13–21 A few showers, mild. 22–31 Scattered showers, turning hot.

AUG. 2022: Temp. 19°C (1°C above avg.); precip. 115mm (avg. north, 50mm above south). 1–5 Sunny, turning cool. 6–16 A few showers, warm. 17–24 Scattered showers, turning hot. 25–31 A few showers, cooler.

SEPT. 2022: Temp. 13°C (1°C below avg.); precip. 190mm (50mm above avg. north, 120mm above south). 1–4 Sunny, cool. 5–9 Rainy, cool. 10–20 Showers, cool. 21–30 Rainy periods, mild.

OCT. 2022: Temp. 9.5°C (1°C above avg.); precip. 90mm (30mm below avg.). 1–2 Showers. 3–5 Hurricane threat. 6–10 A few showers, mild. 11–18 Rainy periods, cool. 19–22 Hurricane threat. 23–31 Sunny; cool, then mild.

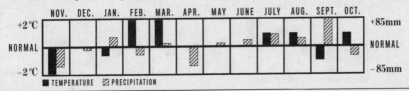

SOUTHERN QUEBEC

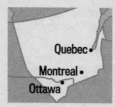

Quebec

Montreal

Ottawa

SUMMARY: Winter temperatures will be slightly above normal in the east and below normal in the west, with the coldest periods in early and mid- to late December; early, mid-, and late January; and mid- to late February. Precipitation will be above normal, with snowfall above normal in the east and below normal in the west. The snowiest periods will be in mid-December, early January, and mid-February. **April** and **May** will be warmer and drier than normal. **Summer** will be slightly cooler as well as rainier than normal, with the hottest periods in mid-July and mid- to late August. **September** and **October** will be cooler and rainier than normal.

NOV. 2021: Temp. –1°C (2°C below avg.); precip. 50mm (30mm below avg.). 1–7 Snow showers, cold. 8–13 Rainy periods, mild. 14–19 Flurries, cold. 20–30 Rain and wet snow, then snow showers, cold.

DEC. 2021: Temp. –9°C (3°C below avg. east, 30mm below west). 1–8 Snow showers, cold. 9–18 Snow showers; mild, then cold. 19–25 Snow, then flurries, cold. 26–31 Snow showers, milder.

JAN. 2022: Temp. –11.5°C (1°C above avg. east, 3°C below west); precip. 105mm (30mm above avg.). 1–3 Snow showers, cold. 4–12 Snowstorm, then flurries, very cold. 13–18 Sunny; mild east, cold west. 19–27 Snowy periods, cold. 28–31 Flurries, cold.

FEB. 2022: Temp. –7°C (2°C above avg.); precip. 70mm (10mm above avg.). 1–8 Snow showers, turning mild. 9–17 Rain and snow showers, mild. 18–21 Snowstorm, then showers, mild. 22–25 Sunny, cold. 26–28 Rain and snow, mild.

MAR. 2022: Temp. –1.5°C (3°C above avg.); precip. 85mm (20mm below avg. east, 40mm above west). 1–10 Showers, warm. 11–19 Snow showers, cold. 20–25 Showers, mild. 26–31 Rain and wet snow, chilly.

APR. 2022: Temp. 6°C (1°C above avg.); precip. 40mm (50mm below avg. east, avg. west). 1–6 Flurries, then sunny, turning warm. 7–13 Showers, then sunny, warm.

14–23 Showers; warm, then cool. 24–30 Scattered showers, cool.

MAY 2022: Temp. 13.5°C (0.5°C above avg.); precip. 55mm (10mm below avg.). 1–4 Showers, cool. 5–11 Showers; cool east, turning hot west. 12–19 Scattered showers, warm. 20–31 Scattered showers, cool.

JUNE 2022: Temp. 18°C (1°C below avg.); precip. 90mm (avg.). 1–9 Scattered showers, turning warm. 10–18 Sunny east, a few showers west; cool. 19–30 Scattered showers, warm.

JULY 2022: Temp. 20°C (avg.); precip. 130mm (30mm above avg.). 1–3 Sunny, warm. 4–11 Scattered t-storms, warm. 12–15 T-storms, hot. 16–22 A few t-storms east, sunny west; warm. 23–31 Scattered t-storms, warm.

AUG. 2022: Temp. 18°C (1°C below avg.); precip. 130mm (30mm above avg.). 1–11 T-storms, then a few showers, cool. 12–19 Scattered t-storms, cool. 20–26 A few showers, turning hot. 27–31 Showers, cool.

SEPT. 2022: Temp. 12°C (2°C below avg.); precip. 130mm (40mm above avg.). 1–6 Scattered showers, cool. 7–13 Sunny east, a few showers west, turning warm. 14–19 Showers, cool. 20–30 Rainy periods, cool.

OCT. 2022: Temp. 9°C (1°C above avg.); precip. 90mm (10mm above avg.). 1–12 A few showers, cool. 13–18 Sunny, turning mild. 19–22 Showers, warm. 23–28 Sunny, warm. 29–31 Showers.

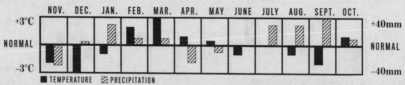

QUÉBEC DU SUD

RÉSUMÉ: L'hiver sera légèrement plus chaud que la normale à l'est et plus froid que la normale à l'ouest. Les périodes les plus froides seront le début et de la mi à la fin décembre et tout le mois de janvier jusqu'à la mi à fin février. Les précipitations seront supérieures à la normale. Les chutes de neige seront supérieures à la normale à l'est et inférieures à la normale à l'ouest. Les périodes les plus neigeuses seront la mi-décembre, début janvier, et mi-février. **Avril** et **mai** seront plus chauds et secs que la normale. **L'été** sera légèrement plus frais que la normale et plus pluvieux. Les périodes les plus chaudes seront la mi-juillet et de la mi à la fin août. **Septembre** et **octobre** seront plus frais et pluvieux que la normale.

NOV. 2021: Temp. −1°C (2°C en dessous de la moy.); précip. 50mm (30mm en dessous de la moy.). 1–7 Chutes de neige, froid. 8–13 Périodes pluvieuses, doux. 14–19 Rafales, froid. 20–30 Pluie et neige mouillée, puis chutes de neige, froid.

DÉC. 2021: Temp. −9°C (3°C en dessous de la moy.); précip. 85mm (40mm au-dessus de la moy. à l'est, 30mm en dessous à l'ouest). 1–8 Chutes de neige, froid. 9–18 Chutes de neige; doux, puis froid. 19–25 Neige, puis rafales, froid. 26–31 Chutes de neige, plus doux.

JAN. 2022: Temp. −11,5°C (1°C au-dessus de la moy. à l'est, 3°C en dessous à l'ouest); précip. 105mm (30mm au-dessus de la moy.). 1–3 Chutes de neige, froid. 4–12 Tempête de neige, puis rafales, très froid. 13–18 Ensoleillé; doux à l'est, froid à l'ouest. 19–27 Périodes de neige, froid. 28–31 Rafales, froid.

FÉV. 2022: Temp. −7°C (2°C au-dessus de la moy.); précip. 70mm (10mm au-dessus de la moy.). 1–8 Chutes de neige, devenant doux. 9–17 Pluie et chutes de neige, doux. 18–21 Tempêtes de neige, puis averses, doux. 22–25 Ensoleillé, froid. 26–28 Pluie et neige, doux.

MARS 2022: Temp. −1,5°C (3°C au-dessus de la moy. à l'est, 40mm au-dessus à l'ouest). 1–10 Averses, chaud. 11–19 Chutes de neige, froid. 20–25 Averses, doux. 26–31 Pluie et neige mouillée, très frais.

AVR. 2022: Temp. 6°C (1°C au-dessus de la moy.); précip. 40mm (50mm en dessous de la moy. à l'est, moy. à l'ouest). 1–6 Rafales, puis ensoleillé, devenant chaud. 7–13 Averses, puis ensoleillé, chaud. 14–23 Averses; chaud, puis frais. 24–30 Averses éparses, frais.

MAI 2022: Temp. 13,5°C (0,5°C au-dessus de la moy.); précip. 55mm (10mm en dessous de la moy.). 1–4 Averses, frais. 5–11 Averses; frais à l'est, devenant très chaud à l'ouest. 12–19 Averses éparses, chaud. 20–31 Averses éparses, frais.

JUIN 2022: Temp. 18°C (1°C en dessous de la moy.); précip. 90mm (moy.). 1–9 Averses éparses, devenant chaud. 10–18 Ensoleillé à l'est, quelques averses à l'ouest; frais. 19–30 Averses éparses, chaud.

JUIL. 2022: Temp. 20°C (moy.); précip. 130mm (30mm au-dessus de la moy.). 1–3 Ensoleillé, chaud. 4–11 Orages épars, chaud. 12–15 Orages, très chaud. 16–22 Quelques orages à l'est, ensoleillé à l'ouest; chaud. 23–31 Orages épars, chaud.

AOÛT 2022: Temp. 18°C (1°C en dessous de la moy.); précip. 130mm (30mm au-dessus de la moy.). 1–11 Orages, puis quelques averses, frais. 12–19 Orages épars, frais. 20–26 Quelques averses, devenant chaud. 27–31 Averses, frais.

SEPT. 2022: Temp. 12°C (2°C en dessous de la moy.); précip. 130mm (40mm au-dessus de la moy.). 1–6 Averses éparses, frais. 7–13 Ensoleillé à l'est, quelques averses à l'ouest, devenant chaud. 14–19 Averses, frais. 20–30 Périodes pluvieuses, frais.

OCT. 2022: Temp. 9°C (1°C au-dessus de la moy.); précip. 90mm (10mm au-dessus de la moy.). 1–12 Quelques averses, frais. 13–18 Ensoleillé, devenant doux. 19–22 Averses, chaud. 23–28 Ensoleillé, chaud. 29–31 Averses.

SOUTHERN ONTARIO

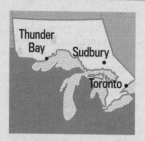

SUMMARY: Winter will be colder than normal, with above-normal precipitation and below-normal snowfall. The coldest periods will be in late November, mid- to late December, and much of January, with the snowiest periods in mid- to late November, early December, and early January. **April** and **May** will be warmer and rainier than normal. **Summer** will be cooler and rainier than normal, with the hottest periods in early to mid-July and mid- to late August. **September** and **October** will be warmer and rainier than normal.

NOV. 2021: Temp. –2°C (4°C below avg.); precip. 55mm (20mm below avg.). 1–6 Snow showers, cold. 7–11 Showers east, sunny west; milder. 12–19 Snow showers, cold. 20–30 Snow, then flurries, very cold.

DEC. 2021: Temp. –7°C (3°C below avg.); precip. 50mm (10mm below avg.). 1–2 Flurries, cold. 3–7 Rain, then snow showers east; snowstorm, then flurries west; mild, then cold. 8–13 Rain and snow showers, mild. 14–21 Flurries, cold. 22–31 Snow showers; very cold, then milder.

JAN. 2022: Temp. –11°C (4°C below avg.); precip. 100mm (20mm above avg.). 1–3 Flurries, very cold. 4–7 Snow, heavy east, then flurries; very cold. 8–16 Snow showers, cold. 17–20 Flurries, mild. 21–31 Snow showers, cold.

FEB. 2022: Temp. –4°C (1°C above avg.); precip. 90mm (30mm above avg.). 1–7 Showers, mild. 8–13 Sunny; cold, then mild. 14–19 Showers east, snowy periods west. 20–28 Rain and snow showers east, flurries west; mild.

MAR. 2022: Temp. 3°C (3°C above avg.); precip. 85mm (30mm above avg.). 1–10 Rainy periods, mild. 11–19 Snow showers east, sunny west; cold. 20–24 Rainy periods, mild. 25–31 Rainy periods, mild east; snow showers, cold west.

APR. 2022: Temp. 10°C (3°C above avg.); precip. 75mm (10mm above avg.). 1–4 Sunny, cool. 5–11 Scattered showers; warm, then cooler. 12–15 Showers, warm. 16–20 T-storms, then rainy, cool east; sunny, mild west. 21–30 A few showers; cool, then warm.

MAY 2022: Temp. 14.5°C (2°C above avg.); precip. 75mm (avg.). 1–5 Sunny, cool. 6–15 Scattered showers, warm. 16–22 T-storms, then sunny, warm. 23–31 A few showers, cool.

JUNE 2022: Temp. 16.5°C (1°C below avg.); precip. 110mm (30mm above avg.). 1–9 Isolated showers, cool. 10–16 T-storms, then sunny, warm. 17–24 Scattered t-storms, warm. 25–30 A few t-storms, warm.

JULY 2022: Temp. 22.5°C (avg.); precip. 100mm (60mm above avg. east, 20mm below west). 1–5 Scattered t-storms, cool. 6–14 Isolated t-storms, hot. 15–17 Sunny, warm. 18–21 T-storms, then sunny, cool. 22–31 A few t-storms, warm.

AUG. 2022: Temp. 19°C (1°C below avg.); precip. 110mm (avg. east, 60mm above west). 1–5 A few t-storms, warm. 6–19 Scattered showers, cool. 20–27 A few t-storms, hot. 28–31 Scattered showers, cool.

SEPT. 2022: Temp. 16°C (1°C above avg.); precip. 170mm (80mm above avg.). 1–4 T-storms, then sunny, cool. 5–14 A few t-storms, cool. 15–25 Rainy periods, mild. 26–30 Sunny, cool.

OCT. 2022: Temp. 11°C (avg. east, 2°C above west); precip. 65mm (10mm below avg.). 1–5 Rainy periods, cool. 6–10 Sunny, cool. 11–17 Showers, cool east; sunny, mild west. 18–31 A few showers; cool, then mild east; mild west.

WEATHER

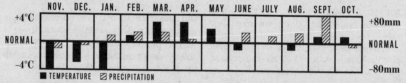

THE PRAIRIES

SUMMARY: Winter will have above-normal temperatures and precipitation, with below-normal snowfall. The coldest periods will be from late December to early January and in mid- to late January, with the snowiest periods in late November, mid-January, and early March. **April** and **May** will be warmer and rainier than normal. **Summer** will be cooler than normal, with the hottest period in mid-July. Rainfall will be below normal in the east and above normal in the west. **September** and **October** will be warmer and rainier than normal.

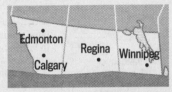

WEATHER

NOV. 2021: Temp. –2.5°C (2°C below avg. east, 3°C above west); precip. 20mm (5mm above avg.). 1–8 Sunny, turning cool. 9–13 Sunny, mild. 14–22 Snow showers, turning cold. 23–30 Snow showers; mild, then cold.

DEC. 2021: Temp. –9°C (2°C below avg. east, 2°C above west); precip. 30mm (15mm above avg.). 1–5 Snow showers; cold east, turning mild west. 6–11 Sunny, mild. 12–20 Flurries; cold, then mild. 21–31 Snow showers, turning very cold.

JAN. 2022: Temp. –13.5°C (3°C below avg. east, 2°C above west); precip. 40mm (20mm above avg.). 1–9 Snow showers, frigid. 10–19 Snow, then sunny, mild. 20–28 Snow showers; frigid, then mild. 29–31 Sunny; cold east, mild west.

FEB. 2022: Temp. –5°C (6°C above avg.); precip. 15mm (avg.). 1–2 Sunny, mild. 3–7 Sunny east; snow, then sunny west; mild. 8–19 Flurries east, sunny west; mild. 20–28 Flurries; cold, then mild east; mild west.

MAR. 2022: Temp. –2°C (2°C above avg.); precip. 10mm (10mm below avg.). 1–7 Sunny east; snow, then flurries west; mild. 8–16 Snow showers, cold. 17–22 Flurries, mild. 23–31 Rain and snow showers, turning mild.

APR. 2022: Temp. 10°C (5°C above avg.); precip. 35mm (5mm above avg.). 1–8 Sunny, warm. 9–15 Scattered showers, cooler. 16–20 Sunny, warm. 21–25 Showers, turning cooler. 26–30 Rainy periods, cool.

MAY 2022: Temp. 14.5°C (6°C above avg. east, 1°C above west); precip. 80mm (30mm above avg.). 1–8 Scattered t-storms, warm. 9–14 Rainy periods, cool. 15–20 Scattered showers, turning warm. 21–31 T-storms, then sunny, turning warm.

JUNE 2022: Temp. 15.5°C (avg.); precip. 60mm (20mm below avg.). 1–9 Scattered t-storms, turning cool. 10–16 Scattered showers; cool east, warm west. 17–24 A few showers, cool. 25–30 Sunny, warm east; showers, cool west.

JULY 2022: Temp. 17.5°C (1°C below avg.); precip. 85mm (10mm above avg.). 1–9 A few showers, cool. 10–21 Isolated t-storms, warm. 22–31 A few showers, cool.

AUG. 2022: Temp. 15°C (2°C below avg.); precip. 80mm (avg. east, 40mm above west). 1–6 A few showers, cool. 7–18 Sunny east, showers west; cool. 19–22 Sunny, cool. 23–31 Showers and a t-storm, cool.

SEPT. 2022: Temp. 10°C (1°C below avg.); precip. 65mm (25mm above avg.). 1–7 Scattered showers, cool. 8–14 A few showers; mild east, cool west. 15–20 Showers, cool. 21–30 Sunny east, a few showers west; cool.

OCT. 2022: Temp. 9°C (3°C above avg.); precip. 25mm (avg.). 1–3 Showers, cool. 4–13 Sunny, turning mild. 14–22 Showers, then sunny, mild. 23–31 A few showers east, sunny west; mild, then colder.

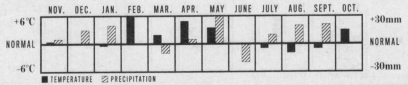

SOUTHERN BRITISH COLUMBIA

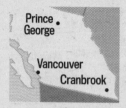

Prince George •

Vancouver •
Cranbrook •

SUMMARY: Winter will be warmer and drier than normal, with below-normal snowfall. The coldest period will be from late December into early January, with the snowiest periods in late November, late December, and early January. **April** and **May** will have near-normal temperatures and be rainier than normal. **Summer** will be warmer and rainier than normal, with the hottest periods in mid- and late July and from early to mid-August. **September** and **October** will have near-normal temperatures and be rainier than normal.

NOV. 2021: Temp. 6°C (1°C above avg.); precip. 110mm (40mm below avg.). 1–6 Showery, mild. 7–18 Rainy coast, rain and snow showers inland; mild. 19–25 Sunny, cool. 26–30 Rain coast, snow inland; cool.

DEC. 2021: Temp. 4°C (2°C above avg.); precip. 160mm (50mm above avg. north, 30mm below south). 1–11 Rainy periods, mild. 12–13 Sunny, cold. 14–18 Misty coast, rain and snow showers inland; mild. 19–26 Rain, then sunny, cold. 27–31 Snow showers, cold.

JAN. 2022: Temp. 0°C (1°C below avg.); precip. 185mm (15mm below avg.). 1–6 Periods of rain and snow coast, snow showers inland; cold. 7–12 Snow showers north, rainy periods south; mild. 13–23 Sunny; mild north, cold south. 24–31 Showers, mild coast; sunny, cold inland.

FEB. 2022: Temp. 4.5°C (7°C above avg. north, 2°C above south); precip. 120mm (20mm below avg.). 1–16 Showers coast, flurries inland; mild. 17–26 Flurries, mild north; showers, cool south. 27–28 Rainy coast, snow showers inland.

MAR. 2022: Temp. 4°C (avg.); precip. 110mm (10mm below avg.). 1–5 Showers coast, snow showers inland; mild. 6–20 Rainy periods coast, flurries inland; cool. 21–31 Sunny, turning mild.

APR. 2022: Temp. 9°C (1°C above avg.); precip. 115mm (40mm above avg. east, 10mm below west). 1–12 Rainy periods, cool. 13–18 Sunny, warm. 19–24 A few showers, mild. 25–30 Rainy periods, cool.

MAY 2022: Temp. 11°C (1°C below avg.); precip. 120mm (30mm above avg.). 1–10 A few showers, cool. 11–14 Sunny, mild. 15–20 Rainy periods, cool. 21–29 Showers, cool. 30–31 Sunny, warm.

JUNE 2022: Temp. 15°C (avg.); precip. 70mm (10mm below avg.). 1–13 Sunny coast, a few showers inland; mild. 14–20 Scattered showers, cool coast; sunny, warm inland. 21–25 Showers north, sunny south; cool. 26–30 A few showers, cool.

JULY 2022: Temp. 17.5°C (0.5°C above avg.); precip. 65mm (10mm above avg.). 1–13 Showery, mild. 14–19 Sunny, warm. 20–24 A few showers, cool. 25–31 Sunny, warm.

AUG. 2022: Temp. 17.5°C (0.5°C above avg.); precip. 95mm (30mm above avg. east, 60mm above west). 1–6 A few showers north, sunny south; hot. 7–14 Sunny, hot. 15–20 Rainy periods, cool. 21–31 Scattered showers, cool.

SEPT. 2022: Temp. 13°C (1°C below avg.); precip. 80mm (20mm above avg.). 1–7 Sunny, cool. 8–15 A few showers, cool. 16–21 Rain, then sunny, cool. 22–30 Showers, then sunny, cool.

OCT. 2022: Temp. 10°C (1°C above avg.); precip. 105mm (5mm above avg.). 1–9 A few showers, cool. 10–14 Sunny, cool. 15–26 Rainy periods, mild. 27–31 Showers, cool.

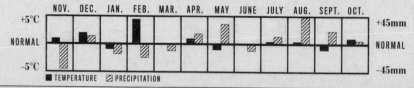

Get your local forecast at Almanac.ca/2022.

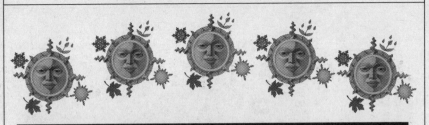

FEAR OF	PHOBIA
Clouds	Nephophobia
Cold	Cheimatophobia Frigophobia Psychrophobia
Dampness, moisture	Hygrophobia
Daylight, sunshine	Heliophobia Phengophobia
Extreme cold, frost, ice	Cryophobia Pagophobia
Floods	Antlophobia
Fog	Homichlophobia Nebulaphobia
Heat	Thermophobia
Hurricanes, tornadoes	Lilapsophobia
Lightning, thunder	Astraphobia Brontophobia Keraunophobia
Northern lights, southern lights	Auroraphobia
Rain	Ombrophobia Pluviophobia
Snow	Chionophobia
Thunder	Ceraunophobia Tonitrophobia
Wind	Ancraophobia Anemophobia

U.S. WEATHER REGIONS

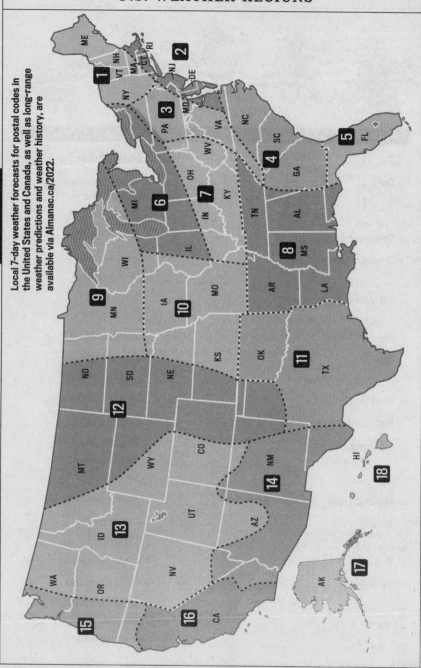

Local 7-day weather forecasts for postal codes in the United States and Canada, as well as long-range weather predictions and weather history, are available via Almanac.ca/2022.

WEATHER

Illustration of U.S. map: Rob Schuster

U.S. REGIONAL WEATHER FORECASTS, 2021–22

1. NORTHEAST

SUMMARY: Winter will be colder than normal, on average, with near- to below-normal snowfall. Precipitation will be above normal in the north and below normal in the south. The coldest periods will be in early December, early to mid- and late January, and mid-February, with the snowiest periods in mid- to late December, early January, and early and mid-February. **April** and **May** will be warmer and drier than normal. **Summer** temperatures will be slightly cooler than normal, on average, with above-normal rainfall. The hottest periods will be in early to mid-July and mid- to late August. **September** and **October** will bring temperatures below normal in the north and above normal in the south and be rainier than normal.

2. ATLANTIC CORRIDOR

SUMMARY: Winter temperatures and precipitation will be below normal, on average, with above-normal snowfall in the north and below-normal in the south. The coldest periods will be in early, mid-, and late December; mid-January; and early to mid-February. The snowiest periods will occur in mid- and late December, from early to mid-January, and in mid-March. **April** and **May** will be warmer than normal, with rainfall near normal in the north and below normal in the south. **Summer** will be hotter and slightly drier than normal, with the hottest periods in mid-June and early to mid-July, from late July into early August, and in late August. **September** and **October** will bring temperatures near normal in the north and above normal in the south and be rainier than normal.

3. APPALACHIANS

SUMMARY: Winter will be colder and drier than normal, with near-normal snowfall. The coldest periods will be in early, mid-, and late December; through much of January; and in early and mid-February. The snowiest periods will be in early December, early January, and mid-February. **April** and **May** will be warmer and drier than normal, with an early hot spell in early to mid-May. **Summer** will be hotter and drier than normal, with the hottest periods in early and mid- to late August. **September** and **October** will bring near-normal temperatures and be rainier than normal.

4. SOUTHEAST

SUMMARY: Winter temperatures will be below normal, on average, with the coldest periods in mid- and late December, throughout much of January, and in early to mid-February. Precipitation will be below normal in the north and above normal in the south. Snowfall will be near normal, with the best chances for snow in mid- to late January and early to mid-February. **April** and **May** will be warmer than normal, with rainfall below normal in the north and above normal in the south. **Summer** will be hotter and drier than normal, with the hottest periods in mid- and late June and early and late July. Watch for a tropical storm in mid- to late August. **September** and **October** will be a bit cooler than normal, with rainfall above normal in the north and below normal in the south. Watch for a hurricane in mid-September.

5. FLORIDA

SUMMARY: **Winter** will be cooler than normal, with the coldest temperatures in mid- and late December and mid-January and from late January into early February. Precipitation will be above normal in the north and below normal in the south. **April** and **May** will be slightly cooler than normal, on average, with near-normal rainfall in the north and well above-normal rainfall in the south. **Summer** will be hotter and slightly drier than normal, with the hottest periods in mid-June, early and late July, and early to mid-August. **September** and **October** will be slightly warmer and much drier than normal, with the hottest period in early September.

6. LOWER LAKES

SUMMARY: **Winter** will be colder and drier than normal, with the coldest temperatures in mid- to late November, through most of December and January, and in early to mid-February. Snowfall will be near-normal in most areas, although a few places south of the Lakes will have much-above-normal snowfall. The snowiest periods will be in late November, mid- and late December, early and mid- to late January, early to mid-February, and mid-March. **April** and **May** will be much warmer and slightly drier than normal. **Summer** will be warmer and slightly rainier than normal, with the hottest periods in mid- and late June, early to mid-July, and mid-August. **September** and **October** will be warmer and rainier than normal.

7. OHIO VALLEY

SUMMARY: **Winter** will be colder than normal, with below-normal precipitation but above-normal snowfall, especially in the west. The coldest periods will occur in mid- to late November and through much of the period from mid-December through January. The snowiest periods will arrive in mid-December, early and mid-January, and mid- to late February. **April** and **May** will be much warmer than normal, with below-normal precipitation. **Summer** will be slightly cooler and drier than normal in the east, with above-normal temperatures and rainfall in the west. The hottest periods will be in late June, early to mid-July, and early August. **September** and **October** will be warmer than normal, with normal precipitation.

8. DEEP SOUTH

SUMMARY: Winter will be colder than normal, on average, with the coldest periods in mid-December, early and mid- to late January, and early to mid-February. Rainfall will be near normal in the north and above normal in the south, with the best threats for snow in the north from late December into early January and in mid- to late January. **April** and **May** will be much warmer than normal, with below-normal rainfall. **Summer** will be hotter and rainier than normal, with the hottest periods in late June, early July, and mid-August. Watch for a tropical storm in mid- to late July. **September** and **October** will bring near-normal temperatures and be rainier than normal. Watch for a tropical storm in late October.

9. UPPER MIDWEST

SUMMARY: Winter temperatures will be below normal, on average, with the coldest periods in early, mid-, and late December; early and late January; and mid-February. Precipitation will be above normal in the east and below normal in the west, while snowfall will be below normal in most areas. The snowiest periods will be in late November, mid- to late December, mid- and late January, mid- and late February, and late March. **April** and **May** will be warmer than normal, with near- to above-normal precipitation. **Summer** will have its hottest period in early to mid-July but

otherwise be slightly cooler than normal and rainer. **September** and **October** will have above-normal temperatures and precipitation.

10. HEARTLAND

SUMMARY: Winter will be colder and drier than normal, on average, with the coldest periods in mid- and late December, early and late January, and early to mid-February. Snowfall will be below normal in the north and above normal in central and southern areas. The snowiest periods will be in late December, early January, and mid-February. **April** and **May** will be warmer and drier than normal. **Summer** will be hotter and rainier than normal, with the hottest periods in early and late June and early to mid-July. **September** and **October** will be slightly warmer and rainier than normal.

11. TEXAS-OKLAHOMA

SUMMARY: Winter will be colder than normal, especially in the south, with the coldest periods in mid- to late November, mid- and late December, and early and late January. Precipitation will be below normal in the north and above normal in the south. Snowfall will be near normal, with the best chances for snow in early and late January, mainly in the north. **April** and **May** will be warmer than normal, with rainfall below normal in the north and above normal in the south. **Summer** will be hotter than normal, with the

WEATHER

hottest periods in late June and from mid-July into mid-August. Rainfall will be slightly above normal in the north and below normal in the south. Watch for a tropical storm in mid- to late June. **September** and **October** will be warmer and drier than normal.

12. HIGH PLAINS

SUMMARY: Winter will be milder than normal, with the coldest periods in mid- to late November, late December, and early and mid- to late January. Precipitation will be near to slightly above normal, with snowfall above normal in the north and below normal in the south. The snowiest periods will be in mid- to late November, late December, early to mid-January, and the last third of March. **April** and **May** will be warmer and drier than normal. **Summer** will be hotter than normal, with the hottest periods in mid-June and throughout the first half of July. The season will be drier than normal in the north and rainier than normal in the south. **September** and **October** will be warmer and slightly drier than normal.

13. INTERMOUNTAIN

SUMMARY: Winter will be slightly colder than normal as well as drier, with below-normal snowfall in most areas. The coldest periods will be in late November, late December, and early and late January, with the snowiest periods in late December,

late January, and early March. **April** and **May** will have above-normal temperatures, with slightly above-normal precipitation. **Summer** temperatures will be hotter than normal, with slightly above-normal rainfall. The hottest periods will be in mid-June, mid- and late July, and early to mid-August. **September** and **October** temperatures will be near normal in the north and above normal in the south, with near-normal precipitation.

14. DESERT SOUTHWEST

SUMMARY: Winter will be colder than normal in the east, with above-normal precipitation, while the west will be slightly warmer and drier than normal. The coldest periods will be in mid- to late November, from late December into early January, and in late February. Snowfall will be above normal in most areas that normally receive snow, with the snowiest periods in late November, early December, and early January. **April** and **May** will be slightly warmer than normal, with near-normal rainfall. **Summer** will be hotter than normal, with below-normal rainfall. The hottest periods will occur in mid-June, through much of July, and in mid-August. **September** and **October** will be warmer than normal, with near-normal precipitation.

15. PACIFIC NORTHWEST

SUMMARY: Winter temperatures will be milder than normal, with below-

U.S. REGIONAL WEATHER FORECASTS, 2021–22

normal precipitation and snowfall. The coldest periods will occur in early December, from late December into early January, and in mid-January and early March. The snowiest periods will occur in late December and early March. **April** and **May** will be slightly warmer and rainier than normal. **Summer** will have above-normal temperatures and rainfall. The hottest periods will be in late July and early August. **September** and **October** will be slightly cooler and rainier than normal.

16. PACIFIC SOUTHWEST

SUMMARY: Winter will be warmer and drier than normal, with below-normal mountain snows. The coldest temperatures will occur from mid-December into mid-January, in mid-February, and in early March. The stormiest period will be in late December. **April** and **May** will be slightly cooler than normal, with rainfall below normal in the north and above normal in the south. **Summer** temperatures will be hotter than normal, with generally above-normal rainfall. The hottest periods will be in mid-June, mid- to late July, and mid- to late August. **September** and **October** will bring temperatures close to normal and be a bit drier than usual.

17. ALASKA

SUMMARY: Winter temperatures will be milder than normal, with the coldest periods in mid- to late January, late February, and early March. Precipitation will be near normal north and above normal south. Snowfall will be above normal in all areas but the south, with the snowiest periods in early November and mid- to late January. **April** and **May** will be warmer than normal, with near-normal precipitation. Watch for snow in late April. **Summer** will be warmer and drier than normal, with the hottest periods from mid-July into mid-August. **September** and **October** will be milder than normal, with precipitation below normal north and above normal south.

18. HAWAII

SUMMARY: Winter temperatures will be warmer than normal, with the coolest periods in mid- to late December and mid- to late March. Rainfall will be below normal, with the stormiest periods in early December, late January, and early March. **April** and **May** will be warmer and rainier than normal. **Summer** will be warmer than normal, with the hottest periods from mid-July into early August and in late August. Rainfall will be below normal east and above normal west. **September** and **October** will be warmer than normal, with the hottest periods in early September and from late September into early October. Rainfall will be below normal despite a stormy period in mid-October. ∎

SECRETS OF THE ZODIAC

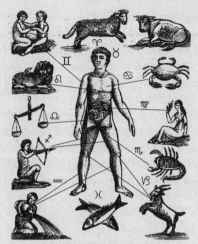

The Man of the Signs

Ancient astrologers believed that each astrological sign influenced a specific part of the body. The first sign of the zodiac—Aries—was attributed to the head, with the rest of the signs moving down the body, ending with Pisces at the feet.

♈ Aries, head	**ARI**	*Mar. 21–Apr. 20*
♉ Taurus, neck	**TAU**	*Apr. 21–May 20*
♊ Gemini, arms	**GEM**	*May 21–June 20*
♋ Cancer, breast	**CAN**	*June 21–July 22*
♌ Leo, heart	**LEO**	*July 23–Aug. 22*
♍ Virgo, belly	**VIR**	*Aug. 23–Sept. 22*
♎ Libra, reins	**LIB**	*Sept. 23–Oct. 22*
♏ Scorpio, secrets	**SCO**	*Oct. 23–Nov. 22*
♐ Sagittarius, thighs	**SAG**	*Nov. 23–Dec. 21*
♑ Capricorn, knees	**CAP**	*Dec. 22–Jan. 19*
♒ Aquarius, legs	**AQU**	*Jan. 20–Feb. 19*
♓ Pisces, feet	**PSC**	*Feb. 20–Mar. 20*

ASTROLOGY VS. ASTRONOMY

Astrology is a tool we use to plan events according to the placements of the Sun, the Moon, and the planets in the 12 signs of the zodiac. In astrology, the planetary movements do not cause events; rather, they explain the path, or "flow," that events tend to follow. *The Moon's astrological place is given on the next page.* **Astronomy** is the study of the actual placement of the known planets and constellations. The Moon's astronomical place is given in the **Left-Hand Calendar Pages, 120–146.** *(The placement of the planets in the signs of the zodiac is not the same astrologically and astronomically.)*

The dates in the **Best Days** table, **pages 226–227,** are based on the astrological passage of the Moon.

WHEN MERCURY IS RETROGRADE

Sometimes the other planets appear to be traveling backward through the zodiac; this is an illusion. We call this illusion *retrograde motion.*

Mercury's retrograde periods can cause our plans to go awry. However, intuition is high during these periods and coincidences can be extraordinary.

When Mercury is retrograde, stay flexible, allow more time for travel, and don't sign contracts. Review projects and plans but wait until Mercury is direct again to make final decisions.

In 2022, Mercury will be retrograde during January 13–February 3, May 10–June 2, September 9–October 1, and December 28–(January 18, 2023).

–Celeste Longacre

GARDENING BY THE MOON'S SIGN

USE CHART ON NEXT PAGE TO FIND THE BEST DATES FOR THE FOLLOWING GARDEN TASKS . . .

PLANT, TRANSPLANT, AND GRAFT: Cancer, Scorpio, Pisces, or Taurus

HARVEST: Aries, Leo, Sagittarius, Gemini, or Aquarius

BUILD/FIX FENCES OR GARDEN BEDS: Capricorn

CONTROL INSECT PESTS, PLOW, AND WEED: Aries, Gemini, Leo, Sagittarius, or Aquarius

PRUNE: Aries, Leo, or Sagittarius. During a waxing Moon, pruning encourages growth; during a waning Moon, it discourages it.

Chicks take about 21 days to hatch. Those born under a waxing Moon in Cancer, Scorpio, or Pisces are healthier and mature faster. To ensure that chicks are born during these times, "set eggs" (place eggs in an incubator or under a hen) 21 days before the desired hatching dates.

EXAMPLE:
The Moon is new on April 30 and full on May 16 (EDT). Between these dates, the Moon is in the sign of Cancer on May 5 and 6. To have chicks born on May 5, count back 21 days; set eggs on April 14.

Below are the best days to set eggs in 2022, using only the fruitful dates between the new and full Moons, and counting back 21 days:

JAN.: 12, 13, 22, 23
FEB.: 9, 10, 18–20
MAR.: 17–19

APR.: 14, 15, 23, 24
MAY: 11–13, 21, 22
JUNE: 7–9, 17, 18

JULY: 14, 15
AUG.: 10–12, 19, 20
SEPT.: 7, 8, 15, 16

OCT.: 4, 5, 13, 14
NOV.: 2, 9, 10
DEC.: 6, 7, 16

The Moon's Astrological Place, 2021–22

	NOV.	DEC.	JAN.	FEB.	MAR.	APR.	MAY	JUNE	JULY	AUG.	SEPT.	OCT.	NOV.	DEC.
1	VIR	SCO	SAG	AQU	AQU	ARI	TAU	CAN	LEO	VIR	SCO	SAG	AQU	PSC
2	LIB	SCO	CAP	PSC	PSC	TAU	GEM	CAN	LEO	LIB	SCO	CAP	AQU	ARI
3	LIB	SAG	CAP	PSC	PSC	TAU	GEM	CAN	VIR	LIB	SAG	CAP	PSC	ARI
4	SCO	SAG	AQU	ARI	ARI	TAU	GEM	LEO	VIR	SCO	SAG	AQU	PSC	TAU
5	SCO	CAP	AQU	ARI	ARI	GEM	CAN	LEO	VIR	SCO	CAP	AQU	ARI	TAU
6	SAG	CAP	PSC	ARI	TAU	GEM	CAN	VIR	LIB	SAG	CAP	PSC	ARI	TAU
7	SAG	AQU	PSC	TAU	TAU	CAN	LEO	VIR	LIB	SAG	AQU	PSC	TAU	GEM
8	CAP	AQU	ARI	TAU	TAU	CAN	LEO	LIB	SCO	SAG	AQU	ARI	TAU	GEM
9	CAP	PSC	ARI	GEM	GEM	CAN	LEO	LIB	SCO	CAP	PSC	ARI	GEM	CAN
10	AQU	PSC	TAU	GEM	GEM	LEO	VIR	LIB	SAG	CAP	PSC	ARI	GEM	CAN
11	AQU	PSC	TAU	GEM	CAN	LEO	VIR	SCO	SAG	AQU	ARI	TAU	GEM	CAN
12	PSC	ARI	TAU	CAN	CAN	VIR	LIB	SCO	CAP	AQU	ARI	TAU	CAN	LEO
13	PSC	ARI	GEM	CAN	CAN	VIR	LIB	SAG	CAP	PSC	TAU	GEM	CAN	LEO
14	ARI	TAU	GEM	LEO	LEO	VIR	SCO	SAG	AQU	PSC	TAU	GEM	LEO	VIR
15	ARI	TAU	CAN	LEO	LEO	LIB	SCO	CAP	AQU	ARI	TAU	CAN	LEO	VIR
16	ARI	TAU	CAN	LEO	VIR	LIB	SAG	CAP	PSC	ARI	GEM	CAN	LEO	VIR
17	TAU	GEM	CAN	VIR	VIR	SCO	SAG	AQU	PSC	TAU	GEM	CAN	VIR	LIB
18	TAU	GEM	LEO	VIR	LIB	SCO	CAP	AQU	ARI	TAU	CAN	LEO	VIR	LIB
19	GEM	CAN	LEO	LIB	LIB	SAG	CAP	PSC	ARI	GEM	CAN	LEO	LIB	SCO
20	GEM	CAN	VIR	LIB	SCO	SAG	AQU	PSC	ARI	GEM	CAN	VIR	LIB	SCO
21	GEM	CAN	VIR	SCO	SCO	CAP	AQU	ARI	TAU	GEM	LEO	VIR	LIB	SAG
22	CAN	LEO	VIR	SCO	SCO	CAP	PSC	ARI	TAU	CAN	LEO	VIR	SCO	SAG
23	CAN	LEO	LIB	SAG	SAG	AQU	PSC	TAU	GEM	CAN	VIR	LIB	SCO	CAP
24	LEO	VIR	LIB	SAG	SAG	AQU	PSC	TAU	GEM	LEO	VIR	LIB	SAG	CAP
25	LEO	VIR	SCO	CAP	CAP	PSC	ARI	TAU	CAN	LEO	LIB	SCO	SAG	AQU
26	LEO	LIB	SCO	CAP	CAP	PSC	ARI	GEM	CAN	LEO	LIB	SCO	CAP	AQU
27	VIR	LIB	SAG	CAP	AQU	ARI	TAU	GEM	CAN	VIR	LIB	SAG	CAP	PSC
28	VIR	LIB	SAG	AQU	AQU	ARI	TAU	CAN	LEO	VIR	SCO	SAG	AQU	PSC
29	LIB	SCO	CAP	—	PSC	ARI	GEM	CAN	LEO	LIB	SCO	CAP	AQU	ARI
30	LIB	SCO	CAP	—	PSC	TAU	GEM	CAN	LEO	LIB	SAG	CAP	PSC	ARI
31	—	SAG	AQU	—	ARI	—	GEM	—	VIR	SCO	—	AQU	—	TAU

BEST DAYS FOR 2022

This chart is based on the Moon's sign and shows the best days each month for certain activities. –*Celeste Longacre*

	JAN.	FEB.	MAR.	APR.	MAY	JUNE	JULY	AUG.	SEPT.	OCT.	NOV.	DEC.
Quit smoking	22, 26	18, 23	22, 30	18, 27	24, 29	20, 25	17, 22	14, 19	15, 25	12, 22	18, 23	15, 16
Bake	15–17	12, 13	11–13	7–9	5, 6	1–3, 28–30	25–27	22, 23	18–20	15–17	12, 13	9–11
Brew	25, 26	21, 22	20–22	17, 18	14, 15	11, 12	8, 9	4, 5, 31	1, 2, 28, 29	25, 26	22, 23	19, 20
Dry fruit, vegetables, or meat	27, 28	23, 24	23, 24	19, 20	25, 26	21, 22	18–20	15, 16	21, 22	18, 19	14–16	12, 13
Make jams or jellies	6, 7	2, 3	2, 3, 29, 30	25, 26	22–24	19, 20	16, 17	13, 14	9, 10	6, 7	3, 4, 30	1, 27, 28
Can, pickle, or make sauerkraut	25, 26	21, 22	20–22	25, 26	22–24	19, 20	16, 17	22, 23	18–20	15–17	12, 13	9–11
Begin diet to lose weight	22, 26	18, 23	22, 30	18, 27	24, 29	20, 25	17, 22	14, 19	15, 25	12, 22	18, 23	15, 16
Begin diet to gain weight	7, 12	4, 8	3, 8	4, 9	1, 11	8, 12	5, 31	1, 6	2, 10	8, 26	4, 30	1, 6, 28
Cut hair to encourage growth	10–12	7, 8	6–8	2–4	12, 13	9, 10	6, 7	2, 3	9, 10	6, 7	3, 4, 7	4–6
Cut hair to discourage growth	23, 24	19, 20	19, 29, 30	25, 26	27, 28	23–25	21, 22	17, 18	13–15	11, 12	19–21	17, 18
Perm hair	4, 5, 31	1, 28	1, 27, 28	23, 24	20, 21	17, 18	14, 15	11, 12	7, 8	4, 5, 31	1, 2, 28, 29	25, 26
Color hair	10–12	7, 8	6–8	2–4, 30	1, 27, 28	23–25	21, 22	17, 18	13–15	11, 12	7, 8	4–6, 31
Straighten hair	1, 27, 28	23, 24	23, 24	19, 20	16, 17	13, 14	10, 11	6–8	3, 4, 30	1, 27, 28	24, 25	21, 22
Have dental care	20–22	17, 18	16, 17	12–14	10, 11	6, 7	3–5, 31	1, 27, 28	23, 24	20–22	17, 18	14–16
Start projects	3	2	3	30	1	1	1	28	26	26	24	24
End projects	1	1	1	2	30	27	27	26	24	24	22	22
Demolish	25, 26	21, 22	20–22	17, 18	14, 15	11, 12	8, 9	4, 5, 31	1, 2, 28, 29	25, 26	22, 23	19, 20
Lay shingles	18, 19	14–16	14, 15	10, 11	7–9	4, 5	1, 2, 28–30	24–26	21, 22	18, 19	14–16	12, 13
Paint	23, 24	19, 20	18, 19	15, 16	12, 13	8–10	6, 7	2, 3, 29, 30	25–27	23, 24	19–21	17, 18
Wash windows	8, 9	4–6	4, 5, 31	1, 27–29	25, 26	21, 22	18–20	15, 16	11, 12	8–10	5, 6	2, 3, 29, 30
Wash floors	6, 7	2, 3	2, 3, 29, 30	25, 26	22–24	19, 20	16, 17	13, 14	9, 10	6, 7	3, 4, 30	1, 27, 28
Go camping	1, 27, 28	23, 24	23, 24	19, 20	16, 17	13, 14	10, 11	6–8	3, 4, 30	1, 27, 28	24, 25	21, 22

See what to do when via Almanac.ca/2022.

	JAN.	FEB.	MAR.	APR.	MAY	JUNE	JULY	AUG.	SEPT.	OCT.	NOV.	DEC.
Entertain	18, 19	14–16	14, 15	10, 11	7–9	4, 5	1, 2, 28–30	24–26	21, 22	18, 19	14–16	12, 13
Travel for pleasure	18, 19	14–16	14, 15	10, 11	7–9	4, 5	1, 2, 28–30	24–26	21, 22	18, 19	14–16	12, 13
Get married	23, 24	19, 20	18, 19	15, 16	12, 13	8–10	6, 7	2, 3, 29, 30	25–27	23, 24	19–21	17, 18
Ask for a loan	25, 26	21, 22	20, 21	17, 18	27, 28	23–25	21, 22	17, 18	13, 14	11, 12	12, 13, 22	19, 20
Buy a home	10–12	7, 8	6–8	2–4	14, 15	11, 12	8, 9	4, 5	1, 2, 29	6, 7, 26	7, 8	4–6
Move (house/household)	13, 14	9–11	9, 10	5, 6	2–4, 29–31	26, 27	23, 24	19–21	16, 17	13, 14	9–11	7, 8
Advertise to sell	10–12	7, 8	6–8	2–4, 30	14, 15	11, 12	8, 9	4, 5	1, 2, 28, 29	2, 3, 26	7, 8	4–6
Mow to promote growth	8, 9	4–6	4, 5	1, 12–14	14, 15	11, 12	8, 9	4, 5	1, 2, 28, 29	8, 9	7, 8	2, 3, 29, 30
Mow to slow growth	25, 26	21, 22	20–22	17, 18	27, 28	21, 22	21, 22	17, 18	13–15	11, 12	15, 16	19, 20
Plant aboveground crops	6, 7	2, 3	2, 3	7–9	5, 6	1–3	8, 9	4, 5	1, 2, 28, 29	6, 7	3, 4, 30	1, 27, 28
Plant belowground crops	25, 26	21, 22	20–22	25, 26	22–24	19, 20	25–27	22, 23	18–20	15–17	12, 13	9–11
Destroy pests and weeds	8, 9	4–6	4, 5, 31	1, 27–29	25, 26	21, 22	18–20	15, 16	11, 12	8–10	5, 6	2, 3, 29, 30
Graft or pollinate	15–17	12, 13	11–13	7–9	5, 6	1–3, 28–30	25–27	22, 23	18–20	15–17	12, 13	9–11
Prune to encourage growth	8, 9	4–6	4, 5	10, 11	7–9	4, 5	10, 11	6–8	3, 4	27, 28	5, 6	2, 3, 29, 30
Prune to discourage growth	27, 28	23, 24	23, 24	19, 20	25, 26	21, 22	18–20	24–26	21, 22	18, 19	14–16	12, 13
Pick fruit	20–22	17, 18	16, 17	12–14	10, 11	6, 7	3–5	1, 27, 28	23, 24	20–22	17, 18	14–16
Harvest aboveground crops	10–12	7, 8	6–8	2–4	10, 11	6, 7	3–5	1, 4, 5	1, 2	2, 3	7, 8	4–6
Harvest belowground crops	20–22	17, 18	20–22	17, 18	27, 28	23–25	21, 22	17, 18	23, 24	20–22	17, 18	14–16
Cut hay	8, 9	4–6	4, 5	1, 27–29	25, 26	21, 22	18–20	15, 16	11, 12	8–10	5, 6	2, 3, 29, 30
Begin logging, set posts, pour concrete	2, 3, 29, 30	25–27	25, 26	21, 22	18, 19	15, 16	12, 13	9, 10	5, 6	2, 3, 29, 30	26, 27	23, 24
Purchase animals	15–17	12, 13	11–13	7–9	5, 6	1–3, 28–30	25–27	22, 23	18–20	15–17	12, 13	9–11
Breed animals	25, 26	21, 22	20–22	17, 18	14, 15	11, 12	8, 9	4, 5, 31	1, 2, 28, 29	25, 26	22, 23	19, 20
Wean	22, 26	18, 23	22, 30	18, 27	24, 29	20, 25	17, 22	14, 19	15, 25	12, 22	18, 23	15, 16
Castrate animals	4, 5, 31	1, 28	1, 27, 28	23, 24	20, 21	17, 18	14, 15	11, 12	7, 8	4, 5, 31	1, 2, 28, 29	25, 26
Slaughter livestock	25, 26	21, 22	20–22	17, 18	14, 15	11, 12	8, 9	4, 5, 31	1, 2, 28, 29	25, 26	22, 23	19, 20

BEST FISHING DAYS AND TIMES

The best times to fish are when the fish are naturally most active. The Sun, Moon, tides, and weather all influence fish activity. For example, fish tend to feed more at sunrise and sunset, and also during a full Moon (when tides are higher than average). However, most of us go fishing simply when we can get the time off. But there are best times, according to fishing lore:

■ One hour before and one hour after high tides, and one hour before and one hour after low tides. The times of high tides for Halifax are given on **pages 120–146;** also see **pages 238–239.** (Inland, the times for high tides correspond with the times when the Moon is due south. Low tides are halfway between high tides.)

GET TIDE TIMES AND HEIGHTS NEAREST TO YOUR LOCATION VIA ALMANAC.CA/2022.

■ During the "morning rise" (after sunup for a spell) and the "evening rise" (just before sundown and the hour or so after).

■ During the rise and set of the Moon.

■ When the barometer is steady or on the rise. (But even during stormy periods, the fish aren't going to give up feeding. The clever angler will find just the right bait.)

■ When there is a hatch of flies—caddis flies or mayflies, commonly.

■ When the breeze is from a westerly quarter, rather than from the north or east.

■ When the water is still or slightly rippled, rather than during a wind.

THE BEST FISHING DAYS FOR 2022, WHEN THE MOON IS BETWEEN NEW AND FULL

January 2–17
February 1–16
March 2–18
April 1–16
April 30–May 16
May 30–June 14
June 28–July 13
July 28–August 11
August 27–September 10
September 25–October 9
October 25–November 8
November 23–December 7
December 23–31

Dates based on Eastern Time.

HOW TO ESTIMATE THE WEIGHT OF A FISH

Measure the fish from the tip of its nose to the tip of its tail. Then measure its girth at the thickest portion of its midsection.

The weight of a fat-bodied fish (bass, salmon) = (length x girth x girth)/800

The weight of a slender fish (trout, northern pike) = (length x girth x girth)/900

EXAMPLE: If a trout is 20 inches long and has a 12-inch girth, its estimated weight is (20 x 12 x 12)/900 = 2,880/900 = 3.2 pounds

SALMON

TROUT

CATFISH

GESTATION AND MATING TABLES

	PROPER AGE OR WEIGHT FOR FIRST MATING	PERIOD OF FERTILITY (YRS.)	NUMBER OF FEMALES FOR ONE MALE	PERIOD OF GESTATION (DAYS) AVERAGE	RANGE
CATTLE: Cow	15–18 mos.[1]	10–14		283	279–290[2] 262–300[3]
Bull	1 yr., well matured	10–12	50[4] / thousands[5]		
GOAT: Doe	10 mos. or 85–90 lbs.	6		150	145–155
Buck	well matured	5	30		
HORSE: Mare	3 yrs.	10–12		336	310–370
Stallion	3 yrs.	12–15	40–45[4] / record 252[5]		
PIG: Sow	5–6 mos. or 250 lbs.	6		115	110–120
Boar	250–300 lbs.	6	50[6] / 35–40[7]		
RABBIT: Doe	6 mos.	5–6		31	30–32
Buck	6 mos.	5–6	30		
SHEEP: Ewe	1 yr. or 90 lbs.	6		147 / 151[8]	142–154
Ram	12–14 mos., well matured	7	50–75[6] / 35–40[7]		
CAT: Queen	12 mos.	6		63	60–68
Tom	12 mos.	6	6–8		
DOG: Bitch	16–18 mos.	8		63	58–67
Male	12–16 mos.	8	8–10		

[1]Holstein and beef: 750 lbs.; Jersey: 500 lbs. [2]Beef; 8–10 days shorter for Angus. [3]Dairy. [4]Natural. [5]Artificial. [6]Hand-mated. [7]Pasture. [8]For fine wool breeds.

INCUBATION PERIOD OF POULTRY (DAYS)

Chicken	21
Duck	26–32
Goose	30–34
Guinea	26–28
Turkey	28

AVERAGE LIFE SPAN OF ANIMALS IN CAPTIVITY (YEARS)

Cat (domestic)	14	Goose (domestic)	20
Chicken (domestic)	8	Horse	22
Dog (domestic)	13	Pig	12
Duck (domestic)	10	Rabbit	6
Goat (domestic)	14	Turkey (domestic)	10

	ESTRAL/ESTROUS CYCLE (INCLUDING HEAT PERIOD) AVERAGE	RANGE	LENGTH OF ESTRUS (HEAT) AVERAGE	RANGE	USUAL TIME OF OVULATION	WHEN CYCLE RECURS IF NOT BRED
Cow	21 days	18–24 days	18 hours	10–24 hours	10–12 hours after end of estrus	21 days
Doe goat	21 days	18–24 days	2–3 days	1–4 days	Near end of estrus	21 days
Mare	21 days	10–37 days	5–6 days	2–11 days	24–48 hours before end of estrus	21 days
Sow	21 days	18–24 days	2–3 days	1–5 days	30–36 hours after start of estrus	21 days
Ewe	16½ days	14–19 days	30 hours	24–32 hours	12–24 hours before end of estrus	16½ days
Queen cat		15–21 days	3–4 days, if mated	9–10 days, in absence of male	24–56 hours after coitus	Pseudo-pregnancy
Bitch	24 days	16–30 days	7 days	5–9 days	1–3 days after first acceptance	Pseudo-pregnancy

PLANTING BY THE MOON'S PHASE

ACCORDING TO THIS AGE-OLD PRACTICE, CYCLES OF THE MOON AFFECT PLANT GROWTH.

Plant annual flowers and vegetables that bear crops above ground during the light, or waxing, of the Moon: from the day the Moon is new to the day it is full.

Plant flowering bulbs, biennial and perennial flowers, and vegetables that bear crops below ground during the dark, or waning, of the Moon: from the day after it is full to the day before it is new again.

The Planting Dates columns give the safe periods for planting in areas that receive frost. (See **page 232** for frost dates in your area.) The Moon Favorable columns give the best planting days within the Planting Dates based on the Moon's phases for 2021. (See **pages 120–146** for the exact days of the new and full Moons.)

The dates listed in this table are meant as general guidelines only. For seed-sowing dates based on frost dates in your local area, go to **Almanac.ca/2022.**

Aboveground crops are marked *.
(E) means early; (L) means late.

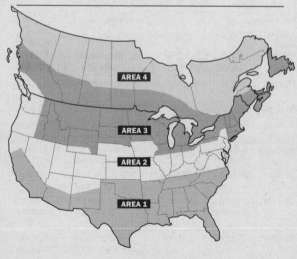

* Barley	
* Beans	(E)
	(L)
Beets	(E)
	(L)
* Broccoli plants	(E)
	(L)
* Brussels sprouts	
* Cabbage plants	
Carrots	(E)
	(L)
* Cauliflower plants	(E)
	(L)
* Celery plants	(E)
	(L)
* Collards	(E)
	(L)
* Corn, sweet	(E)
	(L)
* Cucumbers	
* Eggplant plants	
* Endive	(E)
	(L)
* Kale	(E)
	(L)
Leek plants	
* Lettuce	
* Muskmelons	
* Okra	
Onion sets	
* Parsley	
Parsnips	
* Peas	(E)
	(L)
* Pepper plants	
Potatoes	
* Pumpkins	
Radishes	(E)
	(L)
* Spinach	(E)
	(L)
* Squashes	
Sweet potatoes	
* Swiss chard	
* Tomato plants	
Turnips	(E)
	(L)
* Watermelons	
* Wheat, spring	
* Wheat, winter	

	AREA 1	AREA 2		AREA 3		AREA 4	
PLANTING DATES	MOON FAVORABLE	PLANTING DATES	MOON FAVORABLE	PLANTING DATES	MOON FAVORABLE	PLANTING DATES	MOON FAVORABLE
5-3/7	2/15-16, 3/2-7	3/15-4/7	3/15-18, 4/1-7	5/15-6/21	5/15-16, 5/30-6/14	6/1-30	6/1-14, 6/28-30
5-4/7	3/15-18, 4/1-7	4/15-30	4/15-16, 4/30	5/7-6/21	5/7-16, 5/30-6/14	5/30-6/15	5/30-6/14
-31	8/7-11, 8/27-31	7/1-21	7/1-13	6/15-7/15	6/28-7/13	—	—
-28	2/17-28	3/15-4/3	3/19-31	4/25-5/15	4/25-29	5/25-6/10	5/25-29
-30	9/11-24	8/15-31	8/15-26	7/15-8/15	7/15-27, 8/12-15	6/15-7/8	6/15-27
5-3/15	2/15-16, 3/2-15	3/7-31	3/7-18	5/15-31	5/15-16, 5/30-31	6/1-25	6/1-14
-30	9/7-10, 9/25-30	8/1-20	8/1-11	6/15-7/7	6/28-7/7	—	—
4-3/20	2/11-16, 3/2-18	3/7-4/15	3/7-18, 4/1-15	5/15-31	5/15-16, 5/30-31	6/1-25	6/1-14
4-3/20	2/11-16, 3/2-18	3/7-4/15	3/7-18, 4/1-15	5/15-31	5/15-16, 5/30-31	6/1-25	6/1-14
5-3/7	2/17-3/1	3/7-31	3/19-31	5/15-31	5/17-29	5/25-6/10	5/25-29
-9/7	8/12-26	7/7-31	7/14-27	6/15-7/21	6/15-27, 7/14-21	6/15-7/8	6/15-27
5-3/7	2/15-16, 3/2-7	3/15-4/7	3/15-18, 4/1-7	5/15-31	5/15-16, 5/30-31	6/1-25	6/1-14
'-31	8/7-11, 8/27-31	7/1-8/7	7/1-13, 7/28-8/7	6/15-7/21	6/28-7/13	—	—
5-28	2/15-16	3/7-31	3/7-18	5/15-6/30	5/15-16, 5/30-6/14, 6/28-30	6/1-30	6/1-14, 6/28-30
5-30	9/25-30	8/15-9/7	8/27-9/7	7/15-8/15	7/28-8/11	—	—
3-3/20	2/11-16, 3/2-18	3/7-4/7	3/7-18, 4/1-7	5/15-31	5/15-16, 5/30-31	6/1-25	6/1-14
'-30	9/7-10, 9/25-30	8/15-31	8/27-31	7/1-8/7	7/1-13, 7/28-8/7	—	—
5-31	3/15-18	4/1-17	4/1-16	5/10-6/15	5/10-16, 5/30-6/14	5/30-6/20	5/30-6/14
'-31	8/7-11, 8/27-31	7/7-21	7/7-13	6/15-30	6/28-30	—	—
'-4/15	3/7-18, 4/1-15	4/7-5/15	4/7-16, 4/30-5/15	5/7-6/20	5/7-16, 5/30-6/14	5/30-6/15	5/30-6/14
'-4/15	3/7-18, 4/1-15	4/7-5/15	4/7-16, 4/30-5/15	6/1-30	6/1-14, 6/28-30	6/15-30	6/28-30
5-3/20	2/15-16, 3/2-18	4/7-5/15	4/7-16, 4/30-5/15	5/15-31	5/15-16, 5/30-31	6/1-25	6/1-14
15-9/7	8/27-9/7	7/15-8/15	7/28-8/11	6/7-30	6/7-14, 6/28-30	—	—
1-3/20	2/11-16, 3/2-18	3/7-4/7	3/7-18, 4/1-7	5/15-31	5/15-16, 5/30-31	6/1-15	6/1-14
'-30	9/7-10, 9/25-30	8/15-31	8/27-31	7/1-8/7	7/1-13, 7/28-8/7	6/25-7/15	6/28-7/13
15-4/15	2/17-3/1, 3/19-31	3/7-4/7	3/19-31	5/15-31	5/17-29	6/1-25	6/15-25
15-3/7	2/15-16, 3/2-7	3/1-31	3/2-18	5/15-6/30	5/15-16, 5/30-6/14, 6/28-30	6/1-30	6/1-14, 6/28-30
15-4/7	3/15-18, 4/1-7	4/15-5/7	4/15-16, 4/30-5/7	5/15-6/30	5/15-16, 5/30-6/14, 6/28-30	6/1-30	6/1-14, 6/28-30
15-6/1	4/15-16, 4/30-5/16, 5/30-6/1	5/25-6/15	5/30-6/14	6/15-7/10	6/28-7/10	6/15-7/7	6/28-7/7
4-28	2/17-28	3/1-31	3/1, 3/19-31	5/15-6/7	5/17-29	6/1-25	6/15-25
20-3/15	3/2-15	3/1-31	3/2-18	5/15-31	5/15-16, 5/30-31	6/1-15	6/1-14
5-2/4	1/18-31	3/7-31	3/19-31	4/1-30	4/17-29	5/10-31	5/17-29
5-2/7	1/15-17, 2/1-7	3/7-31	3/7-18	4/15-5/7	4/15-16, 4/30-5/7	5/15-31	5/15-16, 5/30-31
15-30	9/25-30	8/7-31	8/7-11, 8/27-31	7/15-31	7/28-31	7/10-25	7/10-13
4-20	3/2-18	4/1-30	4/1-16, 4/30	5/15-6/30	5/15-16, 5/30-6/14, 6/28-30	6/1-30	6/1-14, 6/28-30
10-28	2/17-28	4/1-30	4/17-29	5/1-31	5/17-29	6/1-25	6/15-25
7-20	3/7-18	4/23-5/15	4/30-5/15	5/15-31	5/15-16, 5/30-31	6/1-30	6/1-14, 6/28-30
21-3/1	1/21-31, 2/17-3/1	3/7-31	3/19-31	4/15-30	4/17-29	5/15-6/5	5/17-29
'1-21	10/10-21	9/7-30	9/11-24	8/15-31	8/15-26	7/10-31	7/14-27
7-3/15	2/7-16, 3/2-15	3/15-4/20	3/15-18, 4/1-16	5/15-31	5/15-16, 5/30-31	6/1-25	6/1-14
'1-21	10/1-9	8/1-9/15	8/1-11, 8/27-9/10	7/17-9/7	7/28-8/11, 8/27-9/7	7/20-8/5	7/28-8/5
15-4/15	3/15-18, 4/1-15	4/15-30	4/15-16, 4/30	5/15-6/15	5/15-16, 5/30-6/14	6/1-30	6/1-14, 6/28-30
23-4/6	3/23-31	4/21-5/9	4/21-29	5/15-6/15	5/17-29, 6/15	6/1-30	6/15-27
'3-15	2/7-16, 3/2-15	3/15-4/15	3/15-18, 4/1-15	5/1-31	5/1-16, 5/30-31	5/15-31	5/15-16, 5/30-31
7-20	3/7-18	4/7-30	4/7-16, 4/30	5/15-31	5/15-16, 5/30-31	6/1-15	6/1-14
20-2/15	1/20-31	3/15-31	3/19-31	4/7-30	4/17-29	5/10-31	5/17-29
4-10/15	9/11-24, 10/10-15	8/1-20	8/12-20	7/1-8/15	7/14-27, 8/12-15	—	—
15-4/7	3/15-18, 4/1-7	4/15-5/7	4/15-16, 4/30-5/7	5/15-6/30	5/15-16, 5/30-6/14, 6/28-30	6/1-30	6/1-14, 6/28-30
15-28	2/15-16	3/1-20	3/2-18	4/7-30	4/7-16, 4/30	5/15-6/10	5/15-16, 5/30-6/10
15-12/7	10/25-11/8, 11/23-12/7	9/15-10/20	9/25-10/9	8/11-9/15	8/11, 8/27-9/10	8/5-30	8/5-11, 8/27-30

FROSTS AND GROWING SEASONS

Dates given are normal averages for a light freeze; local weather and topography may cause considerable variations. The possibility of frost occurring after the spring dates and before the fall dates is 33 percent. The classification of freeze temperatures is usually based on their effect on plants. **Light freeze:** –2° to 0°C (29° to 32°F)—tender plants killed. **Moderate freeze:** –4° to –2°C (25° to 28°F)—widely destructive to most plants. **Severe freeze:** –4°C (24°F and colder)—heavy damage to most plants.   –dates courtesy Environment Canada

PROV.	CITY	GROWING SEASON (DAYS)	LAST SPRING FROST	FIRST FALL FROST	PROV.	CITY	GROWING SEASON (DAYS)	LAST SPRING FROST	FIRST FALL FROST
AB	Athabasca	103	May 28	Sept. 9	NT	Fort Simpson	81	May 31	Aug. 21
AB	Calgary	99	May 29	Sept. 6	NT	Norman Wells	91	May 29	Aug. 29
AB	Edmonton	123	May 15	Sept. 16	NT	Yellowknife	102	May 31	Sept. 11
AB	Grande Prairie	106	May 22	Sept. 6	ON	Barrie	147	May 12	Oct. 7
AB	Lethbridge	108	May 25	Sept. 11	ON	Brantford	151	May 5	Oct. 4
AB	Medicine Hat	118	May 18	Sept. 14	ON	Hamilton	160	May 3	Oct. 11
AB	Peace River	96	May 28	Sept. 2	ON	Kapuskasing	75	June 18	Sept. 2
AB	Red Deer	108	May 24	Sept. 10	ON	Kingston	161	Apr. 28	Oct. 7
BC	Abbotsford	168	Apr. 30	Oct. 16	ON	London	141	May 15	Oct. 4
BC	Castlegar	141	May 8	Sept. 27	ON	Ottawa	135	May 13	Sept. 26
BC	Chilliwack	191	Apr. 19	Oct. 28	ON	Owen Sound	147	May 14	Oct. 9
BC	Coombs	139	May 13	Sept. 30	ON	Peterborough	137	May 12	Sept. 27
BC	Dawson Creek	76	June 8	Aug. 24	ON	Sudbury	124	May 21	Sept. 23
BC	Kamloops	152	May 3	Oct. 3	ON	Timmins	86	June 13	Sept. 8
BC	Kelowna	150	May 8	Oct. 6	ON	Toronto	161	May 4	Oct. 13
BC	Nanaimo	163	May 4	Oct. 15	ON	Wawa	97	June 6	Sept. 12
BC	Prince George	120	May 20	Sept. 18	ON	Windsor	172	Apr. 28	Oct. 18
BC	Prince Rupert	145	May 14	Oct. 7	PE	Alberton	122	May 31	Oct. 1
BC	Vancouver	180	Apr. 21	Oct. 19	PE	Charlottetown	142	May 20	Oct. 10
BC	Victoria	208	Apr. 14	Nov. 9	PE	Summerside	154	May 13	Oct. 15
MB	Brandon	92	June 6	Sept. 7	QC	Baie-Comeau	103	June 2	Sept. 14
MB	Lynn Lake	87	June 10	Sept. 6	QC	La Tuque	101	June 5	Sept. 15
MB	The Pas	106	May 31	Sept. 15	QC	Magog	129	May 19	Sept. 26
MB	Thompson	58	June 18	Aug. 16	QC	Montréal	168	Apr 25	Oct. 11
MB	Winnipeg	116	May 21	Sept. 15	QC	Québec	129	May 17	Sept. 24
NB	Bathurst	101	June 4	Sept. 14	QC	Rimouski	140	May 18	Oct. 6
NB	Fredericton	125	May 22	Sept. 25	QC	Roberval	117	May 25	Sept. 20
NB	Miramichi	115	May 27	Sept. 20	QC	Thetford Mines	128	May 20	Sept. 26
NB	Moncton	103	June 3	Sept. 15	QC	Trois-Rivières	128	May 19	Sept. 25
NB	Saint John	165	Apr. 30	Oct. 13	SK	Moose Jaw	110	May 24	Sept. 12
NL	Corner Brook	129	May 27	Oct. 4	SK	North Battleford	108	May 26	Sept. 12
NL	Gander	115	June 6	Sept. 30	SK	Prince Albert	88	June 7	Sept. 4
NL	Grand Falls	105	June 8	Sept. 22	SK	Regina	91	June 1	Sept. 1
NL	St. John's	117	June 11	Oct. 7	SK	Saskatoon	126	May 15	Sept. 19
NS	Halifax	164	May 8	Oct. 20	SK	Weyburn	107	May 26	Sept. 11
NS	Kentville	122	May 26	Sept. 26	SK	Yorkton	106	May 26	Sept. 10
NS	Sydney	135	May 27	Oct. 10	YT	Dawson	62	June 9	Aug. 11
NS	Truro	103	June 7	Sept. 19	YT	Watson Lake	83	June 6	Aug. 29
NS	Yarmouth	162	May 4	Oct. 14	YT	Whitehorse	72	June 12	Aug. 24

PHENOLOGY: NATURE'S CALENDAR

Study nature, love nature, stay close to nature. It will never fail you.
–Frank Lloyd Wright, American architect (1867–1959)

For centuries, farmers and gardeners have looked to events in nature to tell them when to plant vegetables and flowers and when to expect insects. Making such observations is called "phenology," the study of phenomena. Specifically, this refers to the life cycles of plants and animals as they correlate to weather and temperature, or nature's calendar.

VEGETABLES

- Plant peas when forsythias bloom.
- Plant potatoes when the first dandelion blooms.
- Plant beets, carrots, cole crops (broccoli, brussels sprouts, collards), lettuce, and spinach when lilacs are in first leaf or dandelions are in full bloom.
- Plant corn when oak leaves are the size of a squirrel's ear (about ½ inch in diameter). Or, plant corn when apple blossoms fade and fall.
- Plant bean, cucumber, and squash seeds when lilacs are in full bloom.
- Plant tomatoes when lilies-of-the-valley are in full bloom.
- Transplant eggplants and peppers when bearded irises bloom.
- Plant onions when red maples bloom.

FLOWERS

- Plant morning glories when maple trees have full-size leaves.
- Plant zinnias and marigolds when black locusts are in full bloom.
- Plant pansies, snapdragons, and other hardy annuals when aspens and chokecherries have leafed out.

INSECTS

- When purple lilacs bloom, grasshopper eggs hatch.
- When chicory blooms, beware of squash vine borers.
- When Canada thistles bloom, protect susceptible fruit; apple maggot flies are at peak.
- When foxglove flowers open, expect Mexican beetle larvae.
- When crabapple trees are in bud, eastern tent caterpillars are hatching.
- When morning glory vines begin to climb, Japanese beetles appear.
- When wild rocket blooms, cabbage root maggots appear.

If the signal plants are not growing in your area, notice other coincident events; record them and watch for them in ensuing seasons.

GROW UP!

Do you, too, have a weakness for vigorous climbing annuals? Every year, I seek out varieties known for their rampant growth—'Kentucky Wonder' pole beans, 'Scarlet Runner' beans, 'Tall Telephone' ('Alderman') peas. I've even grown to love lima beans, so that I can justify a row of 'Christmas' limas. And I can't resist the ornamental hyacinth bean, which I once saw

PEA STAKES

■ This is an old-time method for supporting climbing peas, beans, and flowers. Best of all, it's free. Cut branches about 4 feet long from trees or shrubs on your property. (Estimate the height of your plants and add an extra 8 to 12 inches to compensate for the part of the branch that goes into the ground.) Leave the twigs on to give your plants lots of places to grab hold. With a hatchet, sharpen the thick ends of the branches and drive them into the ground. Or, if you can, just push them in next to your plants.

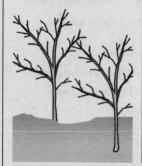

TWINE TRELLIS

■ Set two posts 8 feet apart with a crossbar running along the top. Tie a taut string between the two posts at ground level, then weave a grid of untreated biodegradable twine between the two posts and between the crossbar and the ground-level string. Let your plants ramble at will on this web. When the season is over, cut down the plants and twine and toss them into the compost pile.

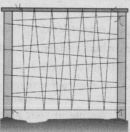

INVERTED-V FRAME

■ Use 12 slender bamboo poles or branches at least 6 feet long and a 13th pole that is 12 feet long. Push the 12 poles into the ground in pairs, with about 3 feet between their bottom ends and at a slant so that the tops meet, as shown. Leave about 2 feet between the pairs. Lash the top of each inverted "V" to the 13th pole, placed horizontally. Plant two or three seeds around each pole. This makes a wonderful tunnel for small children to crawl through.

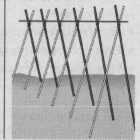

on an arbor at Monticello, or blue morning glories and moonflowers. Vertical garden plants need a good place to climb. I prefer to get the support into place and then plant my peas or flowers. For beans, however, I often wait until the first two leaves have opened and then position the stakes. Here are a few ideas for supports that you can put together yourself. *–Jessica Barlow*

TEPEE

■ To secure plants growing in a circle, push eight to ten bamboo poles (each about 5 to 6 feet long) into the ground following the circle of plants. Slant the poles in toward the center of the circle and tie them together at the top to form a tepee. Run a circle of twine or wire around the bottom of the poles, attach strings to the twine or wire between the poles, and run the strings to the top of the tepee for additional climbing space.

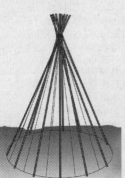

CHICKEN-WIRE FENCE

■ Buy 48- or 60-inch-wide chicken wire with a 2-inch mesh, and support it by nailing or fastening it to posts driven into the ground about 6 feet apart. Try the metal fence posts sold at lumberyards and also at hardware stores. The wedge-shape plate attached to the bottom of the post makes it easy to pound into cold ground, and the posts have little "fingers" that hold the chicken wire in place. When your harvest is over, peel off the vines and roll up the wire for another year.

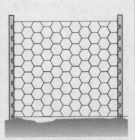

WALL SUPPORT

■ If you want plants to cover a shed or garage wall, attach two 1x4s (approximately 6 feet long) horizontally to the wall about 8 to 10 feet apart. Screw hooks at 10-inch intervals along the two boards and run string vertically between the hooks. Plant a seed near each string.

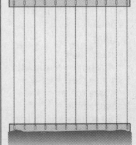

TABLE OF MEASURES

LINEAR

1 hand = 4 inches
1 link = 7.92 inches
1 span = 9 inches
1 foot = 12 inches
1 yard = 3 feet
1 rod = 5½ yards
1 mile = 320 rods = 1,760
  yards = 5,280 feet
1 international nautical
  mile = 6,076.1155 feet
1 knot = 1 nautical mile
  per hour
1 fathom = 2 yards = 6 feet
1 furlong = ⅛ mile =
  660 feet = 220 yards
1 league = 3 miles =
  24 furlongs
1 chain = 100 links =
  22 yards

SQUARE

1 square foot =
  144 square inches
1 square yard =
  9 square feet
1 square rod =
  30¼ square yards =
  272¼ square feet =
  625 square links

1 square chain =
  16 square rods
1 acre = 10 square chains
  = 160 square rods =
  43,560 square feet
1 square mile =
  640 acres = 102,400
  square rods

CUBIC

1 cubic foot = 1,728 cubic
  inches
1 cubic yard = 27 cubic
  feet
1 cord = 128 cubic feet
1 U.S. liquid gallon =
  4 quarts = 231 cubic
  inches
1 imperial gallon =
  1.20 U.S. gallons =
  0.16 cubic foot
1 board foot = 144 cubic
  inches

DRY

2 pints = 1 quart
4 quarts = 1 gallon
2 gallons = 1 peck
4 pecks = 1 bushel

LIQUID

4 gills = 1 pint
63 gallons = 1 hogshead
2 hogsheads =
  1 pipe or butt
2 pipes = 1 tun

KITCHEN

3 teaspoons = 1 tablespoon
16 tablespoons = 1 cup
1 cup = 8 ounces
2 cups = 1 pint
2 pints = 1 quart
4 quarts = 1 gallon

AVOIRDUPOIS

(for general use)

1 ounce = 16 drams
1 pound = 16 ounces
1 short hundredweight =
  100 pounds
1 ton = 2,000 pounds
1 long ton = 2,240 pounds

APOTHECARIES'

(for pharmaceutical use)

1 scruple = 20 grains
1 dram = 3 scruples
1 ounce = 8 drams
1 pound = 12 ounces

METRIC CONVERSIONS

LINEAR

1 inch = 2.54 centimeters
1 centimeter = 0.39 inch
1 meter = 39.37 inches
1 yard = 0.914 meter
1 mile = 1.61 kilometers
1 kilometer = 0.62 mile

SQUARE

1 square inch =
  6.45 square centimeters
1 square yard = 0.84
  square meter
1 square mile =
  2.59 square kilometers

1 square kilometer =
  0.386 square mile
1 acre = 0.40 hectare
1 hectare = 2.47 acres

CUBIC

1 cubic yard = 0.76 cubic
  meter
1 cubic meter = 1.31 cubic
  yards

HOUSEHOLD

½ teaspoon = 2.46 mL
1 teaspoon = 4.93 mL
1 tablespoon = 14.79 mL
¼ cup = 59.15 mL

⅓ cup = 78.86 mL
½ cup = 118.29 mL
¾ cup = 177.44 mL
1 cup = 236.59 mL
1 liter = 1.057 U.S. liquid
  quarts
1 U.S. liquid quart =
  0.946 liter
1 U.S. liquid gallon =
  3.78 liters
1 gram = 0.035 ounce
1 ounce = 28.349 grams
1 kilogram = 2.2 pounds
1 pound = 0.45 kilogram

TO CONVERT CELSIUS AND FAHRENHEIT: °C = (°F − 32)/1.8; °F = (°C × 1.8) + 32

There's more of everything at Almanac.ca

TIDAL GLOSSARY

APOGEAN TIDE: A monthly tide of decreased range that occurs when the Moon is at apogee (farthest from Earth).

CURRENT: Generally, a horizontal movement of water. Currents may be classified as tidal and nontidal. Tidal currents are caused by gravitational interactions between the Sun, Moon, and Earth and are part of the same general movement of the sea that is manifested in the vertical rise and fall, called tide. Nontidal currents include the permanent currents in the general circulatory systems of the sea as well as temporary currents arising from more pronounced meteorological variability.

DIURNAL TIDE: A tide with one high water and one low water in a tidal day of approximately 24 hours.

MEAN LOWER LOW WATER: The arithmetic mean of the lesser of a daily pair of low waters, observed over a specific 19-year cycle called the National Tidal Datum Epoch.

NEAP TIDE: A tide of decreased range that occurs twice a month, when the Moon is in quadrature (during its first and last quarters, when the Sun and the Moon are at right angles to each other relative to Earth).

PERIGEAN TIDE: A monthly tide of increased range that occurs when the Moon is at perigee (closest to Earth).

RED TIDE: Toxic algal blooms caused by several genera of dinoflagellates that usually turn the sea red or brown. These pose a serious threat to marine life and may be harmful to humans.

RIP CURRENT: A potentially dangerous, narrow, intense, surf-zone current flowing outward from shore.

SEMIDIURNAL TIDE: A tide with one high water and one low water every half-day. East Coast tides, for example, are semidiurnal, with two highs and two lows during a tidal day of approximately 24 hours.

SLACK WATER (SLACK): The state of a tidal current when its speed is near zero, especially the moment when a reversing current changes direction and its speed is zero.

SPRING TIDE: A tide of increased range that occurs at times of syzygy each month. Named not for the season of spring but from the German *springen* ("to leap up"), a spring tide also brings a lower low water.

STORM SURGE: The local change in the elevation of the ocean along a shore due to a storm, measured by subtracting the astronomic tidal elevation from the total elevation. It typically has a duration of a few hours and is potentially catastrophic, especially on low-lying coasts with gently sloping offshore topography.

SYZYGY: The nearly straight-line configuration that occurs twice a month, when the Sun and the Moon are in conjunction (on the same side of Earth, at the new Moon) and when they are in opposition (on opposite sides of Earth, at the full Moon). In both cases, the gravitational effects of the Sun and the Moon reinforce each other, and tidal range is increased.

TIDAL BORE: A tide-induced wave that propagates up a relatively shallow and sloping estuary or river with a steep wave front.

TSUNAMI: Commonly called a tidal wave, a tsunami is a series of long-period waves caused by an underwater earthquake or volcanic eruption. In open ocean, the waves are small and travel at high speed; as they near shore, some may build to more than 30 feet high, becoming a threat to life and property.

VANISHING TIDE: A mixed tide of considerable inequality in the two highs and two lows, so that the lower high (or higher low) may appear to vanish. ∎

HIGH TIDE TIMES AND HEIGHTS

This table lists the biweekly times and heights of high tide at Churchill, Manitoba, and Vancouver, British Columbia. (A dash indicates that high tide occurs on or after midnight and is recorded on the next day.) Tide times for other days can be interpolated; low tides occur about 6 hours before and after high tides. In addition, the **Calendar Pages, 120–147,** list times and some heights of high tides at Halifax, Nova Scotia. This table is *not* meant to be used for navigation. To get accurate tide times and heights by postal code, go to **Almanac.ca/2022.**

Standard time shown, except for Daylight Saving Time between 2:00 A.M., Mar. 13, and 2:00 A.M., Nov. 6.

	CHURCHILL					VANCOUVER			
DATE	CST/CDT	HEIGHT (FT.)	CST/CDT	HEIGHT (FT.)	DATE	PST/PDT	HEIGHT (FT.)	PST/PDT	HEIGHT (FT.)
SAT., JAN. 1	6:03	13.5	**6:17**	14.0	SAT., JAN. 1	5:37	15.8	**2:51**	15.5
TUES., JAN. 4	8:49	14.9	**8:57**	15.0	TUES., JAN. 4	7:53	16.7	**5:36**	14.6
SAT., JAN. 8	**12:07**	14.3	—	—	SAT., JAN. 8	10:25	16.2	**10:16**	10.8
TUES., JAN. 11	2:10	12.2	**2:35**	12.5	TUES., JAN. 11	2:01	11.6	11:59	14.6
SAT., JAN. 15	6:21	12.2	**6:26**	12.4	SAT., JAN. 15	5:41	15.1	**2:32**	13.6
TUES., JAN. 18	8:24	13.3	**8:24**	13.3	TUES., JAN. 18	7:17	15.5	**4:39**	13.7
SAT., JAN. 22	10:41	13.7	**10:47**	13.5	SAT., JAN. 22	9:08	15.7	**8:07**	12.0
TUES., JAN. 25	12:11	12.9	**12:39**	13.2	TUES., JAN. 25	10:30	15.4	—	—
SAT., JAN. 29	4:25	12.2	**4:47**	12.6	SAT., JAN. 29	4:36	15.2	**1:36**	14.8
TUES., FEB. 1	7:46	14.0	**7:56**	14.2	TUES., FEB. 1	6:45	16.3	**4:46**	14.6
SAT., FEB. 5	10:52	14.6	**11:04**	14.1	SAT., FEB. 5	8:55	16.0	**8:49**	12.0
TUES., FEB. 8	12:27	12.8	**12:47**	12.9	TUES., FEB. 8	10:15	14.4	—	—
SAT., FEB. 12	4:24	10.9	**4:42**	11.0	SAT., FEB. 12	4:37	14.4	**1:15**	12.7
TUES., FEB. 15	7:23	12.4	**7:27**	12.5	TUES., FEB. 15	6:09	15.0	**4:04**	13.4
SAT., FEB. 19	9:39	13.9	**9:48**	13.8	SAT., FEB. 19	7:48	15.2	**7:24**	13.0
TUES., FEB. 22	11:25	13.8	**11:44**	13.3	TUES., FEB. 22	9:03	15.0	**11:00**	12.6
SAT., FEB. 26	2:35	11.7	**3:02**	11.8	SAT., FEB. 26	3:19	14.7	**12:15**	13.5
TUES., MAR. 1	6:41	13.0	**6:55**	13.2	TUES., MAR. 1	5:32	15.7	**4:01**	13.9
SAT., MAR. 5	9:42	14.4	**9:55**	14.2	SAT., MAR. 5	7:30	15.4	**7:49**	13.2
TUES., MAR. 8	11:23	13.4	**11:42**	12.8	TUES., MAR. 8	8:39	13.9	**11:04**	12.7
SAT., MAR. 12	2:03	10.9	**2:23**	10.7	SAT., MAR. 12	3:04	13.8	11:08	11.7
TUES., MAR. 15	7:00	11.4	**7:12**	11.5	TUES., MAR. 15	5:48	14.5	**4:17**	12.5
SAT., MAR. 19	9:35	13.8	**9:47**	13.9	SAT., MAR. 19	7:27	14.7	**7:43**	13.6
TUES., MAR. 22	11:20	14.3	**11:43**	14.0	TUES., MAR. 22	8:39	14.6	**10:48**	13.9
SAT., MAR. 26	2:08	12.3	**2:28**	12.0	SAT., MAR. 26	2:38	14.6	11:45	12.4
TUES., MAR. 29	6:24	12.2	**6:47**	12.3	TUES., MAR. 29	5:13	15.2	**4:17**	12.6
SAT., APR. 2	9:35	14.1	**9:51**	14.0	SAT., APR. 2	7:08	14.8	**8:02**	13.8
TUES., APR. 5	11:12	13.8	**11:35**	13.4	TUES., APR. 5	8:11	13.4	**10:35**	13.9
SAT., APR. 9	1:25	11.8	**1:33**	11.4	SAT., APR. 9	1:48	13.8	—	—
TUES., APR. 12	4:56	11.0	**5:26**	10.8	TUES., APR. 12	4:12	14.1	**3:12**	11.1
SAT., APR. 16	8:25	13.5	**8:43**	13.6	SAT., APR. 16	6:02	14.5	**6:58**	13.8
TUES., APR. 19	10:16	14.6	**10:45**	14.5	TUES., APR. 19	7:17	14.6	**9:50**	15.0
SAT., APR. 23	1:05	13.2	**1:19**	12.9	SAT., APR. 23	12:59	15.1	**10:21**	11.8
TUES., APR. 26	4:51	12.2	**5:23**	12.0	TUES., APR. 26	3:45	15.0	**3:25**	11.4
SAT., APR. 30	8:29	13.7	**8:51**	13.6	SAT., APR. 30	5:46	14.3	**7:21**	14.0
TUES., MAY 3	10:08	13.9	**10:35**	13.7	TUES., MAY 3	6:49	13.3	**9:37**	14.7
SAT., MAY 7	12:23	12.8	**12:26**	12.4	SAT., MAY 7	8:17	11.3	—	—
TUES., MAY 10	3:01	11.5	**3:23**	11.0	TUES., MAY 10	2:22	14.3	**1:29**	10.1
SAT., MAY 14	7:05	13.1	**7:31**	13.1	SAT., MAY 14	4:31	14.4	**6:09**	13.5
TUES., MAY 17	9:12	14.6	**9:46**	14.6	TUES., MAY 17	5:57	14.9	**8:57**	15.5
SAT., MAY 21	12:13	14.2	**12:24**	13.8	SAT., MAY 21	9:13	12.2	—	—
TUES., MAY 24	3:20	12.9	**3:50**	12.3	TUES., MAY 24	2:10	15.2	**2:12**	10.6
SAT., MAY 28	7:19	13.3	**7:50**	13.1	SAT., MAY 28	4:21	14.0	**6:40**	13.9
TUES., MAY 31	9:11	13.6	**9:44**	13.7	TUES., MAY 31	5:34	13.3	**8:47**	14.9
SAT., JUNE 4	11:37	13.1	—	—	SAT., JUNE 4	7:37	11.9	**11:19**	14.9
TUES., JUNE 7	1:40	12.6	**1:51**	11.9	TUES., JUNE 7	12:38	14.7	11:16	10.0

Bold = P.M.   Light = A.M.

	CHURCHILL					VANCOUVER			
DATE	CST/CDT	HEIGHT (FT.)	CST/CDT	HEIGHT (FT.)	DATE	PST/PDT	HEIGHT (FT.)	PST/PDT	HEIGHT (FT.)
SAT., JUNE 11	5:29	12.8	6:04	12.7	SAT., JUNE 11	2:52	14.5	5:16	13.0
TUES., JUNE 14	8:04	14.3	8:45	14.4	TUES., JUNE 14	4:40	15.1	8:01	15.6
SAT., JUNE 18	11:31	14.7	—	—	SAT., JUNE 18	8:13	13.0	11:09	15.9
TUES., JUNE 21	2:02	14.1	2:25	13.3	TUES., JUNE 21	12:34	15.5	12:31	10.4
SAT., JUNE 25	5:54	12.9	6:35	12.7	SAT., JUNE 25	2:50	13.8	5:53	13.7
TUES., JUNE 28	8:18	13.2	8:56	13.4	TUES., JUNE 28	4:27	13.3	7:57	14.9
SAT., JULY 2	10:49	13.6	11:22	13.8	SAT., JULY 2	6:56	12.6	10:07	15.0
TUES., JULY 5	12:37	13.5	12:45	13.0	TUES., JULY 5	9:50	10.8	11:38	14.8
SAT., JULY 9	3:43	12.9	4:18	12.5	SAT., JULY 9	1:11	14.6	4:10	12.5
TUES., JULY 12	6:48	13.7	7:35	13.8	TUES., JULY 12	3:23	15.0	7:00	15.3
SAT., JULY 16	10:32	15.2	11:11	15.5	SAT., JULY 16	7:17	13.9	9:50	15.8
TUES., JULY 19	12:49	15.1	1:07	14.4	TUES., JULY 19	10:48	11.1	11:34	15.2
SAT., JULY 23	4:10	12.8	4:53	12.3	SAT., JULY 23	1:13	13.6	4:54	13.3
TUES., JULY 26	7:13	12.7	7:59	13.0	TUES., JULY 26	3:24	13.0	7:00	14.6
SAT., JULY 30	10:00	13.8	10:30	14.1	SAT., JULY 30	6:21	13.1	8:56	14.7
TUES., AUG. 2	11:46	13.8	—	—	TUES., AUG. 2	8:54	11.8	10:11	14.7
SAT., AUG. 6	2:09	13.4	2:38	12.8	SAT., AUG. 6	2:39	12.2	—	—
TUES., AUG. 9	5:18	12.9	6:15	13.0	TUES., AUG. 9	2:04	14.3	5:55	14.9
SAT., AUG. 13	9:31	15.1	10:08	15.6	SAT., AUG. 13	6:24	14.2	8:31	15.6
TUES., AUG. 16	11:55	15.2	—	—	TUES., AUG. 16	9:31	12.2	10:01	15.1
SAT., AUG. 20	2:26	13.2	3:00	12.5	SAT., AUG. 20	3:28	12.8	—	—
TUES., AUG. 23	5:39	11.9	6:39	12.2	TUES., AUG. 23	2:15	12.2	5:53	14.2
SAT., AUG. 27	9:06	13.7	9:34	14.1	SAT., AUG. 27	5:45	13.1	7:40	14.4
TUES., AUG. 30	10:47	14.4	11:10	14.7	TUES., AUG. 30	8:10	13.3	8:48	14.5
SAT., SEPT. 3	12:53	14.1	1:20	13.5	SAT., SEPT. 3	12:55	12.8	10:40	13.8
TUES., SEPT. 6	3:39	12.5	4:40	12.4	TUES., SEPT. 6	12:42	13.2	4:40	14.7
SAT., SEPT. 10	8:31	14.7	9:05	15.3	SAT., SEPT. 10	5:37	13.8	7:11	15.3
TUES., SEPT. 13	10:47	15.4	11:09	15.6	TUES., SEPT. 13	8:33	13.3	8:32	14.7
SAT., SEPT. 17	12:58	13.9	1:27	13.3	SAT., SEPT. 17	1:16	13.0	10:09	12.2
TUES., SEPT. 20	3:34	11.6	4:31	11.7	TUES., SEPT. 20	12:31	11.3	4:27	13.9
SAT., SEPT. 24	8:01	13.2	8:27	13.9	SAT., SEPT. 24	5:02	12.7	6:18	14.2
TUES., SEPT. 27	9:46	14.6	10:04	14.9	TUES., SEPT. 27	7:27	13.5	7:24	14.3
SAT., OCT. 1	12:16	14.3	—	—	SAT., OCT. 1	11:31	14.0	9:10	13.6
TUES., OCT. 4	2:10	13.0	3:05	12.7	TUES., OCT. 4	3:07	14.7	—	—
SAT., OCT. 8	7:26	14.1	7:58	14.8	SAT., OCT. 8	4:56	13.1	5:50	15.1
TUES., OCT. 11	9:42	15.2	9:58	15.5	TUES., OCT. 11	7:46	14.1	7:05	14.5
SAT., OCT. 15	12:13	14.0	—	—	SAT., OCT. 15	11:23	14.2	8:28	12.2
TUES., OCT. 18	1:43	12.2	2:32	12.1	TUES., OCT. 18	2:30	14.1	—	—
SAT., OCT. 22	6:35	12.3	7:03	13.2	SAT., OCT. 22	4:13	11.8	4:49	14.3
TUES., OCT. 25	8:40	14.2	8:55	14.7	TUES., OCT. 25	6:45	13.9	5:57	14.5
SAT., OCT. 29	11:16	15.0	11:22	14.9	SAT., OCT. 29	10:25	15.4	7:51	13.8
TUES., NOV. 1	12:59	13.7	1:48	13.5	TUES., NOV. 1	1:28	15.4	11:22	11.2
SAT., NOV. 5	6:08	13.3	6:40	14.1	SAT., NOV. 5	4:15	12.3	4:25	15.1
TUES., NOV. 8	7:39	14.6	7:51	14.9	TUES., NOV. 8	6:07	14.6	4:41	14.4
SAT., NOV. 12	10:09	14.4	10:12	14.1	SAT., NOV. 12	9:11	15.3	6:11	12.6
TUES., NOV. 15	12:06	13.0	—	—	TUES., NOV. 15	11:27	14.9	—	—
SAT., NOV. 19	3:35	11.5	4:12	12.4	SAT., NOV. 19	2:07	10.7	2:09	14.6
TUES., NOV. 22	6:25	13.4	6:38	14.0	TUES., NOV. 22	5:01	13.8	3:27	14.9
SAT., NOV. 26	9:16	15.1	9:22	15.1	SAT., NOV. 26	8:27	16.3	5:45	14.5
TUES., NOV. 29	11:45	14.4	11:57	13.8	TUES., NOV. 29	10:58	16.2	8:56	11.5
SAT., DEC. 3	3:33	12.8	4:07	13.5	SAT., DEC. 3	2:21	11.5	1:52	15.3
TUES., DEC. 6	6:34	13.6	6:44	13.9	TUES., DEC. 6	5:28	14.7	3:18	14.4
SAT., DEC. 10	9:13	14.2	9:14	14.1	SAT., DEC. 10	8:13	15.9	5:14	13.2
TUES., DEC. 13	11:02	13.6	11:03	13.1	TUES., DEC. 13	9:59	15.7	7:11	11.4
SAT., DEC. 17	1:28	11.8	2:07	12.4	SAT., DEC. 17	12:00	10.0	12:18	15.0
TUES., DEC. 20	4:42	12.3	5:02	13.0	TUES., DEC. 20	4:13	13.4	1:52	15.1
SAT., DEC. 24	8:14	14.6	8:20	14.9	SAT., DEC. 24	7:27	16.5	4:47	15.2
TUES., DEC. 27	10:43	14.9	10:54	14.6	TUES., DEC. 27	9:38	16.7	7:51	12.6
SAT., DEC. 31	1:50	12.9	2:23	13.4	SAT., DEC. 31	12:50	11.0	12:12	15.5

TIME CORRECTIONS

Astronomical data for Ottawa (45°25' N, 75°42' W) are given on **pages 104, 106, 108–109,** and **120–146.** Use the Key Letters shown on those pages with this table to find the number of minutes that you must add to or subtract from Ottawa time to get the approximate time for your locale. Time zone codes represent standard time. Newfoundland is –1½, Atlantic is –1, Eastern is 0, Central is 1, Mountain is 2, Pacific is 3. For more information on the use of Key Letters, see **How to Use This Almanac, page 116.**

GET EXACT TIMES EASILY: Download astronomical times calculated for your postal code and presented as Left-Hand Calendar Pages via **Almanac.ca/2022.**

PROVINCE	CITY	NORTH LATITUDE °	NORTH LATITUDE '	WEST LONGITUDE °	WEST LONGITUDE '	TIME ZONE CODE	A	B	C	D	E
AB	Athabasca	54	43	113	17	2	–18	+9	+28	+51	+71
AB	Banff	51	10	115	34	2	+12	+27	+38	+51	+62
AB	Calgary	51	5	114	5	2	+6	+21	+32	+45	+56
AB	Edmonton	53	33	113	28	2	–10	+13	+29	+48	+65
AB	Fort McMurray	56	45	111	27	2	–41	–3	+21	+49	+75
AB	Fort Vermilion	58	24	116	0	2	–38	+9	+38	+73	+105
AB	Grande-Prairie	55	10	118	48	2	0	+30	+50	+74	+95
AB	Lethbridge	49	42	112	50	2	+8	+19	+27	+37	+45
AB	Medicine Hat	50	3	110	40	2	–1	+10	+19	+29	+38
AB	Peace River	56	14	117	17	2	–14	+21	+44	+71	+96
AB	Red Deer	52	16	113	48	2	–1	+17	+31	+46	+60
BC	Dawson Creek	55	46	120	14	2	+1	+34	+56	+81	+105
BC	Fort Nelson	58	49	122	39	3	–75	–26	+5	+41	+75
BC	Kamloops	50	40	120	20	3	–26	–12	–2	+9	+19
BC	Nelson	49	30	117	17	3	–32	–21	–14	–5	+2
BC	Port Alice	50	23	127	27	3	+3	+16	+26	+37	+46
BC	Prince George	53	55	122	45	3	–35	–10	+6	+26	+44
BC	Prince Rupert	54	19	130	19	3	–8	+18	+36	+58	+77
BC	Telegraph Creek	57	55	131	10	3	–32	+11	+39	+72	+102
BC	Trail	49	6	117	42	3	–28	–19	–12	–4	+2
BC	Vancouver	49	16	123	7	3	–7	+1	+9	+17	+24
BC	Victoria	48	25	123	21	3	–2	+4	+10	+16	+22
MB	Brandon	49	50	99	57	1	+16	+28	+36	+46	+54
MB	Churchill	58	46	94	10	1	–68	–19	+11	+47	+80
MB	Flin Flon	54	46	101	53	1	–4	+23	+43	+65	+85
MB	Gillam	56	21	94	43	1	–45	–9	+14	+41	+66
MB	Gimli	50	38	96	59	1	0	+14	+24	+35	+45
MB	Gypsumville	51	47	98	38	1	0	+18	+30	+45	+57
MB	Norway House	53	59	97	50	1	–15	+9	+27	+47	+65
MB	Portage-la-Prairie	49	59	98	18	1	+9	+21	+29	+39	+48
MB	The Pas	53	50	101	15	1	–1	+23	+40	+60	+78
MB	Winnipeg	49	53	97	9	1	+5	+16	+25	+34	+43
NB	Bathurst	47	36	65	39	–1	+10	+15	+19	+24	+28
NB	Chatham	47	2	65	28	–1	+11	+16	+19	+22	+25
NB	Fredericton	45	58	66	39	–1	+21	+22	+23	+25	+26
NB	Moncton	46	6	64	47	–1	+13	+15	+16	+17	+19
NB	Saint John	45	16	66	3	–1	+21	+21	+21	+21	+21
NL	Corner Brook	48	57	57	57	–1½	+3	+12	+18	+26	+32
NL	Gander	48	57	54	37	–1½	–10	–1	+5	+13	+19
NL	Goose Bay	53	20	60	25	–1	–11	+12	+27	+46	+62
NL	Grand Falls	48	56	55	40	–1½	–6	+3	+9	+17	+23

PROVINCE/STATE	CITY	NORTH LATITUDE °	'	WEST LONGITUDE °	'	TIME ZONE CODE	A	B	C	D	E
NL	St. John's	47	34	52	43	−1½	−11	−5	−1	+2	+6
NL	Stephenville	48	33	58	35	−1½	+7	+15	+21	+28	+33
NS	Halifax	44	39	63	36	−1	+14	+12	+11	+10	+9
NS	Sydney	46	9	60	11	−1	−5	−3	−1	0	0
NS	Yarmouth	43	50	66	7	−1	+27	+24	+21	+19	+16
ON	Fort Severn	56	0	87	38	0	−10	+23	+46	+72	+96
ON	Hamilton	43	15	79	51	0	+24	+20	+16	+13	+9
ON	Kapuskasing	49	25	82	26	0	+8	+19	+26	+35	+42
ON	Kingston	44	15	76	30	0	+7	+5	+3	+1	0
ON	London	42	59	81	14	0	+31	+26	+22	+18	+14
ON	Pembroke	45	49	77	7	0	+3	+4	+5	+6	+7
ON	Peterborough	44	18	78	19	0	+14	+12	+10	+8	+7
ON	Port Arthur	48	30	89	17	0	+40	+48	+53	+60	+66
ON	Sault Sainte Marie	46	31	84	20	0	+29	+32	+34	+36	+38
ON	Sioux Lookout	50	6	91	55	1	−16	−4	+4	+14	+23
ON	Sudbury	46	30	81	0	0	+16	+19	+21	+23	+25
ON	Thunder Bay	48	23	89	15	0	+40	+48	+53	+60	+65
ON	Timmins	48	28	81	20	0	+8	+16	+22	+28	+34
ON	Toronto	43	39	79	23	0	+21	+17	+15	+11	+9
ON	Waterloo	43	28	80	31	0	+26	+22	+19	+16	+13
ON	Windsor	42	18	83	1	0	+40	+34	+29	+24	+19
PE	Charlottetown	46	14	63	8	−1	+6	+8	+9	+11	+13
QC	Chicoutimi	48	26	71	4	0	−32	−24	−18	−12	−6
QC	Fort George	53	50	79	0	0	−30	−4	+12	+31	+49
QC	Gaspé	48	50	64	29	0	−60	−51	−45	−37	−31
QC	Montréal	45	31	73	34	0	−9	−8	−8	−8	−7
QC	Québec	46	49	71	11	0	−24	−20	−18	−15	−12
QC	Schefferville	54	48	66	50	0	−85	−56	−36	−14	+5
QC	Sept-Îles	50	12	66	23	0	−59	−46	−37	−27	−18
QC	Sherbrooke	45	25	71	54	0	−15	−15	−15	−14	−14
QC	Trois-Rivières	46	21	72	33	0	−16	−14	−12	−10	−8
QC	Val-d'Or	48	7	77	47	0	−3	+3	+8	+13	+18
SK	Estevan	49	7	103	5	1	+32	+42	+49	+57	+63
SK	Moose Jaw	50	37	105	32	1	+34	+48	+58	+70	+79
SK	North Battleford	52	47	108	17	2	−26	−5	+9	+26	+41
SK	Prince Albert	53	12	105	46	1	+21	+43	+59	+77	+93
SK	Regina	50	25	104	39	1	+32	+45	+55	+66	+75
SK	Saskatoon	52	7	106	38	1	+31	+49	+62	+77	+91
SK	Swift Current	50	17	107	50	1	+45	+58	+67	+78	+87
SK	Uranium City	59	34	108	36	2	−79	−24	+9	+47	+84
SK	Yorkton	51	13	102	28	1	+19	+35	+46	+59	+70

SELECTED U.S. CITIES

PROVINCE/STATE	CITY	NORTH LATITUDE °	'	WEST LONGITUDE °	'	TIME ZONE CODE	A	B	C	D	E
AL	Decatur	34	36	86	59	1	+20	+1	−13	−31	−45
AL	Mobile	30	42	88	3	1	+35	+10	−9	−32	−50
AR	Little Rock	34	45	92	17	1	+41	+22	+7	−10	−23
CA	Palm Springs	33	49	116	32	3	+21	0	−16	−35	−50
CA	Redding	40	35	122	24	3	+24	+14	+7	−1	−7
CO	Grand Junction	39	4	108	33	2	+33	+21	+11	+1	−7
CT	New Haven	41	18	72	56	0	+4	−4	−10	−17	−23
DE	Wilmington	39	45	75	33	0	+19	+8	0	−9	−17
GA	Macon	32	50	83	38	0	+72	+49	+32	+12	−2
IA	Dubuque	42	30	90	41	1	+10	+4	0	−4	−9
ID	Boise	43	37	116	12	2	+48	+44	+42	+38	+36
ID	Pocatello	42	52	112	27	2	+36	+31	+27	+22	+19
IL	Chicago-Oak Park	41	52	87	38	1	0	−6	−11	−18	−23

(continued)

STATE	CITY	NORTH LATITUDE		WEST LONGITUDE		TIME ZONE CODE	KEY LETTERS (MINUTES)				
		°	′	°	′		A	B	C	D	E
IL	Springfield	39	48	89	39	1	+15	+4	−3	−13	−21
IN	Fort Wayne	41	4	85	9	0	+53	+44	+38	+30	+24
IN	South Bend	41	41	86	15	0	+55	+48	+42	+36	+30
IN	Terre Haute	39	28	87	24	0	+67	+56	+47	+37	+28
KS	Oakley	39	8	100	51	1	+62	+50	+41	+30	+21
KS	Topeka	39	3	95	40	1	+42	+29	+20	+9	0
LA	Lake Charles	30	14	93	13	1	+57	+31	+11	−12	−30
LA	Shreveport	32	31	93	45	1	+53	+30	+13	−7	−23
MA	Boston	42	22	71	3	0	−6	−13	−17	−23	−27
MD	Hagerstown	39	39	77	43	0	+28	+17	+8	−1	−9
MD	Salisbury	38	22	75	36	0	+24	+10	0	−11	−21
MI	Cheboygan	45	39	84	29	0	+33	+34	+35	+35	+36
MI	Ironwood	46	27	90	9	1	−6	−4	−2	0	+1
MI	Jackson	42	15	84	24	0	+46	+40	+35	+29	+24
MN	Bemidji	47	28	94	53	1	+7	+12	+16	+20	+24
MO	St. Joseph	39	46	94	50	1	+36	+25	+17	+7	0
MO	Springfield	37	13	93	18	1	+38	+22	+11	−2	−13
MS	Biloxi	30	24	88	53	1	+39	+13	−5	−29	−47
MS	Tupelo	34	16	88	34	1	+28	+7	−7	−25	−39
MT	Glasgow	48	12	106	38	2	−8	−1	+3	+9	+14
MT	Miles City	46	25	105	51	2	−3	−1	0	+2	+4
NC	Raleigh	35	47	78	38	0	+44	+26	+12	−3	−15
NC	Wilmington	34	14	77	55	0	+45	+25	+9	−8	−22
ND	Minot	48	14	101	18	1	+29	+36	+42	+48	+53
ND	Williston	48	9	103	37	1	+39	+46	+51	+57	+62
NE	Lincoln	40	49	96	41	1	+40	+31	+24	+16	+9
NE	North Platte	41	8	100	46	1	+55	+47	+40	+33	+27
NJ	Trenton	40	13	74	46	0	+14	+4	−3	−12	−19
NM	Las Cruces	32	19	106	47	2	+46	+23	+5	−15	−31
NV	Elko	40	50	115	46	3	−3	−12	−19	−27	−33
NY	Binghamton	42	6	75	55	0	+13	+6	+1	−4	−9
NY	Ogdensburg	44	42	75	30	0	+1	0	0	−1	−2
OH	Columbus	39	57	83	1	0	+48	+38	+29	+20	+12
OH	Toledo	41	39	83	33	0	+45	+37	+31	+25	+19
OK	Tulsa	36	9	95	60	1	+52	+35	+22	+6	−5
OR	Pendleton	45	40	118	47	3	−8	−8	−7	−7	−6
OR	Salem	44	57	123	1	3	+10	+9	+9	+8	+8
PA	Reading	40	20	75	56	0	+19	+9	+1	−7	−14
PA	Scranton–Wilkes-Barre	41	25	75	40	0	+14	+6	0	−6	−12
SC	Columbia	34	0	81	2	0	+58	+38	+22	+4	−10
SC	Spartanburg	34	56	81	57	0	+59	+40	+26	+8	−4
SD	Sioux Falls	43	33	96	44	1	+31	+27	+24	+21	+18
TN	Knoxville	35	58	83	55	0	+64	+47	+33	+18	+5
TX	Amarillo	35	12	101	50	1	+78	+59	+45	+28	+15
TX	El Paso	31	45	106	29	2	+46	+22	+4	−17	−33
TX	San Antonio	29	25	98	30	1	+80	+53	+32	+8	−11
UT	Moab	38	35	109	33	2	+39	+26	+16	+4	−4
UT	Ogden	41	13	111	58	2	+40	+31	+25	+18	+12
VA	Norfolk	36	51	76	17	0	+31	+15	+3	−11	−22
VA	Roanoke	37	16	79	57	0	+44	+29	+17	+4	−6
VA	Winchester	39	11	78	10	0	+31	+19	+10	0	−8
WA	Bellingham	48	45	122	29	3	−7	0	+6	+13	+19
WI	Oshkosh	44	1	88	33	1	−3	−6	−8	−10	−12
WI	Wausau	44	58	89	38	1	−2	−3	−4	−4	−5
WV	Charleston	38	21	81	38	0	+48	+34	+24	+12	+2
WY	Sheridan	44	48	106	58	2	+7	+5	+5	+4	+3

GLOSSARY OF TIME

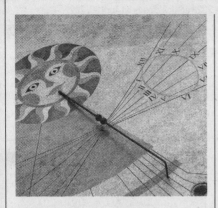

ATOMIC TIME (TA) SCALE: A time scale based on atomic or molecular resonance phenomena. Elapsed time is measured by counting cycles of a frequency locked to an atomic or molecular transition.

DATE: A unique instant defined in a specified time scale. NOTE: The date can be conventionally expressed in years, months, days, hours, minutes, seconds, and fractions.

GREENWICH MEAN TIME (GMT): A 24-hour system based on mean solar time plus 12 hours at Greenwich, England. Greenwich Mean Time can be considered approximately equivalent to Coordinated Universal Time (UTC), which is broadcast from all standard time and frequency radio stations. However, GMT is now obsolete and has been replaced by UTC.

INTERNATIONAL ATOMIC TIME (TAI): An atomic time scale based on data from a worldwide set of atomic clocks. It is the internationally agreed-upon time reference conforming to the definition of the second, the fundamental unit of atomic time in the International System of Units (SI).

LEAP SECOND: An intentional time step of one second used to adjust UTC. An inserted second is called a positive leap second, and an omitted second is called a negative leap second. We currently need to insert a leap second about once per year.

MEAN SOLAR TIME: Apparent solar time corrected for the effects of orbital eccentricity and the tilt of Earth's axis relative to the ecliptic plane; that is, corrected by the equation of time, which is defined as the hour angle of the true Sun minus the hour angle of the mean Sun.

SECOND: The basic unit of time or time interval in the International System of Units (SI), which is equal to 9,192,631,770 periods of radiation corresponding to the transition between the two hyperfine levels of the ground state of cesium-133 as defined at the 1967 Conférence Générale des Poids et Mesures.

SIDEREAL TIME: The measure of time defined by the apparent diurnal motion of the vernal equinox; hence, a measure of the rotation of Earth with respect to the reference frame that is related to the stars rather than the Sun. A mean solar day is about 4 minutes longer than a sidereal day.

–(U.S.) National Institute of Standards and Technology (NIST)

GENERAL STORE CLASSIFIEDS

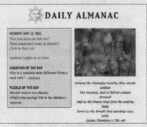
The Old Farmer's Almanac has no liability whatsoever for any third-party claims arising in connection with such advertisements or any products or services mentioned therein.

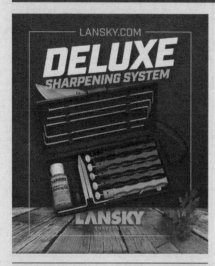
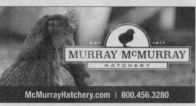
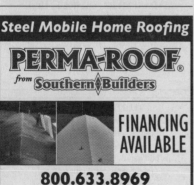

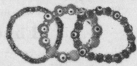

2021 ESSAY CONTEST WINNERS

"A Kindness I Will Always Remember"

We received hundreds of entries for this contest—possibly the most ever! Thank you to all who entered and shared a heartfelt tribute.

First Prize: $300

My husband and I were expecting our first baby. We were young, naïve, and poor as can be. Close to the birth of our daughter, with not a single item of baby "anything" having been purchased, a guardian angel introduced us to a local church group. After attending a few Sundays, we found the acceptance heartwarming. One Sunday, the pastor and his wife invited us to supper. When it was done, they "remembered" a couple of chores at the church and asked if we would be willing to lend a hand. We folded pamphlets, updated the calendar, had a tour, and then proceeded to the basement. Pastor led the way, opened the door, and turned on the light, where almost everyone in the congregation cheered, "Surprise!" There before us was everything needed for a newborn: clothes, bath and personal care items, a crib, a high chair, and a buggy. I was overwhelmed. The following day, they delivered everything to our door, plus a rocking chair for us to relax in while holding our precious new arrival.

–Vicki Thome, Medicine Hat, Alberta

Second Prize: $200

It was May 1982, and two small-town girls had arrived in New York City for a fun-filled weekend! Upon our arrival at the Hotel Edison on 47th, we met Johnny, our bellman, who had a big, genuine smile. He said that if we had any trouble, we should call the hotel and he would be there to help us. Long story short: We did need to borrow $20 from him to get back to the airport. Fast-forward to June 2010. I was back in NYC with my teenage daughter and determined to find Johnny, as I never forgot him and his kindness. At the Hotel Edison, I was advised that Johnny was retired. The staff thought that I was a bit crazy but also was rather intrigued and said that they would help. I wrote him a letter on hotel stationery explaining that I had never forgotten him and enclosed the $20. Two weeks later, Johnny called! His voice was breaking as he said that this was the nicest thank-you gesture that he had ever received. Johnny and his kindness live on forever through this story, which is just one of many about him, I am sure.

–Suzanne Cascanette, Halifax, Nova Scotia

Third Prize: $100

I was an only child, and my mother always tried her best to fill my absent father's shoes. When I was 8 years old, my Cub Scout pack was having their annual "Father and Son Dinner." This was one time when my mom could not step in, and I remember feeling both sad and embarrassed that I did not have a father to go with. Unbeknownst to me, the Cub leaders had made arrangements with an older gentleman to be my "stand-in" father for the dinner.

I remember how good it felt to have a man around me, and I felt incredibly special when he asked me about school and my hobbies. When dessert arrived, there were two flavors of pie: apple and cherry. I told the gentleman that I couldn't decide what kind of pie to have—I liked them both. To my surprise, he said, "Why don't you have both?," and he got up and returned with two plates of pie! I may not have been the only boy with two slices of pie that night, but I sure felt special. Sixty years later, I have never forgotten this act of kindness from my "father for a night."

–Joe Hargitt, Powell River,
British Columbia

Honorable Mention

I was feeling lonely in a world where everyone seemed to be my opponent.

"People are cruel—I do not trust them anymore," I told him.

"No, sweetheart: There is kindness in this world," he replied.

I looked at him with disbelief.

"Look!" he continued. "I've been through many situations. When I was about your age, I felt invincible. I owned a car and felt like the 'boss' of the road. However, God decided to change my mind. It was early in the morning after I had finished my night shift and fallen asleep while driving. A vehicle coming from the opposite side crashed into me. I fainted. The car driver who crashed into me came closer when he realized that I was not moving. He dragged me out of the open window, and a few seconds later, my car exploded. My life was saved. Remember that when you feel alone, there will always be a hand to drag you out of the window."

"Grandpa, what if there is nobody there for me?" I asked.

"Then be that somebody," he smiled.

–Eirini Giantsi, Regina, Saskatchewan

ANNOUNCING THE 2022 ESSAY CONTEST TOPIC:
MY MOST MEMORABLE WILDLIFE EXPERIENCE
SEE CONTEST RULES ON PAGE 251.

MADDENING MIND-MANGLERS

Tennessee Teasers for '22!

Which one does not belong?

1. Alligator • Cockroach • Crocodile • Hippopotamus • Iguana • Octopus

2. 1 • 7 • 11 • 13 • 14 • 17

3. Creek • Dam • Lake • Ocean • Pond • River • Snow

4. Chevrolet • Dodge • Ford • Nissan • Toyota • Volkswagen

–Morris Bowles, Cane Ridge, Tennessee

Virginia Vexer

One Devil of a Puzzle

5. __ __ __ __ __ __ __ __
   1 2 3 4 5 6 7 8

I am a word of eight letters.

According to *The Devil's Dictionary* (1906) by Ambrose Bierce:

My 1, 7, 2, 4 is "a preparation that renders the hook more palatable."

My 5, 8, 6, 3, 7 is "a kind of animal that the ancients catalogued under many heads."

My 1, 7, 4, 5 is "a kind of mystic ceremony substituted for religious worship, with what spiritual efficacy has not been determined."

My 5, 8, 1, 3, 2, 6 is "a pooled issue."

My 6, 2, 7, 3, 8 is "a daily record of that part of one's life, which he can relate to himself without blushing."

My 5, 7, 1, 2, 4 is "a shackle for the free."

–Monty Gilmer, Rosedale, Virginia

Types of Municipalities

What do the names of these six places have in common?

6. Asbury Park • Billings • Biloxi • Fresno • Louisville • Sitka

The Farmer's Herd

7. A farmer in Arkansas passed away and left his 17 cows to his children, as follows: to his elder son, he left one-half; to his daughter, one-third; to his younger son, one-ninth. How did the children divide up the herd without killing or cutting up a cow?

A Matter of Perspective

8. Here are top and side views of a solid object. What are two possible front views??

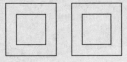

Do you have a favorite puzzler for "Maddening Mind-Manglers" that you'd like to share? Send it to us at Mind-Manglers, The Old Farmer's Almanac, P.O. Box 520, Dublin, NH 03444, or via Almanac.ca/Feedback, Subject: Mind-Manglers.

ANSWERS

1. Iguana: only one with a repeating vowel pronounced in the same way, e.g., alligator has both short and long "a" sounds, while iguana has only the short "a" sound. **2.** 13: only one with a rounded digit. **3.** Ocean: only one not associated with fresh water. **4.** Nissan: only one with no letter "o". **5.** Bait, Hydra, Bath, Hybrid, Diary, Habit, BIRTHDAY. **6.** They are all names of typefaces (fonts). **7.** They borrowed a cow from a neighbor, making 18 in total. The elder son got nine; the daughter, six; the younger son, two. They then returned the extra cow. **8.**

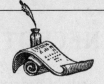

ESSAY AND RECIPE CONTEST RULES

Cash prizes (first, $300; second, $200; third, $100) will be awarded for the best essays in 200 words or less on the subject "My Most Memorable Wildlife Experience" and the best recipes in the category "Bananas." Entries must be yours, original, and unpublished. Amateur cooks only, please. One recipe per person. All entries become the property of Yankee Publishing, which reserves all rights to the material. The deadline for entries is Friday, January 28, 2022. Enter at Almanac.ca/EssayContest or at Almanac.ca/RecipeContest or label "Essay Contest" or "Recipe Contest" and mail to The Old Farmer's Almanac, P.O. Box 520, Dublin, NH 03444. Include your name, mailing address, and email address. Winners will appear in *The 2023 Old Farmer's Almanac Canadian Edition* and on Almanac.ca. ∎

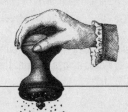

ANECDOTES & PLEASANTRIES

A sampling from the thousands of letters, clippings, articles, and emails sent to us during the past year by our Almanac family in the United States and Canada.

ILLUSTRATIONS BY TIM ROBINSON

THIS YEAR'S ANIMAL NEWS

A moment of silence, please, for Maurice, a raucous rooster in western France whose owners were once sued because of his "noise pollution." The crowing cockerel's case—which he won—became a cause célèbre that led to greater appreciation for and protection of that nation's countryside sounds. Alas, a respiratory infection recently claimed the cock-a-doodle-dooer, although laryngitis has been secretly suspected in some quarters. Maurice was survived by three hens and thousands of *omelettes françaises.*   *–C. M. N., Sherbrooke, Quebec*

Satellite dishes have been sprouting atop beaver lodges across Canada. The work

of pranksters or the sign of more fans for *Hockey Night in Canada?* As far as we know, no one has yet squeezed into a den to find out for sure, but come to think of it, who would better know "streaming" than the clever castors?

–J. W., Yellowknife, Northwest Territories

Don't look now (especially if you're a cow, sheep, or pig!), but in a striking blow to animal privacy rights, facial recognition technology is now being used for livestock management through tracking individual animals' drinking, eating, and "other" habits. It also can ID suspects that are acting strangely, like kicking up their heels about being facially monitored.

–M. G., Ames, Iowa

Why Grandparents Play Silly Games With Grandchildren

On the first day, God created the dog and said, "Sit all day by the door of your house and bark at anyone who comes in or walks past. For this, I will give you a life span of 20 years." The dog replied, "That's a long time to be barking—how about only 10 years and I'll give you back the other 10?" And God saw that this was good.

On the second day, God created the monkey and said, "Entertain people, do tricks, and make them laugh. For this, I will give you a 20-year life span." The monkey replied, "Monkey tricks for 20 years? That's a pretty long time to perform. How about I give you back 10 like the dog did?" And again, God saw that this was good.

On the third day, God created the cow and said, "You must go into the field with the farmer all day long and suffer in the sun, have calves, and give milk to support the farmer's family. For this, I will give you a life span of 60 years." The cow replied, "That's kind of a tough life that you want me to live for 60 years. How about 20 and I'll give back the other 40?" And again, God agreed that this was good.

On the fourth day, God created the human and said, "Eat, sleep, play, marry, and enjoy your life. For this, I will give you 20 years." But the human replied, "Only 20 years? Could you possibly give me my 20, the 40 that the cow gave back, the 10 the monkey gave back, and the 10 the dog gave back—that would make 80, right?" And God said, "Okay, it shall be as you ask."

This is why for our first 20 years, we eat, sleep, play, and enjoy ourselves. For the next 40, we slave in the sun to support our family. For the next 10, we do monkey tricks to entertain the grandchildren. And for the last 10, we sit on the front porch and bark at everyone.

–W. W., Taos, New Mexico
(continued)

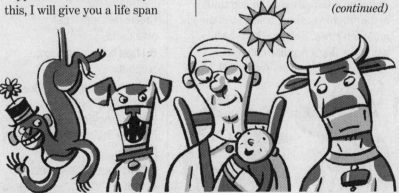

Riddle Us These

Ever wonder why . . .

• the sun lightens our hair but darkens our skin?

• you never see the headline "Psychic Wins Lottery"?

• "abbreviated" is such a long word?

• doctors call what they do "practice"?

• you have to click "Start" to stop Windows?

• packaged lemon juice is made with artificial flavor, while dishwashing liquid is made with real lemon juice?

• the man who invests all your money is called a "broker"?

• there isn't mouse-flavor cat food?

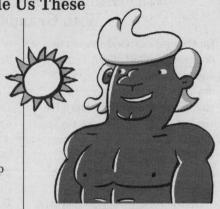

• an airplane is not made from the same material as the indestructible black box?

• they are called apartments when they are all stuck together?

–G. W. S., Marlborough, New Hampshire

How to De-Skunk a Dog

According to the Purdue University College of Medicine: For small to medium dogs (and other pets), use 2 ounces of Massengill douche with 1 gallon of water. For large dogs, double the amount of water and Massengill. Pour the mixture over the dog until it is thoroughly soaked, wait 15 minutes, and then rinse. Follow with a bath using the dog's regular shampoo.

–A. B., Indianapolis, Indiana

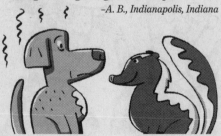

WHY YOU SHOULD PAINT YOUR BATHROOM PURPLE*

As most people know, colors can impart or signify certain qualities.

Black: drama, formality, security

Brown: dependability, simplicity, trustworthiness

Green: freshness, healing, naturalness

Orange: bravery, confidence, sociability

Pink: compassion, sincerity, sweetness

Purple: luxury, royalty (*it's the "throne room," after all!), spirituality

Red: energy, love, strength

Yellow: creativity, happiness, warmth

–M. B., Lorton, Virginia

When the Cat Doesn't Notice the Mouse

Pay attention to these old-time signs and omens around the house if you know what's good for you! (We think.) (Well, maybe.)

Chairs back to back—If chairs have accidentally been placed back to back, a stranger will arrive.

Falling cup—If a cup falls from your hand and does not break, you will be asked to witness a stranger's wedding.

Last piece of pie—The person who is asked to have the last piece of pie will have a handsome husband or wife.

Mouse unnoticed by cat—If a mouse should cross your room unnoticed by the cat, it is a sure sign of a visit from one you love.

Overflowing water—If a pail or tub overflows while you are filling it, you will be overrun with callers.

Raising an empty glass—This will bring unexpected news.

Torn napkin—This foretells a fortunate journey.

Window blind rolls up askew—This is a sign of impending disappointment.

–The Book of Signs and Omens: or How to Avoid Ill-Luck *(Toronto, 1905)*

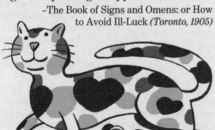

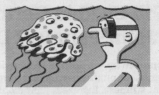

THANKS, BUT I'LL STICK WITH PEANUT BUTTER

I hope that I shall never see
A jellyfish as big as me.
The little ones are bad enough,
All filled with pulsing purple stuff;
A giant one might well deliver
Stings to make a strong man quiver.
I don't fear squids or octopuses–
Count me not among such wusses.
With equanimity I've viewed a
Toothsome tribe of barracuda,
Met with quiet heart the dreaded
Shark (both white and hammer-headed),
Mastered mantas without quail
And cowed the hulking killer whale.
But all my strength and skills desert me
When faced with squishy things that hurt me.

–*Tim Clark, Dublin, New Hampshire* ■

Send your contribution for *The 2023 Old Farmer's Almanac* by January 28, 2022, to "A & P," The Old Farmer's Almanac, P.O. Box 520, Dublin, NH 03444, or email it to AlmanacEditors@ yankeepub.com (subject: A & P).

Now available in the U.S. without a prescription!

Pill Used in Germany For 53 Years Relieves Joint Pain In 7 Days Without Side Effects

Approved by top doctors nationwide. Active ingredient numbs nerves that trigger pain. Relieves joint stiffness. Increases joint mobility and freedom.

By J.K. Roberts
Interactive News Media

INM — A pill that relieves joint pain and stiffness in 7 days without side effects has been used safely in Germany for 53 years. It is now available in the United States.

This pill contains an active ingredient that not only relieves pain quickly, but also works to rebuild damaged cartilage between bones for greater range of motion.

It can cut your pain relief costs up to 82% less than using pain relief drugs and pain relief cream and heat products.

An improved version of this pill is now being offered in the United States under the brand name FlexJointPlus.

FlexJointPlus relieves joint pain, back pain, neck pain, carpal tunnel, sprains, strains, sports injuries, and more. With daily use, users can expect to feel 24-hour relief.

"Relief in pain and stiffness is felt in as quickly as 7 days," said Roger Lewis, Chief Researcher for FlexJointPlus.

"And with regular use, you can expect even more reduction in the following 30-60 days," added Lewis.

WHAT SCIENTISTS DISCOVERED

FlexJointPlus contains an amazing compound with a known ability to rebuild damaged cartilage and ligaments associated with joint pain.

This compound is not a drug. It is the active ingredient in FlexJointPlus.

Studies show it naturally reduces inflammation while repairing bone and cartilage in the joint.

Many joint pain sufferers see an increase in flexibility and mobility. Others are able to get back to doing the things they love.

With so much positive feedback, it's easy to see why sales for this newly approved joint pain pill continue to climb every day.

IMPRESSIVE BENEFITS FOR JOINT PAIN SUFFERERS

The 8 week clinical study was carried out by scientists across six different clinic sites in Germany. The results were published in the Journal of Arthritis in July 2014.

The study involved patients with a variety of joint pain conditions associated with osteoarthritis. They were not instructed to change their daily routines. They were only told to take FlexJointPlus's active ingredient every day.

The results were incredible.

Taking FlexJointPlus's active ingredient just once daily significantly reduced both joint pain and stiffness compared to placebo at 7, 30, and 60 days.

In fact, many patients experienced greater than 50% reduction in pain and stiffness at 60 days.

They also enjoyed an improvement in stiffness when first getting out of the bed in the morning, and an improvement in pain when doing light household chores.

The findings are impressive, no doubt, but results will vary.

But with results like these it's easy to see why thousands of callers are jamming the phone lines trying to get their hands on FlexJointPlus.

HOW IT REBUILDS DAMAGED JOINTS

Scientists have discovered that after the age of 40 the body is no longer able to efficiently repair bone and cartilage in the joint. This results in deterioration and inflammation in the joint, leading to pain.

The natural compound found in FlexJointPlus contains the necessary ingredients needed for the body to rebuild damaged bone and cartilage.

This compound is known as NEM®.

"Essentially, it contains the same elements found in your joints, which are needed to repair and rebuild cartilage and ligaments," explains chief researcher Roger Lewis.

There also have been no adverse side effects reported with the use of NEM®.

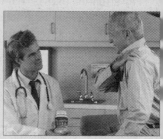

Approved by U.S. Doctors: U.S. medical doctors are now recommending the powerful new pill FlexJointPlus. Participants in clinical studies reported noticeable results in just days.

This seems to be another reason why FlexJointPlus's release has triggered such a frenzy of sales.

RECOMMENDED BY U.S. MEDICAL DOCTORS

"Based on my 20 years of experience treating people with osteoarthritis, FlexJointPlus receives my highest recommendation to any person suffering from joint pain and stiffness," said Dr. David Vallance, Rheumatologist from Ann Arbor, MI.

"I use FlexJointPlus every day for my stiff and aching joints. I also have my wife and daughter taking it regularly as well," said Dr. Oozer, G.P. from LaSalle, CA.

OLD FARMER'S ALMANAC READERS GET SPECIAL DISCOUNT SUPPLY

This is the official release of FlexJointPlus and so for a limited time, the company is offering a special discount supply to our readers. An Order Hotline has been set up for our readers to call, but don't wait. The special offer will not last forever. All you have to do is call TOLL FREE **1-800-540-7740**. The company will do the rest.

IMPORTANT: Due to FlexJoint's recent media exposure, phone lines are often busy. If you call, and do not immediately get through, please be patient and call back. Current supplies of FlexJoint are limited, so consumers that don't get through to the order hotline will have to wait until more inventory is available. Call **1-800-540-7740** today!